A Neurologist's Tale

# A Neurologist's Tale

*by*

EDMUND CRITCHLEY

The Memoir Club

© Edmund Critchley 2001

First published in 2001 by
The Memoir Club
Whitworth Hall
Spennymoor
County Durham

All rights reserved.
Unauthorised duplication
contravenes existing laws.

British Library Cataloguing in
Publication Data.
A catalogue record for this book
is available from the
British Library.

ISBN: 1 84104 035 5

Typeset by George Wishart & Associates, Whitley Bay.
Printed by Bookcraft (Bath) Ltd.

*To my Grandchildren*

**Also by Edmund Critchley**

*Speech Origins and Development*
*A Pocket Guide to Migraines and Headaches*
*Neurological Emergencies*
*Hallucinations and their Impact on Art*
*Language and Speech Disorders*
*Diseases of the Spinal Cord*
*The Neurological Boundaries of Reality*
*Spinal Cord Disease*

# Contents

Foreword ............................................... xi

## Part I
### Early Years

My Early Life ............................................. 1
Bury St Edmunds .......................................... 5
Huntington's Disease in East Anglia and Elsewhere ............. 7
Back to Bury St Edmunds .................................. 11
Bath and Buckinghamshire ................................. 12
Baghdad ................................................ 19
Early Experience ......................................... 24
House-Surgeon .......................................... 27
House-Physician ......................................... 31
National Service ......................................... 32
Leptospirosis ............................................ 36
Away from Taiping ....................................... 38
B.M.H. Kluang .......................................... 40
My Incursion into Neurology ............................... 41
Parkinson's Disease ....................................... 44
Wilson's Disease ......................................... 51
Neurological Aspects of Tuberculosis ........................ 51
The Royal Free Hospital .................................. 53
University College Hospital ................................ 55
Deafness and Hearing Children of Deaf Parents ............... 57
Dyslexia and the Drift into Delinquency ..................... 62
Bedford ................................................ 66
America – Kentucky ...................................... 67
Neuro-acanthocytosis ..................................... 71
The Second Family ....................................... 74
Abetalipoproteinaemia and Related Syndromes ............... 76
Back to Kentucky ........................................ 78
Johns Hopkins Hospital ................................... 79

Charcot's Hysteria Renaissant ............................... 83
Kentucky Again ............................................. 90
Early American English ..................................... 92

## Part II
## Neurological Consultant

Preston and the Surrounding Area ........................... 96
Epilepsy .................................................. 101
Pain ...................................................... 113
Speech .................................................... 119
Hallucinations ............................................ 127
Unusual Auditory Hallucinations ........................... 133
A. Musical Hallucinations ................................. 133
B. Hallucinations in Prelingually Deaf Schizophrenic Patients ........ 135
The Role of the Neurologist ............................... 141
Cerebro-vascular Disease .................................. 144
Parietal Lobes, Rehabilitation and Disability ............. 149
Migraine .................................................. 153
Sleep Singing, Watches, and Bioelectrical Phenomena ....... 160
Drug-induced Neurological Disease ......................... 163
Motor Neurone Disease and Disorders of the Spinal Cord .... 169
The Motivation of Mouth- and Foot-Painting Artists ........ 172
The Spectrum of Mouth- and Foot-Painters .................. 179
Sarah Biffin .............................................. 181

## Part III
## Wider Horizons

Examining for Membership .................................. 187
Aspects of Art ............................................ 195
Sleep Disorders ........................................... 199
Medico-legal Work ......................................... 203
Lecture Tours ............................................. 209
Neurological Emergencies .................................. 213
Multiple Sclerosis ........................................ 217
Diagnostic Puzzles ........................................ 221
Muscle Neurology .......................................... 222
Botulism .................................................. 225
The Public Health Story ................................... 234

The Other Affected Patients ................................ 235
Illustrative Histories ...................................... 236
Historical Aspects ........................................ 240
The Ghillie's Farewell ..................................... 242
Toxico-infective Forms of Botulism .......................... 243
Long-term Symptoms Following Botulism .................... 245
Ecological Factors and Animal Botulism ...................... 249
Putting Botulinum to Good Use ............................. 254
Future Experimental Applications of Botulinum Toxins ......... 260

# Part IV
## The Finale of the Neurologist's Tale

Looking Back ............................................ 263
Life After Neurology ..................................... 265

Index .................................................. 269

# Foreword

THE PURPOSE OF THIS idiosyncratic volume is to prove that the jobbing neurologist has the opportunity to see a great variety of interesting patients, and as many really fascinating ones as someone such as Oliver Sacks, who has written brilliantly on just a few patients. The text includes a description of a patient with the 'crown of thorns' in his blood stream, prelingually deaf schizophrenic patients who have auditory hallucinations, patients with botulism, and the medical conditions of mouth- and foot-painting artists. Conditions such as Huntington's disease, parkinsonism and epilepsy can be the source of great fascination, as can the neurology of language. The basis of the story is a varied career, including paediatric neurology, tropical conditions such as leptospirosis and rickettsiae, medico-legal problems, Creutzfeld-Jakob disease, chronic fatigue syndrome as originally seen at the Royal Free Hospital, bio-electric phenomena associated with watches, hearing children of deaf parents, hysteria, sleep disorders including sleep singing, and much else besides. There are explanations of the use of botulinum toxin to treat neurological conditions and its future potential, how drugs may induce neurological disease, of trauma to the spinal cord, and how our knowledge of neurology provides insight into the philosophical discussion of reality.

Part I

# EARLY YEARS

**My Early Life**

It has been my good fortune to enter Neurology at a time when it was possible to know all the other neurologists in one's own country and a good many elsewhere in the world. In an earlier more austere era, neurologists, by nature obsessional and introspective, were commonly aloof and, depending purely on clinical skills, were almost invariably pitted against each other in intellectual combat.

In my early days neurologists were thinly spread. I was just one of two neurologists appointed to consultant posts in 1968, and, being away from the major centres, found myself covering every conceivable branch of the subject. A neurologist even then had to be established in his post for a year or two before joining, by election, the select band of the Association of British Neurologists. Entry became progressively easier, imaging techniques meant that clinical findings could be supported by hard, agreed evidence, and a camaraderie grew up among all within the speciality. Today everyone is appointed with a special interest, and even in neighbouring centres I cannot claim to know all the occupants.

The joy, the interest in neurology, stems from the fact that we, almost uniquely, have the opportunity to look at the workings of the human brain, and to adapt our techniques of examination to the personality, the intelligence and the state of awareness of our patients. Critics might disagree: there are neurologists whose primary interest is in the blood supply to the brain, others interested in its electrical activity, and yet others who confine their expertise primarily to the peripheral nervous system, or even to the body's musculature – 'muscle neurologists'! We work on what exists, on the nerves of the body, the spinal cord, and the brain, its metabolism, its chemistry, its reality. Psychiatrists work on something more nebulous – the mind. As the joke has it, the neurotic builds castles in the air, the psychotic lives in them, and the psychiatrist collects the rent. Alternatively, Psychiatry is the care of the id by the odd.

That man should know himself, his mind, his brain, has increasingly become a subject of universal and popular interest. This interest has been fed expertly by such exponents as Oliver Sacks and Harold Klawans, and by psychologists such as Anthony Storr. Storr and Klawans have analysed the illnesses of the famous – Churchill, Kafka, Snow, Jung, Toscanini's fumble, Newton's madness – leading on to studies of the elect among their patients. Sacks, with brilliant idiosyncrasy, has interwoven his personality with the unusual problems of his patients. Sacks and Storr I know. I have yet to have the privilege of meeting Klawans. But it is my contention that a neurologist, even if his career has been much more mundane than that of Oliver Sacks, has similar opportunities, if he is observant and interested, to study the bizarre and unusual – hence this volume.

I will begin my story in Oxford, where the spirit of Sir Charles Sherrington reigned over the medical school, embracing neurophysiology and the reflex arc. There were still professors and lecturers from Sherrington's day, though much of the research had dried up. Sherrington's prose was always regarded as convoluted: 'it is as if . . .' His progeny were no more direct in their teaching, in fact most of them were poor teachers. Liddell, the Professor, would drone on verbatim then suddenly turn to his notes before exclaiming, 'and then the whole caboose goes bang'. A pause, and he would continue as before. Sir John Eccles, a former doyen of the department, came over from New Zealand to write his seminal book on *The Self and its Brain* with Karl Popper and to give a series of lectures. We were told that he would start on one theme and end on something quite contrary to that with which he began. He did just that.

Other departments had good teachers and there was even a suggestion of organization of the course. Florey and the others in pathology, responsible for the development of penicillin, Abraham, Heatley, etc, were excellent, as was Burn for pharmacology. Anatomy combined great characters with excellent instruction. The Professor was Le Gros Clark, exposer of the Piltdown man, to whom he bore a certain resemblance, captured in a Maudy Littlehampton cartoon in which the professor asks Maudy, 'What makes you think there are descendants of the Piltdown man alive today?' He would enter the anatomy lab followed by his spaniel. Gray's *Anatomy* would be quickly hidden from view and Le Gros Clark's *Tissues of the Body* would receive pride of place. In his lectures he would read from the unabridged *Water Babies* of Charles Kingsley, that 'everybody has a hippopotamus minor in their brain'. The slightly austere but friendly Sinclair, Weddell and Darcus were anatomists of note. My favourite was Paul Glees, who was also my tutor and a brilliant histologist. To my amazement, when my son went to Cambridge, he also had anatomy lectures from Dr Glees. One was usually happy to be viva-d by any of them, but to do well on a viva from Alice Carleton was a real boost to the ego. She was formidable. She was a clinical dermatologist but could draw any bit of anatomy from every angle to demonstrate its relationships. Less certain teaching came from Bunny Peters' crew in biochemistry. The department was strengthened just after my time by the arrival of Krebs, famous for his carboxylic cycle.

However, physiology was the major subject of the preclinical medical school, and we were left much to our own devices, struggling in practicals with unwieldy Douglas bags, looking over our shoulders for assistance from Cunningham or even the then physiology instructor, Roger Bannister. We relied upon our weekly essays and tutorials, often by dons not directly linked with the department. The modern educationalist would decry our system of learning – at least we learnt the value of using a reference library – but a better taught, more directed course would rightly be expected. Would people like Liddell, or Creed, with his encyclopaedic knowledge of anything to do with the eyes, or even Charles Phillips, be banished to be replaced by lesser people who were better teachers? I hope there will still be a place for both, because although they may not have helped everyone with their exams, they disseminated a diffuse inspiration through apprenticeship, which has meant that many who did not achieve at the time have nonetheless gone on to make advances in medicine and perhaps in particular in the field of neurology.

It was decided that some awareness of the application of anatomy to medical problems would be of benefit and so once a week we would traipse off to the Radcliffe Infirmary to receive a lecture demonstration from Dr Ritchie Russell, Professor of Neurology, or Joe Pennybacker, a much more extrovert Professor of Neurosurgery. The highlight of these demonstrations came when Prof. Pennybacker attempted to show the benefits of frontal lobectomy, illustrated by the success he had had in overcoming his chauffeur's obsessional neurosis. Unfortunately, his driver, noted for his reliability, failed to show up.

There were characters also to be found among the students. One from Eastern Europe arrived in Oxford a few days early, and after testing the water, changed his name by deed poll to Sherrington. He would be seen, whenever the exam results were displayed, telling others how well they had done. He would have failed on several occasions, but eventually was probably more successful than the majority as a medical journalist and translator. David Negus, now a consultant surgeon at St Thomas', would arrive for a practical dressed as Master of the Christ Church and New College Beagles. His father, Sir Victor Negus, shared with Andrew Sherrington the distinction of multiple failures – usually because he produced hospital pantomimes – before becoming world-famous as an anatomist of the nasal pathways. He would begin his lectures at King's College Hospital by pointing out the uselessness of clearing one's throat with a slight cough. The students would remain alert throughout, checking whether he needed to clear his throat. He never did.

Two other students also stood out – fat, big, and rounded, Tweedledum and Tweedledee. They were Oliver Sacks and his anatomy and physiology partner, Michael Tarsh. I always assumed that they were cousins, but they were unrelated. Michael Tarsh became Psychiatrist to Hope Hospital in Manchester. He once wrote an article about his attempts to control his weight. He had part of his small bowel removed, as did his son. But on occasions his flesh was weak. Having wired his mouth to reduce his food intake, he sent his secretary out to buy Mars Bars, which he would melt before eating. Oliver Sacks, I am told, controlled his weight more successfully, initially by psychotherapy and later by swimming daily. I renewed acquaintance with Oliver Sacks in 1993. He was a star at the World Federation of Neurology Conference in Vancouver, British Columbia. His critics, who questioned the accuracy of some of his statements on famous migraineurs, said that this was the reacceptance of Oliver as a neurologist. He had gone to the United States after doing just one neurology job at his teaching hospital without being exposed to British neurology as a whole. He is, as anyone who has watched his television performances would agree, a likeable character, highly intelligent but modest and slightly shy. He told my wife a lovely story of how, when his mother, who was an obstetrician at the Royal Free Hospital, was lecturing on breast feeding, a bundle was produced from under a chair and the young Oliver put to her breast.

I have only vague recollections of Roger Bannister at Oxford, though I have met Sir Roger and Lady Moira on many occasions since. What I do remember from Oxford was his world breaking 4-minute mile. I was in the Parks watching Fred Trueman bowl. He was not flat out but using the gusts of wind to swing the ball in by as much as a yard. Bannister was running at the Iffley ground supported by Brasher and Chataway. The wind calmed as the event was broadcast and listened to by a small crowd on a portable radio. Bannister's progress neurologically has been almost as fast. After working at the Brompton, producing a paper on mitral stenosis and a further paper whilst doing National Service on heat stroke in a dry climate, he worked his way through St Mary's and the National Hospital for Nervous Diseases and as a consultant continued work he had started in Oxford on the autonomic nervous system. Latterly he has been Master of Pembroke College, Oxford. I had the opportunity to review Bannister and Brain's *Clinical Neurology* – better known as the readable Brain, as opposed to Brain's other textbook, which Walton took over. Bannister had thoroughly revised *Clinical Neurology*, bringing the technology up-to-date and making it a practical text for exam students. His family originate from the Burnley and Pendle area, which at one time was part of my neurological 'patch'.

My liking for characters with whom I've worked brings me to another expert on the Autonomic Nervous System who is also a runner of note. I first met Otto Appenzeller when he was a research fellow at the National. He was then a small, rather fat Australian of Swiss extraction, who played the occasional game of squash and was doing research on migraine, examining the peripheral changes with a plethysmograph. I was roped in as a normal subject and given an early beta-blocker, which was potentially carcinogenic. He also did studies on skin fold thickness, assessing obesity. He then went to the USA, working under Denny-Brown, the famous Neurologist from New Zealand. After sustaining a fractured ankle in his forties, he took up jogging, often, in the era before every American took up jogging, to the vocal abuse of motorists. He has since then run 100 marathons, four 100-mile races, run at altitude in the Himalayas to see the effect on encephalins, and edited the *Annals of Sport's Medicine*. No longer is he small and rotund, but skinny with a huge handlebar moustache. I was particularly intrigued by his description of the 'Diving response', whereby an endurance-trained athlete with predominantly parasympathetic tone is liable to faint if cooled rapidly, douched by a cold shower of water from a sympathetic observer as he crosses the finishing line, as a result of bradycardia without vasoconstriction. When I visited Otto in Albuquerque I offered a choice of lectures. He insisted I spoke on all three topics. My son Hugo did an elective with Otto, studying an unusual form of peripheral neuropathy among the Navajo Indians.

## Bury St Edmunds

I associate the town of Bury St Edmunds with two neurologists, Sir David Ferrier and my uncle, Macdonald Critchley. Ferrier came to Bury St Edmunds from Edinburgh where he had been an assistant to Thomas Laycock, the Professor of Practical Medicine. He disliked the necessity of earning a living from private tuition and decided to enter general practice with William Edmund Image, a polymath and aristocratic practitioner, FRCS and Bachelier des lettres, noted in Bury St Edmunds for his fascinating garden. Whilst dabbling in family medicine, Ferrier's energies were deployed in writing his gold medal M.D. thesis on the Corpora Quadrigemina, describing how lesions placed superiorly in the brainstem affected the swimming action of fishes, and their function in rabbits and frogs.

Ferrier left Bury in 1870 and two years later, at the age of 29, was appointed to the Chair of Forensic Medicine at Kings College Hospital, acting as a hack to revise his predecessor's *Principles of Forensic Medicine*. Two years later he was appointed Junior Physician to the West London Hospital, Assistant Physician to the Hospital for Epilepsy and Paralysis in Regent's Park and Consultant at Kings College Hospital. In 1873 he commenced his experimental researches on cerebral physiology and pathology in animals, dividing his time between laboratories at King's and the Asylum at Wakefield in Yorkshire where James Crichton-Browne was superintendent. His experiments, demonstrating the localization of sensory and motor functions in the cerebral cortex by electrical stimulation, were correlated with meteorological data from Kew Gardens. On the basis of his work, he pleaded with surgeons to operate on the brain, inspired by a crusading zeal which bordered on the fanatical. He stressed the 'inviolability of the peritoneal cavity till very recently, why not the dura!' Sir William McEwen in Glasgow was the first surgeon to take up the challenge, operating for intracranial disease. In London, Sir Rickman Godlee (Lister's nephew) removed a cerebral tumour 'the size of a walnut', the position of which had been correctly localized. Hearing that the patient was a Scotsman, a wag asked, why he had not taken the opportunity to insert a joke before closing the skull!

Ferrier was a small man, slim, dapper, always erect, quiet of manner but crisp of speech, with a trace of an Aberdonian accent which added flavour to his words. He was less kindly described as perky and ambitious, of diminutive stature, combining a powerful drive with the habits of a cold perfectionist – an investigator rather than a teacher, a physiologist perhaps, more than a clinician. Although he secured a fashionable practice, he was uneasy and undistinguished as a clinician. Nonetheless, he introduced one clinical sign which at the time gave the most accurate localization of a transverse lesion of the spinal cord. The rim of the guinea coin was pressed against the skin and drawn down the spine, producing a wheal above the lesion but at most a white mark below, where sweating and vital reactions were in abeyance. Sam Nevin used to relate a story which certainly does not flatter Ferrier. In the course of his ward round, accompanied by distinguished visitors, he sought to demonstrate sensory loss in tabes dorsalis on a heavily built sailor by running a pin down his trunk. In tabes, alteration of sensation is frequently seen over the nasal area of the face, the breast-plate area of the chest, the ulnar borders of the forearms and outer aspect of the shins. Unfortunately, the patient was at a hyperaesthetic rather than hypoaesthetic stage of the illness, and incensed by the pain, jumped out of bed, seized the diminutive Ferrier and threw him bodily out of the ward. There is a similar story of another consultant anxious to demonstrate his skill at spot diagnosis, who after reading the G.P.s letter, approached the man as he entered the consulting room, sticking a pin into his nose. It was the G.P. himself, accompanying the patient!

**Huntington's Disease in East Anglia and elsewhere**
Macdonald Critchley came to East Anglia, using our house as a base from which to study gravestones in the churchyards of neighbouring villages. The disease, Huntington's chorea, has its greatest concentration in the United States, whence appeared many of the earliest clinical descriptions, including the pioneer observations of the Rev. C.O. Waters, I.W. Lyon, Osborn, and the Drs. Huntington (father and son). Although in Scandinavia and elsewhere it is historically a disease seen around coastal regions and sea-ports, P.R. Vessie, in 1932, traced the biggest of the American Family groups back to East Anglia and to the year 1630, when three young men left their native Suffolk village to settle in the American colonies. They travelled on a Puritan ship just ten years after the *Mayflower*. Who were they? 'Just ordinary folk, weavers, farmers and the like from Lincolnshire, Yorkshire and Nottingham. Honest, hard-working, clean-living, thrifty folk. Some of them had been in prison for conscience' sake, others had been in exile in Holland. They just believed in a simple form of worship, not conforming either to the rules of the English Prayer Book or to the authority of the Bishops, of whom King James I had declared, 'I will make them conform. They shall worship as I desire, or I will harry them out of the kingdom.'

We know that not all who sailed from Plymouth on 6th September 1620 in the *Mayflower* were dedicated Puritans. Thirty-five were indeed Puritans who had chosen exile in Leyden in 1608. However they returned, wishing their children to be brought up not as Dutch, but true to their native culture. Most of the 66 others who had joined from London and Southampton seem to have been seeking cheap land much more than freedom from religious persecution. The *Mayflower* itself was an old, scarcely sea-worthy ship of only 180 tons, which had seen service under Queen Elizabeth and had latterly been engaged in the wine trade between England and the Mediterranean ports. The Puritans had returned from Holland in another vessel, the *Speedwell*, which was to travel with the *Mayflower*. However, the Speedwell was in need of repair and they changed ship after several false starts. In mid-Atlantic the *Mayflower* nearly floundered, breaking the main beam. After their arrival in America on 22nd December, the boat was to return to England, where its timbers were broken up some years later and used in the construction of the Mayflower Barn at Jordan's Village, Buckinghamshire.

During the reign of Charles I, Herbert Pelham, a strong Parliamentarian who shared the ideals of the earlier Puritans, became increasingly exasperated with his monarch's repressive and High Church tendencies and declared his determination to quit his home – the Manor of Ferrers, just outside the village of Bures St Mary on the Suffolk-Essex border – and seek a new life in the American Colonies. It was the village where Edmund, East Anglian king and martyr, was crowned at the age of 15 on Christmas Day AD 855. Herbert Pelham embarked in James Winthrop's 'great emigration', taking with him his children and a number of villagers. As with earlier colonizations, the fleet, with over a thousand people on board, gathered in the vicinity of the Isle of Wight and landed three months later in Salem, Massachusetts.* The Rev. White and John Endicott had founded the settlement of Salem in 1628. The place was originally given the Indian name of Naumkeag, but had changed by 1630 to Salem (meaning *Peace*) and received the Massachusetts Bay Charter the same year.

Among the villagers who accompanied Pelham were three men, not ostensibly related: Jeffrey, Nicholas and Wilkie. From what we know of these men, it seems unlikely that they left home simply on account of outraged nonconformity. Quite possibly their psychopathic behaviour had made Bures St Mary too hot to hold them. Nicholas' dishonesty caused him to be thrown into irons aboard ship. Wilkie was arraigned on six occasions – for profanity, for revolutionary talk, for selling beer without a licence, and for keeping a disorderly house. Jeffrey was charged with perjury and being in possession of a stolen calf. The descendants of these three men were also undesirables and ne'er-do-wells. One was severely punished for bestiality by a public whipping and was condemned to wear a halter round his neck for a year.

Much more striking, and particularly germane, is the odium which accrued to the female descendants, known as the Salem witches. The troubles they brought and the violence of the reaction of the early colonists is reflected in the many fanatical anti-witchcraft laws of 1642. Nicholas' wife was hanged in 1653 and no fewer than seven of the daughters or grand-daughters were stigmatized as witches. Two were particularly notorious: Mercy Disborough, the granddaughter of Nicholas, and Elizabeth Knapp, granddaughter of Wilkie. Of Elizabeth Knapp, otherwise known as the Groton Witch, a local pastor testified that:

---

*Another site where the pilgrims landed – Lyme county Connecticut – is also associated with a neurological disease named after an outbreak in the artists' district of Old Lyme. It is a tick-borne spirochaetal disease harboured by deer, mice and household pets affecting the skin, joints, lymphatic system, meninges and nerve roots. As with Huntington Chorea, it probably originated in the Old World, where it was known as Bannwarth's syndrome.

this pore and miserable object was observed to carry herselfe in a strange and unwonted manner, sometimes she would given sudden shriekes and then would burst forth into immoderate and extravagant laughter as sometimes shee fell onto ye ground with it. Shee was violent in bodily motions, leapings, strainings and strange agitations, drawing her tongue out of her mouth most frightfully to an extraordinary length and greatnesse, and many amazing postures of her bodye.

After the fifth generation we meet with unequivocal evidence of Huntington's Chorea, carried down with dominant inheritance through ten, fifteen or more generations.

Macdonald Critchley took Vessie's work as the starting point whereby to examine the possibility that Huntington's Chorea had manifested itself before the emigration of 1630 and that this had been one of the factors which determined the emigrants' departure to the colonies. He was able to assert from church records that the three original migrants were closely related as half-brothers. Baptismal records declare Nicholas to be the base son of Mary Haste; and Haste was indeed the surname of both Jeffrey and Wilkie. Perhaps they were all the children of the same wanton Mary Haste. Another well-known Huntingtonian group of New England is the Peck-Welles family. The first member of this family to emigrate to the American colonies between 1629 and 1630 was Nathaniel Welles, who was a well-to-do shipowner and hotel proprietor from Colchester. 'In other words,' declares Macdonald Critchley, 'he dwelt only ten miles away from Bures and from the sinister charms of Mary Haste.' My uncle was unable to refute or confirm the impression that Huntington's Chorea was already extant in East Anglia before the emigration, but produced figures – albeit limited in numbers – which suggested that in 1933 Huntington's Chorea was twelve times commoner in Suffolk than in Lancashire.

Few of today's neurologists will have heard of Macdonald Critchley's sign in Huntington's Chorea. Older ones – and this certainly includes myself – will have seen him demonstrate the sign on numerous occasions but have never been able to reproduce it themselves. The sign is simple enough in conception: when asked to make a fist, one hand will do so naturally but the thumb in the other hand will be protruded between the index and middle fingers. There may possibly be some sleight of hand we fail to recognize, for, early in his career, with Adie, he had studied primitive signs of frontal lobe dysfunction – the gabella tap, frontal grasping and groping, mouthing reflexes, and the palmo-mental reflex.

There has grown up a common belief worldwide – in Lancashire, Scandinavia and Holland – that the original progenitor of this disease had committed a dreadful murder, and that the victim in his death agonies had called upon Providence to afflict the assailant and his offspring in perpetuity. An alternative explanation, preferred by Bickford and Ellison (1953) and Irving Lyon (1863), was that Huntington's Chorea originated from an infidel who mocked by mime Christ's agony on the Cross. Yet a third legend ascribed the disorder to a curse on those who had persecuted the Rev. Roger Williams – an eccentric parson from Bristol – who had migrated to New England in 1630 and died after a stormy career in 1683. It remains a disease, a curse or hex: secretive, hidden, jerking – and, as the Huntingtons described, with three marked peculiarities: its hereditary nature, a tendency to insanity and suicide, and manifestation as a grave disease during adult life. The rare instances of Huntington's at a younger age can cause diagnostic difficulty, presenting with fits or as a movement disorder, even resembling Parkinsonism. Fresh mutations are rare, so much so that P.K. Thomas tells of a patient, neither of whose parents had the disease, but the mother had been 'raped by a madman'.

Most descendants of the original sufferer have been spared other afflictions; the disease is horrible enough. Other conditions occur so infrequently in association with Huntington's as to be readily accounted for as coincidences, essentially without relation to the chorea itself. Whilst agreeing with the generality of this statement, I will describe in a later chapter a condition, not dissimilar from Huntington's Chorea, wherein the patient 'carries a vestige of the crown of thorns in his blood stream'. And as a senior registrar I came across (the second such reported case) a deaf-mute with Huntington's Chorea. I commented that the patient had always been somewhat simple-minded, had never been able to master any means of communication other than signing, crude finger-spelling, elementary reading and writing, and was still able to be intelligible to his family in the early stages of the Chorea. His eventual breakdown in communication was almost certainly the result of increasing dementia and not due to the severity of his involuntary movements.

When I worked among the poor whites of Kentucky's Appalachia, I certainly gained the impression that Huntington's Chorea was more prevalent in the United States than in the U.K. I was able to see patients in whom the movement disorder had preceded the dementia by many years and vice versa. The disease usually appears after the main reproductive period of life. Thus with dominant inheritance and high penetrance, there is a 50% risk of the disease in any sibship. The disinhibition which is commonly an early and unrecognized feature of the condition may lead to bigger than normal families and a number of illegitimate offspring. Even among the genetically unaffected, living alongside affected brethren, there is a high risk of reactive psychiatric disease. Within the U.K. every neurologist will have a few patients with Huntington's disease on his books. Often we are asked to find long-stay accommodation for patients thrown out of hostels or disruptive in the family home. The movement disorder we try to treat with tetrabenazine or other drugs. Secondary depression often occurs and until recently, with the availability of Prozac, monoamine oxidase inhibitors were the only suitable drugs, though they carried the risk of reactions with certain foods. Stereotactic operations have been used with some success, but many are unwilling to apply a destructive operation to a degenerating brain.

What then is the future for this disease? In the past two years my duties have included regular visits to a special unit for Huntington's disease, replacing more general psychiatric accommodation. This unit acts like a hospice, backing up community care. Among such groups of patients with Huntington's Chorea one sees more clearly their similarities: their use of ritualistic gestures and devices when dressing, moving or eating; and the wide-based gait so many adopt, leaning forward out of plumb. In such a unit new drugs can be examined. Huntington's is the opposite neurochemically to Parkinsonism, and Riluzole, which may retard motorneurone disease, could also retard Huntington's. We now know the genetic configuration of the disease but how should such knowledge be applied? Do we tell a boy of 14 that he will develop the disease when he is 40? There may also be false negatives and false positives. The recognition of trinucleide repeats provides evidence of the likely severity of the condition but there is a grey area of uncertainty whether the disease will develop or not. The most practical application of medical help comes from the pioneering work of Professor Harper in Cardiff, counselling families with the condition, whereby many, without coercion, will limit their desire to procreate potentially affected offspring.

**Back to Bury St Edmunds**
Not every miscreant in East Anglia has Huntington's disease. The best gardener and odd-job man around Bury when my parents first moved there was a former poacher who was alleged to have shot a game-keeper. He was found not guilty on the basis that the guns he owned could never have fired the fatal shot. However, on being released he recovered the said gun from a well.

My parents had moved to Suffolk soon after they had married. My father had been a Casualty Officer at the Royal Free Hospital, where my mother was a fourth year student. None of the grandparents were medical but my mother could claim descent from the herbalists of Myddfai. A farmer had wooed a lady who emerged from a lake, Llyn y Fan, on the Black Mountain (Mynydd Ddu), but lost her back to the lake after touching iron on three occasions. However this occurred after they had produced a family, who in turn gave rise to the herbalists of Myddfai. A possible basis for this legend is that the farmer, a Celt, had married a woman from an earlier, iron-age tribe who was supposed to have mystic powers or expertise, perhaps a blacksmith's daughter! My father had done his Bristol M.D. on a neurological topic – blepharospasm in post-encephalitic parkinsonism. He was an excellent clinician who chose to enter public health. In Suffolk he worked under a chief who, in addition to his normal duties, believed he had a mission to help the poorer inhabitants of the county and at week-ends would tour the villages with a caravan, performing guillotine tonsillectomies on all those he felt were in need of such treatment.

No modern obstetrician would have allowed me to have been born when I was: at home, on Christmas day and at three o'clock in the morning. Furthermore, despite being jolted over hump-back bridges, I was two weeks post-mature. The house we occupied was part of the old Abbey of Bury St Edmund's, Samson's tower, as stated in the Chronicles of Jocelyn de Bracquelon. The Abbot Samson planned to build a central tower to the abbey but he had a dream. Perhaps his feet were sticking out of the bed. In his dream the Lord said 'Look to thy feet, Samson'. As a result he built two round towers at the West End, in one of which we lived. The bedrooms were downstairs, the living room was a large round room at the top with a high ceiling. The tower had been put to other uses in the past. We have a picture of a horse emerging from it when it was a smithy. Today it functions as the visitor centre for the Abbey ruins. Close by the Abbey ruins, in a private garden, is a memorial to the knights who met in Bury St Edmund's. Parliaments met here in 1272, 1296, and 1446, at the last of which Duke Humphrey of Gloucester, called the Good, was arrested, and was found dead in his bed immediately afterwards. It was at Bury that King John first met his rebellious barons before he signed the Magna Charta. The memorial is engraved with the names of the knights who drew up the Magna Charta. Many of these names are no longer in existence in England, but can be found in families in the United States.

## Bath and Buckinghamshire

Flashbacks, other than those provoked by drugs, are decidedly rare. I mention the short time we spent in Bath, where my sister was born, because very many years later when I revisited the city and was walking down a slope by the Assembly Rooms, I had a distinct flashback of myself as a toddler, dressed in coat, cap and gloves, walking down that same slope, holding a lead, restraining, or being pulled by, Paddy, our Irish Red Setter. I can recall no other flashback in my life. The vividness of the occasion was astonishing.

As a toddler in Bath, my photo was used as an advertisement to encourage sun-bathing. I was dressed in shorts and a large sun-hat. My family had – to use the expression of that day – to get rid of a maid because of the publicity she attracted. She was an ex-beauty queen, and as far as I know a reasonable worker, but she would get involved in car accidents with boyfriends, explaining one such accident as occurring because her legs were entangled in the steering wheel when her beau was driving! Enough said, let's move on to the greater part of my childhood spent in Buckinghamshire.

A person's perspective of his/her self within his/her environment has always been a subject of interest to neurologists. When driving a car, cycling, skiing, hand-gliding, snorkelling, even typing, the apparatus one is using enters one's own environment as part of one's self. One's dimensional image, or bodily homunculus, adds on that piece of apparatus. One of the most interesting computer adjustments concerns our hands. Pick up a book. Hold it near-to then further away – its size alters with distance. Regard our hands near-to then outstretched – their size remains unaltered. Many years ago, my then chief was discussing how appreciation of perspective changes from childhood. I wrote out my own experience, which, I believe, he was able to use in a book he wrote on the subject. Twenty-five years later he kindly returned the text to me, which I will reproduce:-

> 'Returning to that part of Buckinghamshire where I spent most of my childhood is, for me, like Gulliver revisiting Lilliput. What I had remembered as roads are like damp, overgrown, extremely narrow lanes. The market square of Winslow, the nearest town, is minute. It will only hold half a dozen cars. The houses there also appear small. It used to be the habit of politicians of Disraeli's era to address the crowds from a hotel balcony. If one were to do so in Winslow, he would physically dominate the place.
> 
> 'The village where I was brought up is a tiny nest of houses in a dip. Like Winslow, my earlier recollection was of something much more vast. The dominant feature is a muddy and, at times, very dirty brook. It was my habit to run right across the tennis court and down to the bottom of a field and there, hidden by a bank, to play in the brook. I felt I was out of sight, out of earshot and well clear of any grownups. To escape still further, I had merely to cross the brook and hide in the spinney beyond. This contained an orchard surrounded by a moat with a waterfall. When some five or seven years ago I followed this trail once again, I found that in a few strides I could be across the field, over the brook and have covered most of the spinney. The moat, the orchard and

the waterfall were certainly not figments of the imagination; but the waterfall, which loomed large in my childhood days, was merely where the brook tumbled over the remains of a dilapidated wall and the trees of the spinney were often no more than hawthorn bushes.

'I knew the distances to the neighbouring villages well: two and a half miles to Winslow, to Mursley, and a little more to Nash, a mile and a half to Gt. Harwood and a mile to Swanbourne station. To go to the station to see the trains was a walk in itself when I was a child. Returning, travelling by car, it seemed to take only seconds from one village to the next.'

One can understand the horror of an old person, whose dementia throws him back in the past, expecting children, and seeing himself surrounded by adults.

Recollections of an easy-going childhood tend to be few, until aged eight, when the War added significance to all events. I remember the village school at the end of our garden, where I went from the age of three and a half, run by the Davies, man and wife. For some obscure reason we had to learn and recite repeatedly Ariel's song from the Tempest, by Mr William Shakespeare – with the emphasis on 'Mister'! . . .

> Where the bee sucks, there suck I
> In a cowslip's bell I lie,
> There, I crouch when owls do cry
> On the bat's back I do fly,
> After summer, merrily,
> Merrily, merrily still I live now
> Under the blossom that hangs on the bough.

Goodness knows why! We were also advised that when the Inspector came to the school, we could count on our fingers but should learn to do so behind our backs. One such school inspector was the Bishop. He picked me out and asked: 'Who was born on Christmas day?' Obviously this was not a chance selection. I naturally answered, 'I was'. 'Who else?', he asked. I gave him the answer he expected in the first place – or did he? He called on my parents and was given lunch on the strength of the story.

We lived in the old vicarage. There were days when the bellringers rang peals of bells, though they had never been tuned and one was broken, before collecting for the bellringers' supper, usually held in the Shoulder of Mutton. There was still a feudal atmosphere in some respects. I remember occasions when our drive was filled by horses and riders from the Whaddon Chase. Because it had once been the vicarage, in the bounty of a local laird, they felt they had the right to call and make use of the place for phone calls and toilets. Our maid, who had been in service to gentry, provided separate towels for each and everyone, and few paid for the long-distance calls. My mother naturally objected to the Master of the hunt and in later years our premises were treated with greater respect and the towels were shared! About this time, Jane, my sister, developed an allergy – I think it was to strawberries, which used to bring her out in spots. As a result she had to have rain-water baths and the out-door vats would be emptied, heated, and she would bath in a huge tub by the kitchen fire.

We were on a caravan holiday in Cornwall when war was declared. My father quickly returned home for call-up as a reservist and was sent to France, returning from St Malo before spending four and a half years in the Middle East. He was responsible for putting Shephard's Hotel in Cairo out of bounds to British troops when its hygiene standards did not come up to scratch, and for placing the Egyptian brothels out of bounds to our troops just before El Alamein, ensuring that they were fit to fight in the forthcoming battle. Readjustment was necessary after the War. He had kept a photo of my sister and myself as we were then He was flabbergasted when I, who only knew schoolmasters among males, called him 'Sir'.

The immediate task of my mother with the onset of war was to qualify, ten years after leaving medical school, and despite the house being filled with refugees. She also acted as an air-raid warden, ensuring that blackout precautions were carried out throughout the village. During raids, when the sirens sounded, the passageway leading from a bolted door into the scullery would be filled with people, but later they preferred to stay within their own homes. However, as we were in the country and within easy reach of London, the village soon doubled in population with refugees. One of the first refugees was a French lady, who came as a governess to look after us whilst my mother worked. She gave me lessons from the upstairs study, which opened on to a veranda overlooking the garden and field. I remember the song – Frère Jacques – and her saying 'mouton is the French for mutton, You see those muttons over there in the field.' It soon transpired she was more than the wife of a soldier called up with little pay to fight on the Maginot Line. Our house was under surveillance. My mother found a radio transmitter hidden up the chimney. Contacts were watched and followed. The French lady was eventually arrested and spent the rest of the War on the Isle of Man.

The feudal aspect of the village was reinforced when the self-appointed squire-ess put on a reception for the arrival of the main intake of refugees from London. She stood at the entrance to the village hall dressed as for Ascot with elbow-length gloves. That was until she heard that they were all unmarried mothers. The gloves came off. The reception was still held but as a more muted affair. On V.E. Day the same lady put on display the only flag she possessed – a red flag used to mark danger when the road was being repaired! Our other refugees were initially family acquaintances and friends. A frequent visitor at weekends to replenish her stock of eggs, fruit and vegetables was Dr Josie Oldfield, my godmother, who had been a fellow student, sharing a basement flat, with my mother. She was a medical officer of health doing maternity and child welfare clinics in South London. Her father, Dr Josiah Oldfield, was a well-known vegetarian, friend of Gandhi and George Bernard Shaw. In his eighties he ran a home for old people in their late 60s and 70s. When he died in his mid-90s, my godmother received a letter saying that if he had been a pure vegetarian, or better still a fruitarian, he would have lived longer. His contribution to the War effort included publicizing the 'Oldfield Bath', an attempt to save water. He built a frame, put my godmother's best blankets over it and claimed he could then have a good bath in three inches of water. Soon the uncertain flood of refugees was replaced by the overflow of a girls' school evacuated from the Isle of Wight. We provided two dormitories and a teacher's bedroom. My sister went as a day girl to the same school, where she and Anthea Askey (daughter of the comedian, Arthur Askey) were the only ones in the class not to be in the choir, though Anthea was later to sing on Television.

My first acquaintance with Neurology was a book on *Shipwrecked Survivors* by my uncle. My sister and I were intrigued by the frontispiece – a photograph of the bottom of a sailor who had been sitting on a rope in a raft for 30 days. Besides the anticipated comments on exposure, dehydration, sleep deprivation and hallucinations, the book contained some of the earliest work on fluid replacement. Apparently my uncle would sit for many hours with his feet emerged in buckets of saline to see what changes occurred. I also remember – and it must have been during the brief period when my father was at home during the War – being driven in the blackout through the Bristol blitz by my uncle, seeing the fires and the barrage balloons.

Did I envisage early in my childhood that I would take up Neurology? The answer is an emphatic 'No'! But equally emphatically, I wished from an early age to do medicine. I had thought about law. I had thought about architecture. But no – I wished to do medicine. My parents wanted to make sure this was really so and sought the help of my housemaster, D.I. Brown, an ex-Scottish International full-back with the broadest shoulders imaginable. So much so that when they put him in the tank corps at the beginning of the War, he was unable to get inside the turret. I reiterated that I wanted to do medicine. If I had been asked what I wanted to specialize in, I would probably have said Paediatrics. Though when I first saw a Paediatric ward at my Teaching Hospital, I was so put off by the unnaturalness of the children there that it was some years before I thought once again of Paediatrics. As for Neurology, I no more expected to follow my uncle than I expected to follow my maternal uncle, who was a Welsh rugby international.

My mother had qualified and spent six months doing a house-job in an E.M.S. hospital in Bath. On her return I saw my first operation. My parents performed a circumcision on the bathroom table. My father was the surgeon and my mother administered the anaesthetic by the rag and bottle method. From then on we were very much a medical household. As my sister used to say, the telephone was always ringing with problems such as threatened abortions. Initially my mother went into practice in Aylesbury; two women taking over the largest practice in town with three times the pre-War population. The hospitals they used were the Royal Bucks in Aylesbury itself and Stoke Mandeville, in part of which Guttmann had set up his paraplegic unit.

After a while, rather than travel to Aylesbury each day, my mother set up practice from home. Much of her work centred on a large hostel for refugees from Poland and elsewhere, mainly doing construction and agricultural work. It was given the glorious name of Hogpound. Scattered among the villages were cipher experts working at Bletchley Park, living on amphetamines and caffeine, suffering from insomnia and occasionally waking with the solution to a problem which had been puzzling them for days. We rarely came into direct contact with the patients but I remember Herbert Gilbert, the chimney sweep, being wheeled into our hall slumped in the wooden box which formed the front part of his tricycle. He had fractured his femur. The problem the hospital had was not sepsis, but removing years of grime. In the fields beyond our village was an aerodrome which became a base for Wellington bombers, often limping back after raids on Germany. One plane, low in the flight path of the main runway, may well have tipped our walnut tree before crashing in the field behind the houses on the opposite side of our road. My mother went to help as the airmen were pulled from the wreckage.

Towards the end of the War, when people began to look to the peace, Beveridge's report on the future welfare state, the return of the heroes to something better than awaited those after the First World War and the possibility of a National Health service were very much to the fore. My father was strongly in favour of a health service. My mother was a gradualist, wanting the panel system which applied to working men extended initially to their families. As a G.P., she had many patients whom she could not charge, to whom she gave her services free.

Just after V.E. Day the medical officer of health for Buckingham and Bletchley, who had taken over my father's post when he went to the War, felt it his duty to work with the Allied forces in Germany and my mother was asked to take over from him and also to become M.O.H. for Aylesbury. On demobilization, my father returned to his pre-war job, taking over from my mother! He was asked to establish whether some children who had moved into the area were mentally defective or not. Realizing where they came from, both parents visited them, finding them to be fluent Welsh speakers who soon adapted to their new surroundings. He was also asked to examine a complaint in Bletchley. A new coffee factory had been opened. Some people objected to the smell, but others had a more serious objection. If they left their baby in a pram in the garden, they would return to find it brown all over from a fine sediment of coffee grounds. A migraine sufferer in that town, a well-known ex-teacher, became suicidal, and taking a gun, shot himself through the head. At the postmortem it was apparent that two bullets had been fired. No further action was taken. In the post-War period all members on Bletchley Council were anxious that Bletchley should become the site of a new town — later to be Milton Keynes. There were uncertainties about the water supply from artesian wells. Was it too hard? And did they need to add fluoride to it? In fact it contained more than the requisite amount of fluoride.

I was becoming aware of social issues as they abutted on to medicine. We had essays on the future Health Service, and to my English master's surprise, I wrote a very lengthy and well argued essay on the subject. It did contain one howler which Portia in the Merchant of Venice would have appreciated: '... including a piece from Nye Bevan himself!' I was fascinated by the social service-type talks given on the radio to service men and their families by the then Barbara Betts, later known as Mrs Castle. I listened to the Radio Doctor, Charles Hill, before he became political, and to other medical broadcasts such as, for example, by Una Ledingham, whose ward rounds I was later to attend at the Royal Free Hospital. This aspect of medicine was also enhanced by my father leaving Public Health to take up Industrial Medicine, making me aware of issues such as safety at work and pollution of the environment from industrial effluence.

The immediate post-war period was the time of greatest restriction. Bread was rationed for the first time. The wartime loaf, grey in colour, had provided more nutrition than white bread. In the country we dug for victory. Eggs and milk were plentiful. I became an expert in cleaning out the hen-houses at the end of term and plucking all manner of poultry: chickens, ducks, geese and turkeys — I preferred to skin rabbits! With mash and grain for chickens in short supply, the local farmers allowed the villagers, including ourselves, to glean the fields after the harvest had been gathered. One food we lacked during the war and immediately afterwards was bananas. Before the war my father used to dote on over-ripe bananas, which he would buy late in the day from Johnsons the fruiterers in Bletchley. Much was made of the novelty of bananas when they eventually arrived. We were told that they could save the lives of children with coeliac disease. What a disappointment the anaemic bananas proved to be! It was years before I felt they were a worthwhile fruit. The story that they were a rich source of potassium came many years later.

**Baghdad**

My father was seconded from the Ministry of Supply (where he inspected Royal Ordnance factories up and down the country) to Baghdad as Professor of Public Health and Industrial Medicine. The medical school had been set up on the lines of Edinburgh University. In teaching Public Health, my father was able to introduce several innovations including giving the students specific projects, which they performed with enthusiasm, often supporting their text with photographs. One such was to follow what happened to the bones from the Anatomy lab. They were traced to a dump where the dogs carried them away.

On arrival in Baghdad, my parents stayed temporarily in a house within the bounds of the then Royal Hospital. A tragedy had occurred: the place was overrun by cats and one had eaten a newborn babe. Apparently they had been fed the placentas and this child was as yet unwashed. Attempts to reduce the cat population by shooting failed but our little Welsh terrier, who had lived peacefully alongside our cat, overcome by the heat, attacked and killed many of the cats before dying of exhaustion.

There was a mosque, belonging to a well-known family with whom my father was on friendly terms. One member of the family – I will refer to him as Qadim – had a testicular tumour with a secondary in the frontal lobe of the brain. This was diagnosed by my uncle and operated upon in London. As a result he became a consummate liar. On a return visit, my father called at the Iraqi Embassy and spoke to Qadim's cousin, who was greatly disturbed. Qadim had come to London claiming to be negotiating an oil deal and had been seen by various Foreign Office officials. He had also claimed to have slept with so-and-so's wife. What news had my father got concerning Qadim? 'Nothing bad! He's as pleased as Punch at his new baby, called Ra'ad.' 'But he is not even living with his wife!' Ra'ad turned out to be his daughter's rag-doll; after which we named a dog.

My parents had another dog in Baghdad called La'ath, which means lion.

The dog caught rabies and had to be destroyed. One of the vets in Baghdad had done a thesis on rabies. It had been submitted but lost in the blitz with the bombing of the Royal College of Surgeons in London. If a dog contracts rabies, the owners are advised to have a course of inoculations – at that time with very painful intraperitoneal injections. A professor of pharmacology who had visited the house, and may have stroked the dog, also insisted on being inoculated. We were advised to let him go ahead as he could develop pseudo-rabies, which in turn can be lethal.

I spent several holidays over the next seven years in Iraq. This covered the time from my last years at school to qualification An alternative in the summer was to fly or hitch-hike to meet up in Trieste, Vienna or Istanbul. I had my own car in Baghdad – a secondhand Jaguar. Some Arabs had bought it to go gazelle hunting in the desert. Gazelles would run in a wide circle at about 30 miles per hour and the so-called sport was to shoot at them from Chevrolets. The anglophile Arabs assumed that a Jaguar would be that much quicker but its low clearance meant that it constantly stuck in wadis, so they sold it to some RAF types in disgust. I was intrigued by the suqs, or bazaars, and by the carpet dealers, particularly by one of them, Qashi, who would clean the carpets, drinking a cup of water and producing a fine spray from his nose.*

My medical education was enhanced by visits to the hospital. In the pathology department, Prof. Mills showed me emboli in the brain from schistosomiasis. I had read his work on gastric acidity acting as a barrier against intestinal disease such as typhoid. My father's advice when we were travelling about Iraq was never to take food which appeared to be swimming in liquid, and if we were given anything suspicious, always to drink a glass of Liban (soured milk), however dirty, to increase the gastric acidity.

I remember three of my father's published works from that time. There were examples of tetanus neonatorum where bleeding from the umbilicus of the newborn had been staunched by the use of infected cow-dung. He described cases of dermatitis from primitive dyeing methods, with the workers standing in huge vats of caustic soda and other mordants. He was only allowed to publish the paper, complete with photographs, by comparing it with a newer factory, claiming then and now! Of great interest was the examination of Kurdish porters, who would walk the whole length of

---

*The nose, and especially inability to sneeze, is related to psychiatric disorders in Eastern culture. In Indian Ayurvedic medicine snuff is used to induce sneezing and African traditional healers believed that mental patients had worms in their head that could be expelled by violent sneezing. In India inability to sneeze is associated not only with the more socio-culturally deprived, but with endogenous depression and schizophrenia. Treatments tried include snuffing tobacco, ammonia or chili powder. Claims are made that improvement in sneezing occurs *pari passu* with clinical improvement and that schizophrenic patients seldom have inhalent allergies and therefore seldom sneeze even during the hayfever season.

Rashid street (three miles or so) carrying boxes or arm-chairs on their backs. They were small men with low blood pressure and slow pulses. When asked what they could carry, they gave a set answer, but if asked 'what if I paid you double', the weight would be enormous. And, indeed at times, we saw a single porter carry a grand piano through the milling street. There had been an outbreak of woolsorter's disease, anthrax, and I was taken to see the women at work carding or combing the fleeces seated on the floor in a dusty atmosphere, stopping every now and again in the same room to put a babe to their breast.

The political situation in Baghdad was never stable but my father had endeared himself to the inhabitants of the bund – the squatter encampment – by installing a supply of piped water. If there was a risk of a riot or uprising, unofficial guards would appear from the bund to protect our property. My parents were nearly thrown out of Baghdad due to the action of my mother. Besides doing a limited general practice among the European population, she also worked voluntarily in Maternity and Child Welfare clinics. A year-old infant was brought to her who had not had a normal bowel motion for six months. In the course of examination she rubbed and palpated its abdomen and – lo and behold – it defaecated. It turned out that the child had been seeing another doctor who was the cousin of a senior cabinet minister and had received regular enemas at great expense.

Needless to say, through working in these clinics, my mother soon gained a facility to speak Arabic, but it was colloquial, feminine Arabic, below the umbilicus! She could, seated next to a Sheikh at a dinner, make fruitful conversation by asking how many children he had. Or how many wives! Often they would take on a second or third, because the first bore no children, or just females, and, on reaching the third or fourth, begin to realize that the fault might lie with themselves, but they would keep the wives for company. My mother's request to the gardener to remove his donkey from the lawn 'because its bowels too full open' caused hilarity. Language differences also caused problems. The word 'na'am' in Arabic means 'yes'; the Welsh word for no, 'nage', caused frequent confusion. That, and the habit of some Indians to answer 'yes' by a roll of the head, led my uncle to write an article on Yes and No in the *King's College Hospital Gazette*, later to be reproduced in Aphasiology and other aspects of language as *The City of Yes and the City of No*.

Her rival in general practice was none other than the professor of medicine. He would never say 'you have such and such a condition' but rather 'I have prevented you from developing pneumonia' or some other complication. There were two 'colonies' of homosexuals who seemed to gravitate towards her practice: one centred around the British Council and the other consisted of Mosleyite, ex-18B internees, who were lecturers in English at the University and included the writer Desmond Stewart. A typical passage from his writings would run as follows: 'I will not describe the beautiful lady but the youth . . .'

During our time in Baghdad we lived in two houses in the Alwiyah district, both bungalows with high ceilings and thick mud walls, built by the British when they initially controlled Iraq. Ventilation was achieved by a central rotating fan and water poured over briars covering the windows. As such they were superior in winter and summer to modern air-conditioned homes, which often required additional humidification. My twenty-first birthday party was gate-crashed by the future dictator of Iraq, Col. Qassim. A neighbour, Mohammed Makia, an architect with an English wife (we have reason to believe that she passed her husband off to some of her relatives as being Scottish) came to the party bringing with him a number of Army officers, including the said colonel. Mr Makia was later to act as interpreter in negotiations with the British Ambassador when Qassim came to power. He has since designed many mosques throughout the Gulf States.

My father's other function was to act as adviser to the Minister of Health. There were several ministers over the seven years but the one I remember was Majid Mustafa, whom I accompanied on a visit to the north of the country. Majid Mustafa, was a Kurd. In fact, Nuri-Es-Said's cabinet consisted of the varied groups within the country. Though mainly Sunni, there was always at least one Shia and one Christian. The stated purpose of the trip was to improve public health and particularly the water supply to the villages and towns along the main routes. The idea was that such changes would be readily seen and hopefully copied by other habitations off the main tracks. It was also an opportunity to see some of the religious minorities in Iraq. Christians formed the largest minority group. In some regards they were despised and possessed the faults inherent in minorities, expecting other nominal Christians such as Europeans to give them preference at all times. They could drink alcohol, eat pork, and were not expected to wash several times a day. There were the followers of John the Baptist, mainly silver-smiths. Mohammed persecuted unbelievers but tolerated and taxed believers of other faiths. So they formed a new religion, the chief feature of which was that they remained uncircumcised. There were the devil worshippers who propitiated the devil who could harm them, hence their epithet. They did not eat lettuce because the devil hid under the leaves. A rarer sect, controlling one of the villages and presided over by a Metropolitan (bishop and ruler, as with the Cypriot, Archbishop Makarios) was the Nestorian Christian or, more accurately, Chaldean. Another village was presided over by a powerful woman called Hapsa Khan.

Our journey took us to Suleimaniya, Kirkuk (the oil town), Arbil (or Erbil), and Mosul. Arbil was of interest as having the highest artifactive mound of any town in the world, formed by years of continuous existence. In Mosul, the capital of the northern province, we met up with the local governor and strong man, an able but tough ruler trying to keep the peace. Then, as now, there was an insurrection for an independent Kurdistan led by Brazzani. The Kurds, the Medes of the Old Testament, had an Indo-European language, and lived in parts of Iraq, Iran, Turkey and Russia. They wore a distinctive head-dress, blouse and baggy trousers, except in Turkey, where they were forced to wear cloth caps. Most of them were Sunni Muslims, similar to the ruling group in Iraq; though numerically the Shia Muslims in the south were in the majority. From Mosul we travelled further north to Saladdin and SurArmadia. SurArmadia was a village of bungalows allotted to ministers of the crown, We stayed there overnight and the next morning, to our astonishment, saw various dignitaries talking to each other, wearing dishdashers or galibias (what we would term night shirts), over the garden walls.

At this stage, Majid Mustafa had to return to Baghdad and my father and I continued travelling by horse and mule along the Turkish border to Zakkho and other villages to study their health problems. One problem immediately evident, because of the narrowness of the valleys, was that rice was grown illegally within a mile of the villages, increasing the risk of malaria. My father asked, 'Did any doctors visit'? The answer was, 'Yes, a year or so ago'. 'What for?' 'To investigate "bites from a dagger".' On his return to Baghdad he looked into the question of medical care. The use of a slow-landing aircraft was not possible because there were no landing strips. A helicopter service was also ruled out. He advertised for a doctor who would have a supporting mule team. The advert was answered by the wife of a mountaineer who had died in the mountains. She herself was very much an out-door type. She flew out from England, arrived in Mosul, unpacked her husband's belongings, broke down weeping and had to be flown home.

The other trip I made with a ministerial delegation was to the Shia Holy Cities of Kerbala and Nejef. Annual pilgrimages occur, particularly from Persia, to reenact the procession through the streets of the headless body of Hussein. The more fanatical flagellants cut themselves and kept the blood flowing by beating their heads. The posher fat-cats walked along tapping their chests and wailing. Several million swell the towns at that time of year, creating a health hazard. My father was adviser to the committee of Muslims, who would officially solve the problem. They met in a cellar where they drank whisky. Mohammed had forbidden the drinking of the juice of the grape on the surface of the earth. Whisky had not been mentioned. There are two lovely stories of young Arabic scholars, sent to different parts of Iraq by the British Embassy, to improve their colloquial Arabic. One returned from Kerbala praising the size and taste of the apples he had bought there. It was explained to him that the apples were used to preserve the bodies brought down from Iran for burial in the holy cities. Another questioned the accuracy of the depiction of river boats on Amara silver-ware, showing several people rowing the boats. He had only seen two at most in a boat. The number of rowers, he was told, depended on the importance of the passenger.

On other trips with my father, Majid Mustafa was always keen to visit prisons. He himself had been a political prisoner and showed the imprint of leg irons around his ankles. In one prison my father recognized that a prisoner had leprosy. He was released and despatched across the border to Iran. Other advice given by my father included the inspection of the brothels in Baghdad. This advice was not taken up, but they pulled down part of the brothel-area to erect a statue to ex-king Rhazi (Ghazi). The site was singularly appropriate! To end with a quotation from my father's lectures: 'When a nomad soils the ground, he moves on: when a townsman does so, he builds a house on it.'

**Early Experience**
King's College Hospital had the reputation for producing good G.P.s, though in fact most of my year became consultants. Many of the students were the children of friends or relatives of the consultants. It was one of the more friendly of the London teaching hospitals. The teaching was sound but the atmosphere rather laid back. The number of students from Oxford and Cambridge was small compared with the intake at a different time of year from King's College in the Strand. There were also fewer house-jobs available to us. In addition to the southern English types, there were always a dozen or so Welsh students, typically hard drinking, rugby playing characters. The doyen of these students was one Johnny Harries, diminutive in stature but fly-half for the hospital, for the United Hospitals and London Welsh. If he had not been half the size of Cliff Morgan, he would most certainly have been a Welsh International. He was unexpected in another way: very bright. He ended his days as Professor of Paediatrics at Great Ormond Street.

Although the N.H.S. had been in existence for ten years, something of the pre-War approach still existed among the consultants. In those days the consultants were Honaries at the teaching hospital. This gave them status but their pay came from private practice. The senior honaries were expected to go abroad for three months of the year, when their Assistant Physician, also a consultant, looked after their private work. There were few intermediate posts above house-officers, promotion often coming via appointment as Physician to out-patients. A newly appointed consultant without private means existed by doing visits to the municipally owned hospitals in various parts of London at £5 per time. The work at the Teaching Hospital was always taken seriously because the students, if duly impressed by the teaching they received, once qualified, would refer private patients to their old chiefs. Most teaching was at the bedside to firms of apprentice students who clerked the patients. Attendance at lectures was regarded as less important.

After a brief but useful introductory course, the Oxford and Cambridge graduates were expected to join Terence East's firm. He was the Senior Physician. If you could hear him you could hear any cardiac murmur. The story goes that a house-physician, invited to dinner at his house, found conversation somewhat difficult. The door opened and a shaggy dog entered the room. 'Nice dog, sir', he said. 'Huh, mitral stenosis!' It transpired that Terence had taken the dog to a vet who had clamped a stethoscope on it and diagnosed mitral stenosis. Terence was, in fact, a first class clinical opinion. His short textbook on cardiology was written in precise, very short, sentences; an excellent introduction to the widely used textbook by Paul Wood. The other Physician on the firm was Bruce Pearson – Dr Spruce Person, of the pantomimes. Like his father, a socialite G.P. in Buckingham, he always wore a carnation in his button-hole. There were some excellent Physicians, notably Sam Oram and Clifford Hoyle, on the other firms and we also had a Medical Tutor in Robert Cutforth, brother of the BBC reporter, René Cutforth. Advancement was particularly difficult just after the War and Dr Cutforth emigrated to Tasmania.

The surgical firm was the Admiral's – Sir Cecil Wakeley, Bart – regarded as the character of the hospital. His teaching was down to earth and basic. There was always a touch of surprise when one learnt that he was President of the Seventh Day Adventists. A testimonial from him was invaluable – two lines on the candidate; two lines of his honorary degrees. Edward Muir, the number two, was an excellent thyroid and rectal surgeon, whose reputation was far in excess of his position at King's. The specialities were even better taught. Wood and Catteral for orthopaedics, Yates Bell and Harland Rees for urology, were outstanding.

Three lecturers had very individual techniques. One could hear Sir Phillip Manson-Barr's lectures on Tropical Medicine all over the Medical School.

His lectures were always packed out; but with a booming voice and risqué stories, he would try to empty the lecture theatre of female students, of whom he disapproved. Denis Hill, later Sir Denis, would fill the lecture theatre on a Saturday morning with a psychiatric demonstration, and then, after a coffee break, with a lecture. He would stand leaning against the blackboard, legs crossed, a half-smile on his face, slightly supercilious, but *the fact is* that he attracted people to attend, voluntarily, on a Saturday morning before they dispersed to play rugby all over south London, or on the sloping home pitch at Dog Kennel Hill. One referee I recall at Dog Kennel Hill was Denis Thatcher. The third lecturer with a special technique was Macdonald Critchley. At the National Hospital for Nervous Diseases, Queen Square, his more usual habitat, he gave theatrical lectures with no notes and skilful timing. In demonstrating a patient with a lesion of the parietal lobe, he would display the carefully selected contents of his pockets on a table in front of the patient. The patient in Poppelreuter's test would be asked to find a named object and would respond far quicker if it lay to his right rather than to the left of his field of vision, thereby demonstrating visual neglect. At King's, the patient would be briefly introduced by the house-officer, key signs elicited, and the patient would then leave. Diagnostic possibilities would be sought from the audience and written up on the blackboard. Then, like a detective sorting out clues, he would explain and eliminate each one in turn until the correct diagnosis was found and enlarged upon.

Domiciliary midwifery was part of our requirement to deliver at least 20 babes. We would be taken out by the midwives to the homes. They took pleasure at dead of night to go through all the traffic lights on red. One of the midwives taught me to play chess whilst waiting. The pocket set would be balanced on the mother's abdomen until the contractions became too vigorous and we had to prepare for delivery. How the babe arrived depended on the lie of the child: left to the Lord, i.e. upwards; right to the road, downwards. We used forceps as necessary and afterwards sewed up any episiotomy. Some of the teaching was done at Dulwich Hospital, notably by renowned medical polymath, Dr Friedman. This was an L.C.C. Hospital where Clement Attlee's father had been the medical director. Obstetrics and Gynaecology there were taught by Lady Burt, estranged wife of Sir Cyril Burt, the controversial Clinical Psychologist. They had apparently written an article on vaginismus together, then parted. Lady Burt had two attributes: a fondness of racing – she would have a radio duly draped with sterile cloth wheeled into the operating theatre to listen to a race meeting – and she was slightly deaf: 'I have not heard a foetal heart all day'.

In Paediatrics we were expected to give our own presentations. I remember discussing the vexed point of growing pains and rheumatism in childhood. One disease we encountered then, which thankfully has disappeared, was known as pink disease, or acrodynia. Children from 4 months to 4 years of age would arrive in hospital moribund with painful, red, swollen hands and feet, flaccid, apathetic, unable to take food or move, with a racing pulse and raised blood pressure. At the time there was no specific treatment. The disease was eliminated when mercuric (calomel) teething powders, diaper rinses, vermifuges, laxatives, tonics and ointments were proscribed. Even so, textbooks of Paediatrics and Medicine, fifteen years later, still debated the possible causes, including its presence in certain localities, possible inheritance, arsenical poisoning, dietary deficiency, adrenal insufficiency, and infection (which explained the raised white cell count). Other diseases such as SMON, due to treatment with clioquinol for travellers' diarrhoea and also producing a peripheral neuropathy, were likewise ascribed to infection etc. long after the causative factor had been withdrawn from circulation.

**House-Surgeon**
My first house job, one of the three available to Oxford and Cambridge graduates, was in ENT (Ears, Nose and Throat). Two aspects of the subject were invaluable in preparation for a career in Neurology. The first was an appreciation that speech comprehension, deafness and dementia can overlap and mask each other; the second that of dizzy turns, vertigo and momentary losses of awareness. Hearing gets scant attention in any discussion of speech pathology, despite the adage, attributed to Epictetus, that Nature has given man one tongue, but two ears; that we hear twice as much as we speak. It is also a truism that in many respects deafness is an abnormality treated less sympathetically than blindness. People do not always recognize that someone is deaf. It may develop insidiously and they feel cut off from the world, misunderstanding and misunderstood. Loss of communication may lead to paranoia. I was later to learn that poor facial expression, or lack of facial expression, can seriously interfere with communication, which is always a two-way process. With the Moebius syndrome, where there is absence of facial musculature, or with some psychological or other awkwardness − where one's face does not fit − people are treated harshly and unsympathetically. Older people, often with coincidental deafness, may develop facial rigidity and lose facial expression because of parkinsonism or strokes. Their feelings in conversations are passed over without recognition, and this can enhance paranoia. Furthermore, as these conditions cause pseudobulbar palsy, the situation may be aggravated by untriggered, uncontrolled and

difficult-to-terminate laughter or weeping. Deaf psychiatric units, which I was later to visit, often contain patients who do not suffer from congenital deafness but instead from central disorders of language.

Dizzy turns swamp ENT as well as neurological and even cardiological clinics. The key is to recognize 'vertigo', an hallucination of movement. The archetype vertiginous syndrome is Meniere's disease. The first attack is usually the most severe and lasts several days, accompanied by some loss of hearing, Subsequent attacks are less severe and fade as hearing is lost in that ear. Between attacks some loss of hearing also occurs. Next is the posterior inferior cerebellar artery syndrome, caused by thrombosis or an insufficiency due to poor vascular flow through the vertebrobasilar arteries and their branches. The onset, once again, is sudden, with vomiting, and with a dissociated sensory loss (loss of pain and temperature sensation but not of light touch) which does not persist. Characteristically when lying down, the room appears on a slant so that the doors appear at an angle. The third common syndrome is benign postural vertigo, said to be due to a virus, though I can never remember a virus ever being recognized. There are two types of postural or positional vertigo: 'peripheral' which occurs after a brief interval on lying the patient back, head below the couch – this form of vertigo will fatigue if repeated several times; and 'central', which occurs immediately on movement and persists. The Hallpike-Cawthorne test is used to confirm the findings, differentiating central disturbances from those of the otolith within the ear, and also showing which otolith (on the same or opposite side) is at fault. Hot water and then cold water are injected into the aperture of the ear and the defects are recognised from the mnemonic: House-surgeon = hot to same side; Casualty-officer = cold to opposite side. Other lesser forms of dizziness are separated mostly by history. We would ask about light-headedness or faint feelings, colour changes and palpitations. We avoided the word 'giddiness', which to many patients implied hysteria or limited intelligence. In Leicestershire there was a useful local expression – half-faint. Many years later I lectured in the States on syncope – momentary loss of consciousness due to imperfect oxygenation or perfusion of the brain – after doing an leading article on the subject with a cardiologist. We had advised keeping accounts of the various episodes. This was unacceptable in the town, where there were many more neurologists per head of population than in the U.K. We were told that there were 15 neurologists per million population and if we did not do the full gamut of invasive tests, someone else would.

 I shared house-officer duties with the youngest of the Admiral's sons, Richard – better known as *foetal* – Wakeley, who left medicine to enter the

Royal Academy of Dramatic Art. One patient I had to prepare for tonsillectomy was the son of my teacher and future boss, Sam Nevin. Sam burst into the room anxious to give the history in person, but we had certain set questions to which he did not know the answers: had the child had a recent infection, recent inoculations or been given the polio virus? He beat a hasty retreat.

The senior surgeon was Bill Daggett, an excellent operator. He never knew precisely what he would do until he was well inside the ear. The number two, Terence Cawthorne, had a set operation, performed rapidly by his registrars, but when he himself was operating, liable to take much longer as invariably he had an audience of overseas surgeons. Sir Terence Cawthorne was later to be President of the Royal Society of Medicine. He could be somewhat pompous, telling his students that people in authority usually talk slowly. 'The Prime Minister, for example, talks at about 80 words a minute. When I talk to you, and what I have to say is important, it is perhaps 60 words per minute!'. Newly qualified doctors have difficulty dealing with the demands of private patients and Cawthorne had plenty. I felt I had the right response when asked by one of them whether Mr Cawthorne was the only one doing this particular operation. I replied that he was training a team. When doing National Service, I sent Sir Terence a Christmas card, receiving the reply that he rarely sent such cards and that he had changed his operation on the stapes (of the middle ear) from rock-and-roll to foot-plate work. Had he joined the wheel tappers club?

I remain grateful to Sir Terence Cawthorne for introducing me to Goya. At the age of 46 Goya succumbed to the Vogt-Koyanagi syndrome of deafness and transient blindness. The eye becomes inflamed and along with the deafness is a loss of pigmentation of the hair and skin. Theories differ whether it is a viral infection or a hypersensitivity reaction of the body's antibodies to melanin and other pigment cells. The onset is accompanied by headache, fever and vertigo. I clerked one such patient for Sir Terence and in nearly 40 years of practice have encountered two others, but it is the character of Goya that I remember. Total deafness was associated with brooding hallucinations, from which, even at their most horrific, he achieved wry amusement, drawing satisfaction from the reckless, masterly way he was able to transform the hideous and nightmarish distortions into his famous Black Paintings. Goya talked of monsters coming into his drawings as though he had no control over them. Despite these hallucinations and the episodes of depression and paranoia which so often attend total, acquired deafness, Goya continued at the height of his creative powers, producing over 700 paintings when he was between 62 and 73 years of age. His court paintings were realistic rather than flattering but his relationship with the court was such that the King learnt sign language to converse with him.

Sir Victor Negus had officially retired, occasionally returning to operate. Scrubbing up for him (preparing to operate) was an extremely complicated affair and had to be done meticulously. We were also expected to ring him to wish him a happy birthday or a happy Christmas. Apparently he was most upset because we sang 'Sir Victor' and not 'Dear Gussie'. These were the days when we decorated the wards and the surgeon (or physician) whose ward it was came in to carve the turkey. The other two surgeons were excellent: Mawson, with whom I had relatively little contact and Rolly Lewis, whose wife was a famous detective novelist, Christiana Brand. Rolly was noted for large operations for cancer of the larynx and many hours were spent holding retractors. Most patients after laryngectomy had a very weak voice but oesophageal speech was taught and two – an ex-sergeant major and a buyer from Harrods – developed excellent loud voices. Many of the patients required heroin, the Brompton cocktail or combinations of pethidine and largactil. I came home one day – my parents had bought us a house in Half Moon Lane, Herne Hill to look after their furniture and provide them with a base on return from Iraq – to find they had engaged a gardener who was a laryngectomized, former patient previously on heroin. He managed to do the mowing etc very well.

The house in Herne Hill had an acre and half of garden stretching to the railway line, on the other side of which was the London Welsh rugby ground. There was a cottage down a lane in the garden with garages underneath. All that later became a building site for new housing, including one house owned by Mrs Thatcher. Nearer the house was a large apple tree. The apples were best used for cooking but if not too bruised, for eating also. They fell from a height of at least 20 feet. It was said that Queen Elizabeth 1st had come down the river Effra and had a picnic under that same tree. My story so far seems to be replete with dog anecdotes. Our dog, a mongrel – quarter this and quarter that, – had been bought by my father from Battersea Dogs Home and although generally intelligent, had been hit by vehicle and developed a temporary paralysis of the hind legs. An hysterical paralysis of that type, we were told by a neighbouring G.P., was not uncommon in dogs.

Out-patients were very much the domain of the House-officer, cleaning out ears, examining tonsils and vocal cords, and crunching at sinuses. One patient insisted that he be seen by the House-Surgeon and no other person! By the end of an afternoon, the oft repeated phrase, 'How long have you been hard of hearing?' became a shout, requiring a cooling off period before normal speech was resumed.

## House-Physician

From now on, no more surgery; though I was always happy to do procedures. My next job was in Leicester. In fact I swapped with Chris Dulake, who was coming back to do a job at King's. My chief, Dr Selwyn Tanner, had one peculiar quirk. On his ward rounds the sister carried an umbrella, which would be opened when he came to examine fundi with an ophthalmoscope. Another of the physicians had recently completed an MD thesis on the cardiographic changes in the dying; so much so that his appearance on a ward with an ECG machine behind closed curtains was regarded as a death sentence. Dr Joan Walker, the diabetologist for whom I also worked, had carried out a pioneering epidemiological study in the village of Ibstock. She had had multiple sclerosis, but apart from a wide-based gait, showed no residual sign of the disease. One also learnt a lot from the Senior Registrar, Bertie Matthews. He had the misfortune of having a paper published, nearly two years after he had done the work in Birmingham, the same week that the co-author, Dr Cort, had escaped from Britain as a spy. The press descended on him, assuming that he had collaborated in more ways than one!

The Infirmary was particularly well designed, with an x-ray department above casualty. One was able to complete the diagnosis of Addison's disease, for example, with x-rays and blood taken before the patient reached the ward. However the medical wards at that time were cluttered with patients who had taken overdosages, mainly of barbiturates. In just 6 months I saw over 100 suicidal (or attention-seeking) attempts.

I did a third job, also medical, at the Whittington Hospital, North London. This was a large, former London County Council hospital occupying three adjacent sites. I worked for Hubert Pearson, a cardiologist, and his assistant, Elio Montuschi – a consultant in his own right at the Italian Hospital. To interest Pearson in anything, one merely had to ask whether there was an equivalent disease in animals. 'Monty' was particularly helpful but smoked heavily and had hypertension, which he never treated adequately.

The advantage of the Whittington Hospital was that it provided the opportunity to work for membership. It ran its own course and the juniors could attend the discussion and presentations. We were also able to attend the membership course run by Pappworth, by far the best known course in London. Pappworth had been Senior Registrar to Lord Cohen in Liverpool. He had fallen out with Henry Cohen. Cohen revelled in his ability to make brilliant spot diagnoses. Pappworth not only tried to trick him but had written up Cohen's collection of Bechet's disease without his permission. Consequently he came down to London but failed to get on at any of the major hospitals, and concentrated on teaching, taking his students to see patients at less noted minor establishments. His method of presenting cases to examiners was distinctive – frowned upon by the examiners, who hated his guts, and his comments – he attacked them all for unethical conduct, particularly for the early work on cardiac catheterisation. However his examination technique became current throughout London, taught by registrars who had benefitted from his teaching. He eventually published his examination crib as a textbook. We would have been ill-advised to have used 'Pappworth's Primer Prepares for Membership' as an alternative to other tongue-twisters such as 'West Register Street', 'The Leith Police Dismisseth us', or Sam Nevin's 'say "Royal Irish Constabulary", ah that's lovely, say it again' (Sam's father had been a chief in the R.U.C.) to check on articulation defects. I attended most of Pappworth's lectures, though not those on neurology, and did not attend his ward rounds. When he realized my relationship to Macdonald Critchley, he told of Macdonald's one and only foray as a membership examiner. He lined up three patients, asking the examinees, to comment on their speech defects. One was dysarthria, one dysphonia, and one aphasia. But the candidates felt they were expected to give more high-falutin' answers: Head's semantic aphasia, Wernicke's jargon aphasia, etc. Some would ask the patient his name, which he was usually able to give without revealing his handicap. He therefore decided the best procedure would be to speak to the patients himself, then ask the candidate to comment on the speech defect. One such candidate, a very Brahmin Indian, after he had spoken for a few minutes, answered 'Very sorry, Sir, did not listen, thought it a private conversation!' Reading Lord Walton's Memoirs, I learnt that he had been taken on the long case by Macdonald Critchley and had passed. His patient had a spastic paraparesis and 'Spik no English'.

**National Service**
I began my National Service with a faux-pas, parking my car in what turned out to be the Major General's car port. We were sent first of all to Crookham, to be taught drill and turned into officers. We had the traditional regimental sergeant major with a big handle-bar moustache and a booming voice that carried across the parade ground. I was to encounter him again after I had been in Malaya for some time. He came out, pasty-faced, moustache shaved, flabby, with 7 or 8 children and a sick wife in tow – not exactly the epitome of the modern mobile army.

Our next posting was to Millbank, where we could slip out at lunch time to the Tate Gallery and look out upon the Chelsea Pensioners. At breakfast each officer had his own butter, marmalade, toast and paper rack set before him. If he had no wish to speak, or to be spoken to, he wore his cap. We received lectures on army medicine. Those from the psychiatrists were particularly boring. A psychiatrist is never any good unless he possesses some unusual characteristics. The Tropical Medicine lectures were of value and were soon to be put to the test. Lectures on the medical hazards of atomic warfare raised our ire. We were given to understand that we would be safe if we were the right side of the hedge! The course ended with a quiz. This consisted in the main of pathological bottles and slides; but there was also a photograph, and loud whispers were heard to ensure that we all recognized the Director General of the Medical Corps, Brigadier General Sir Alexander Drummond. I had already written my answer – Baghdad boil on nose!

I used my embarkation leave to do locums at Grays in Essex and at Lowestoft. Grays was a G.P. locum in a practice run by Scotsmen. The major requirement was to write short clear diagnoses and ensure continuity. I learnt that whatever the public face of the Scots is, within their own homes they could be most generous. My locum in Lowestoft was in Accident and Emergency with anaesthetics thrown in. Although one does some anaesthetics as a student, this experience was to come in handy later in Malaya, when the anaesthetist was stranded 40 miles away and I had to give an anaesthetic using cyclopropane for a Caesarian section to a Gurkha lady when the babe was in foetal distress. The baby unfortunately died but the mother was no worse for her ordeal.

The flight out to Malaya was prolonged as we had to return to Bombay during the monsoon and await repairs to the plane. We were treated to a film on the Flowers of Kashmir – significant because India was engaged in war with Pakistan over Kashmir. In Singapore we were taken to the opulent RAMC Officers Mess, set on a cliff overlooking the harbour and the off-shore islands. As we drank our crushed lime seated on the wall opposite the Mess, we could look out on the sunset, complete with electric storms lighting up the islands as though in a pageant. I was pleased not to be working in B.M.H. (British Military Hospital), Singapore, presided over by a Col. Baird, who insisted on a definitive diagnosis for every patient. Patients would leave hospital with unconfirmed diagnoses such as Cat Scratch Fever!

The timing of my arrival up-country at B.M.H., Kamunting, just outside Taiping (translated as City of Peace), was more accurately known to the Indian tailors than to the military authorities. I did not have to wait long to be kitted out with the standard olive-green uniform. This was the military hospital closest to where the CTs (Communist Terrorists) were said to be hanging out in the 'ulu' (jungle) living alongside the 'Abo' – now known as the first people of Malaysia. The Communist leader, Ching Peng, had his camp just over the Thai border and the last known sighting of him in Malaya was the finding of a bottle of Benedictine. Troops would fly out into the jungle, complete with jungle trackers – recruited from the head-hunters of Borneo – to live alongside the Abo and gain knowledge of the whereabouts of the last remaining C.T.s. The New Zealand forces used Maori trackers as their jungle guides.

We were almost the last group to do National Service and the battle in Malaya had been all but won by the concurrent granting of independence (Merdeka) to the civilian population. Chinese know-how, particularly in the cities, was not to swamp the Malays – described in older editions of the *Encylopaedia Britannica* as a contented people. There were also Tamils who had been brought in to work the rubber plantations and as fishermen on the West coast. The Malay rulers of each state took it in turns to be the supreme head of state – the Yang Di Pertuan Agon. (A drunken official is said to have toasted His Anus the Highgone!). Prosperity was returning to Malaya with exports of rubber, palm oil, and, from Taiping, especially, open-cast tin mining.

With two exceptions, the B.M.H. was run entirely by National Service doctors. The Commanding Officer (C.O.), Col. Young, deserved considerable praise for the way he gave us the necessary opportunity and support. In many ways he was a typical regular officer. 'The Brigadier will be inspecting the unit. He may ask you to identify some of the medal ribbons on his tunic. You will recognize so-and-so because your commanding officer also has that distinction.' He had the D.S.O. (Distinguished Service Order) partly for his work on army toilets but more particularly for saving lives in the jungle. He had supplied airmen with ropes so that, when they had to bale out and parachute on to the high forest canopy, they would be able to descend to the ground safely. A high proportion of the National Service doctors who went out to Malaya ultimately ended up in Neurology. They included Roman Kocen, Ralph Ross Russell, David Perkin, Malcolm Parsons and myself. Ross Russell had the distinction of being placed under open arrest by the then C.O. The C.O. developed an obsessional psychosis, timing vehicles going round the hospital to see they did not exceed any speed limit. He would also call parades at odd times and both the Surgical and Medical (R.R.R.) Officers were late on parade. I am told that this C.O. ended up as records officer at one of the London Teaching Hospitals.

Most of the patients came in from the jungle by helicopter. On one occasion I had to fly out to bring a patient in. Some of the staff thought that

I should have put up an intravenous drip before flying back. I was more concerned that we should return before night-fall as the helicopters only flew in the daytime. The majority of sick soldiers presented with fever and I still have my looseleaf exercise book of procedures. 'PUOs (pyrexias of unknown origin) should not be given paludrine until the diagnosis of malaria has been definitely excluded, i.e. until another diagnosis is made or the temperature has remained down for more than 48 hours.' In addition to cerebral and falciparum malaria, the diagnoses included Rickettsiae, Leptospirosis, Dysentery (amoebic and bacillary), viral encephalitis and typhoid. Again, quoting from my exercise book: 'A large number of cases are bound to remain as PUOs on discharge, e.g. R.S. Kocen found 42% of PUOs still remained PUOs after clinical differentiation and the following battery of serological tests carried out by USAMRU at K.L.' The American Medical Research Unit based at Kuala Lumpur and derived from the Walter Reed Institute examined all specimens of jungle fever, particularly sorting out the Rickettsial diseases.

Our jungle forces included Brits (mainly National Service men), Aussies, New Zealanders, and Gurkhas. There were also some Malay drivers. Australian Army nurses worked alongside the Q.A.s (Queen Alexandra military nurses). They would describe the rigors, as in malaria, somewhat basically – 'so-and-so has had a skin action, doctor'. An ill Gurkha would be curled up in a ball in the foetal position. As soon as he felt better, he would lie at attention on top of the bed with boots, newly cleaned, underneath.

The Gurkhas would be recruited, checked that they were physically fit, and sent out to their camp at Sungei Patani. But they were not immune to Western diseases and every four years there would be an outbreak of mumps. We would receive a few cases of mumps meningitis, even mumps encephalitis, and a large number of cases of the other common complication in adults – mumps orchitis. This can lead to testicular atrophy, usually unilateral. Roman Kocen decided we should do a controlled trial of steroids aimed at decreasing the risk of atrophy (shrinkage of the testes with loss of ability to produce sperm). We had to get permission from the Brigadier, who allowed us to use cortisone but not prednisolone. He also wanted his name on any paper but Roman said 'no'. As Roman left shortly after completing the study he escaped, but the Brigadier retaliated by writing a damaging report for me. Not that it really mattered. More amusingly, we learnt that one of the officers at BMH Singapore had obtained an M.D. Singapore. We thought we should have submitted M.D.s – one on the left testicle, one on the right.

The Rickettsial diseases are caused by micro-organisms which share characteristics partway between bacteria and viruses. They include dengue, scrub and tick typhus and many variants with specific serologies. Less than 20% have an eschar, a tell-tale mark on the skin rather like a cigarette burn, at the site of a tick-bite. The search for an eschar was particularly important in anyone who presented with an unexplained paralysis, as tick-paralysis could be cured by removal of the offending organism. Most of the rickettsiae came with enlarged glands and a rash, which could be fleeting, and over the chest sometimes difficult to determine. Ross Russell suggested a Kamunting triad for rickettsial diseases of fever with rash, epitrochlear glands and a dicrotic pulse. Once diagnosed, they were treated with chloramphenicol. Theoretically, as David Weatherall (later to become Sir David Weatherall, Regius Professor of Medicine in Oxford), who spent 6 weeks with us in Taiping, pointed out, all the tropical fevers we saw could be treated with a combination of chloroquine and chloramphenicol, though at the risk of potentially serious side effects. Cerebral malaria could present with a headache increasing in severity with few other features until the patient lapsed into coma, requiring quinine as the best treatment for a life-threatening situation. In addition to the conditions already mentioned, we were also on the lookout for glandular fever, tropical sprue, hepatitis, filiarisis and snake bites. Sea-snakes around Penang island caused several fatalities each year. In addition to my other duties, I doubled up as V.D. doctor for N. Malaya for 6 weeks when Major Sim-Davies was on leave. This was a simple task in so far as the technician did most of the work.

**Leptospirosis**
Leptospirae are elongated flagellate organisms, larger than bacteria, and similar in most characteristics to the spirochaetes that cause syphilis. They are secreted in the urine of rats and small animals and infection is essentially waterborne. Two types are found in England, L. icterohaemorrhagica which causes jaundice (Weil's disease), and L. canicola. Twenty types occur in Malaya. They are usually milder and few cause jaundice. How they enter the body is a matter of dispute. Dr Vollum, who lectured to us in Oxford, suggested ingestion through the accidental gulping of infected water. A couple necking under a bridge fall in and develop 'lepto' a few days later. Water-skiers losing their balance may be at risk. It is also presumed that they enter through cuts. In tropical countries, jungle sores are thought to be a route of entry.

Jungle sores on the shins of troops working in the swelter of the jungle seem to have an arterial distribution on the fronts of the shins, though venous sores lower down near the ankle can also occur. How they arise is unclear. Friction from the protective clothing, sweating, and balding with loss of hair from the skin are all possible factors.

In the course of my time in Kamunting I saw over 100 cases of Leptospirosis. Ross Russell, who had returned to England before I came to Malaya, did an M.D. on Lepto and many of his dicta on treatment were followed. The presentation was characteristic, with fever, severe headache, conjunctival injection and neck stiffness. There was muscle and liver tenderness, occasionally a palpable spleen, a rash, jaundice or petechiae. The blood pressure might be low and at some stage in the illness there would be a reduction of urinary output and even anuria. The temperature could drop suddenly but kick back in 4 to 5 days.

The diagnosis was made by seeing the spirochaete in the blood, or after growth on Korthof's medium by dark ground illumination, and there were specific agglutination and haemagglutination inhibition tests. In one patient we actually saw the spirochaete in the cerebro-spinal fluid. The white blood cell count could be high or low but usually there was an increase in polymorphs. The kidneys were most at risk with a raised blood urea and the urine containing albumin, red cells and casts. A meningitic reaction occurred in the spinal fluid.

Quoting from my exercise book: 'In the healthy soldier, masterly inactivity is the key to treatment.' In fact this was not strictly true. Meticulous charting of blood pressure and fluid intake and output were required.

'Deaths are usually the result of mismanagement. Fluids should be encouraged until the urinary output falls. Then it is essential that the patient is limited as regards fluids and not overhydrated. Tube feeding or intravenous drip may prove necessary.

'The blood pressure may remain as low as 70/50 for 36 to 48 hours. Raise the bed on blocks unless respiratory distress. Noradrenaline and cortisone have not been shown to be of value in this disease. With a low blood pressure, do not start penicillin therapy for fear of a Herxheimer reaction. However, if started, it may be continued.

'Relieve pain, anxiety, and headache with aspirins or pethidine. Tepid sponge and care of mouth as indicated.

'Penicillin probably does shorten the illness by a small but definite amount. It should not be given if there is the risk of sensitivity reactions or the blood pressure is already low. If used, it must be given in large doses 4-6 hourly over 3 days.'

In practice Roman and I deviated from this regimen, preferring for the most part not to use penicillin. Leptospirae are not natural parasites of man and break down in the blood stream with release of protein. It is this sudden release of protein which causes a Jarisch-Herxheimer reaction with a precipitate drop in blood pressure and blocks the kidneys with oliguria and anuria. The Herxheimer reaction itself is not without risk and is accentuated by the use of penicillin, which speeds the breakdown of Leptospirae. Our policy caused some annoyance to Col Mackay Dick (mucky dick) of B.M.H. Kinrara (near Kuala Lumpur), who had claimed that the Herxheimer reaction following penicillin was a diagnostic test for Leptospirosis. In other spirochaetal diseases, such as syphilis or Lyme disease, there are far fewer spirochaetes in the blood stream and a Herxheimer response after antibiotics is useful confirmation of a response to treatment. But if a Herxheimer reaction goes wrong, especially in Leptospirosis in older, unfit people, recourse to dialysis may be required.

I remember two of Dr Vollum's stories which we heard in Florey's department in Oxford with respect to typhoid, which we also saw in Malaya. There had been an outbreak of typhoid at the American Airforce base at Upper Heyford, which was traced to infected ice-cream. Nothing further happened until an outbreak also occurred in the civilian population. During the War ice-cream was not generally available but it transpired that the Americans would bring the cream mixture into Oxford to be frozen, and then collect the full vats for distribution. They failed to realise that liquids expand on freezing. The shopkeeper in Oxford had removed the top layer and sold it locally. The other story I also heard from my father, because it involved the farm from where we obtained the caravan just before war broke out. The mother had had typhoid in the past and continued, like Typhoid Mary, to be a carrier. She was frightened that her young daughter would contract the disease. She had had her gall-bladder removed and took elaborate precautions with toileting. However the daughter eventually did succumb. The farmyard had frozen over, the sewer pipe had burst, and the child was seen in the yard sucking ice.

**Away from Taiping**
I had a large, third- or fourth-hand American car with a gun-holster by the front seat. It had initially belonged to a planter. This enabled me to travel widely: to Frazer's hill, Penang, Pangkor island, the Cameron Highlands and Malacca. I also went infrequently to K.L. (Kuala Lumpur), where I had two very interesting and influential second cousins. Gerwyn Lewis (G.E.D. Lewis) was head of the Victoria Institute, the main grammar school. He and his brother 'Tiny' Lewis had introduced rugger to Malaya. He had been a P.O.W. on the Burma railway, working as a medical orderly. In his autobiography he lists the rugby skills of former pupils – the various state rulers and ministers.

Tom Critchley was the Australian High Commissioner in Malaya and a low handicap golfer. A major function of his was to partner any visiting dignitary in a foursome against the Prime Minister, Tunku Abdul Rahman (also known as Uncle Hitam [Black Uncle]) and the Deputy Prime Minister.

I was short-listed to go to Borneo to recruit head-hunters as jungle trackers. These primitive people were tattooed from head to foot, with the tattooed outline of the larynx particularly prominent. I was eventually told I could not be released for this purpose. However I was able to take my 6 weeks local leave in one go. This enabled me to travel by a French boat to Saigon, Manila, Hong Kong and Japan. I met up with some other soldiers who had been told they must report to the British consulate in Saigon. So we visited the consulate. At that time the Vietnam war was confined to various skirmishes in the Mekong Delta, though a larger conflagration was expected soon. On entering Manila harbour, the island of Corregidor, where MacArthur had hung out, was like an anchored battleship. On a brief visit ashore we were shown the scars of the Japanese conflict. Arriving in Kobe, Japan, where the whole population appeared to be wearing flip-flops with a divided first toe, I travelled to Tokyo and stayed overnight with one of the British Council, previously from Iraq. He made sure the Japanese 'boy' did not molest me. I then joined the others to explore Nijo, Kyoto and the foothills of Mt Fuyi. We stayed in a Japanese inn, the highlight of our visit being the sunken bath. One washes thoroughly in the boiling water outside, the bath getting really hot before taking a final plunge, followed quickly by jumping out and rubbing down.

The return leg of the journey began on a small Australian cargo vessel which took a few passengers. A plaque stated '13 times round this deck is one mile'. From Hong Kong I flew to Bangkok, exhilarated by the quanta of light reflected from the golden, silver, marble and other Buddhas, and on to Siemreap to visit Angkor Wat and Angkor Thom – the city growing out of the jungle. Finally there was a train journey through the peninsula of Thailand to Butterworth.

Towards the end of my time in Taiping I was transferred briefly to the Hussars in Ipoh as their medical officer. An unusual feature of their mess was that one was not allowed to refer to people by their rank but by their semi-official nickname. There was a hill overlooking the town used by the troops for drill in jungle tactics. Despite this, two or three CTs had lived there undisturbed. By going to Ipoh I was able to venture into the jungle with the troops, travelling by canoe using outboard motors, getting out and hauling the canoe up rapids, and shooting the rapids on the return trip. Although we did not contact the CTs, the trip was exhilarating.

## B.M.H. Kluang

My final posting in Malaya was to Kluang, the scene of much bitter fighting early on in the Emergency, and, though it was presumed to be quiet, no one was quite sure. There were impenetrable jungle forts still possibly occupied, and surrounded by moats and hidden spears of bamboo. Here I was the sole physician and in charge of the path lab, aided by a Chinese technician. Harold Fox, from whom I took over (he is currently Professor of Placental Pathology in Manchester), advised me that I knew enough about electrolytes not to require them. The C.O. (I will refer to him as having an Old Testament name) had an unfortunate experience. Having had polio, he took the sugar-coated pill to encourage the others to be immunized, and as a result developed an allergic reaction in the form of the Guillain-Barre syndrome. Just before I arrived, the doctors paid all their mess bills in cash from money earned doing medical clinics based on pharmacies throughout the state. This had been stopped through the intervention of the Malay Medical Association. However, out of interest, we continued to visit the civilian hospital next door and also went to see interesting cases at the hospital in J.B. (Johore Baru). I remember the dramatic manner in which the Chinese physician there explained how to treat the Anterior Tibial Syndrome in order to prevent tissue necrosis by slashing downwards through the skin and fascia.

Whereas the physician in J.B. had double membership of the Royal College of Physicians (Edinburgh and London), the local civilian hospital was more primitive. The gardener was called upon to give the anaesthetics by the rag and bottle method and children were nursed by their relatives. One grandmother, looking after a child who had had a tracheotomy following diphtheria, got so used to it that she fed the babe down the tube. In Malaya we were all part of 17 Gur. Div., with the 2/7 Gurkhas within walking distance of the B.M.H. in Kluang. The medical officer, Brian Duff, was nominated to be the messing officer responsible for the menus but he damaged his reputation by replacing Mulligatawny soup on the breakfast menu with Brown Windsor. The change did not help the Gurkha officers overcome their hangovers! He followed me to Preston as Consultant ENT surgeon.

Working on my own taught me how to be extremely exact in my procedures; thus no case of malaria was treated until I had seen the parasite on thick or thin films – 'Tick and Tin' films, as they were called by the Chinese technician. I had to perform post-mortems: out of interest on snakes, but for real on a soldier who had died of Addison's disease. The troops were kept busy with manoeuvres. From one such there were two casualties –

the C.O. and his sergeant, who, despite being in the water-logged jungle, had restricted their intake of salt and water. I took over a piece of research from Harry Fox, started, I believe, at the instigation of David Weatherall. Sir David (Captain Weatherall) was based in Singapore but came up to Taiping to cover a leave period. He made full use of his National Service, bringing with him one enzyme to study Thalassaemia. A young Malay child was born with the major form and it was decided to top up his anaemia by intra-peritoneal blood transfusions, at the same time seeing what happened to the ratio of foetal to adult haemaglobin.

Just before leaving Malaya, I visited the Chinese markets with Ivan Polunin in Singapore. He was one of three White Russian brothers. One was a noted botanist, another studied migrations of herdsmen in Asia Minor. Ivan was a community physician with a Chinese wife and had produced a TV documentary on the colourful kites and the dragon festivals of Singapore.

## My Incursion into Neurology

Incursion is the right word, because I had avoided Neurology up to this stage. However, I had applied for a job at Maida Vale because I had had a final viva before setting out for Malaya and felt I needed neurological experience to complete my exam. I landed at Stanstead and was taken, still jet-lagged, to be interviewed. I hardly did myself justice, talking of learning some neurology perhaps to do research in industrial medicine. Nonetheless I got the job; and thereafter neurology got a grip of me and held my continued interest. Maida Vale, since closed, was a small hospital, a junior partner to the National, Queen Square, with traditional links with the London Hospital. The two dominant personalities were Lord Brain, (still known as W.R.B.) and the neurosurgeon, Valentine Logue. Brain was a man of few words – 'the silent areas of the brain'. His forte lay in summarizing his findings. He had wide interests, including art and travel, but one rarely had the opportunity to hear him expand on any topic. I remember being told by a Canadian Neurologist, McNaughten, of a verse written by Lord Brain about a colleague – presumably Sir Francis Walshe:-

> This critic is parasitic.
> He makes his living
> Biting
> Other people's writing.'

Valentine Logue was used by all the physicians as a second opinion. He would rapidly sum up a patient in seven minutes. All house-physicians were expected to clerk his neurosurgical patients and we found him a hard task master, but respected and liked. Even after the houseman's late ward round at 10:15 to 10:30 we could expect a call at 11 pm or later; often from his squash club, but it could equally be that he was on the ward, not satisfied with the state of his patient and prepared to take him back to theatre. Certainly working for a neurosurgeon is essential in the training of a neurologist.

These were the days when the porters would open the doors for a senior consultant. They also did so for the Pathology Registrar, Robin Barnard, who would arrive in winged collar, morning suit and cravat in an old-fashioned open-tourer. He did everything with considerable aplomb and, apparently, like all the other staff in the path. lab., was red-green colour blind but gave an excellent opinion. Another extrovert pathologist was Hilary Grant, a sound opinion but wife of Alick Elithorn, Psychiatrist, for whom we also worked but whom we regarded as lost among the clouds. The other Psychiatrist, RTC Pratt, was more down to earth, but believed, as was current among most doctors at the time, that spasmodic torticollis was a psychiatric syndrome. He would follow his patients with this disorder round and round the table in the doctor's mess, giving them small electric shocks which would cause a sudden turning of the head. However, this stimulated my interest in the condition and after a small trial of Amantadine, which was probably of help, was able to use botulinum along with many other neurologists in easing the condition.

Of the Neurologists, Reg Kelly and Peter Croft were undoubtedly the best teachers, and could be relied upon to teach on the patient in front of them rather than on some hypothetical subject. John Marshall and Ronnie Henson were possibly the best clinicians. In a slightly rarefied hospital, Ronnie was the most experienced on general medicine. He could be somewhat tetchy and difficult, which was understandable. In his youth he had been a good sportsman, particularly so in rugger, but developed bulbar polio, retaining a husky, rather awkward, voice. The change in his voice probably affected him more than it would most people. His wife had been an opera singer and he would invite members of staff to his home to sing madrigals. Fortunately for all concerned, I was not invited.

Helen Dimsdale was also to be my chief at my next hospital, the Royal Free. She always knew 57 causes of every condition and had a tendency to graft the Royal Free Disease – Myalgic Encephalomyelitis – on to other disorders to explain slight differences in reflexes etc. I used to refer to the condition, which has had a multitude of names in the past and is now preferentially known as Chronic Fatigue Syndrome, by her approach to the disorder, 'palindromic pleocytosis with glands in the posterior triangle, responding to piriton and perhaps to prednisolone.' She was noted for one of the cleverest M.D. theses, studying the cell changes in the cerebro-spinal fluid following air encephalography. The shortest M.D. thesis I know was by a haematologist at King's College Hospital, who in one page described the sexing of polymorph cells in the blood. There was no previous work to quote.

I certainly retained a soft spot for Sam Nevin, who also worked at Maida Vale. When giving lecture demonstrations at Queen Square, he always worked himself up into a sweat, pausing for breath mid-sentence but giving an excellent display. He used to extract information from doctors or patients by a long series of questions: 'Tell me, doctor, what is the significance of finger clubbing?' By that means he could extract a whole M.D. thesis. On his ward round, piles of electroencephalograms would be examined at the foot of the bed. 'Tell me, doctor, can the diagnosis of dementia be made from the EEG?' He was responsible for establishing the value of the electroencephalogram in what we now call the Creutzfeld-Jakob disease (CJD). A synonym for the condition is the Nevin-Jones syndrome. I examined several patients with the condition whilst working for him and he would examine closely the histological spongiform changes at post-mortem. Since then (1961) I can claim to have seen approximately one patient with CJD every two years, with more when it became more widely diagnosed, though I have yet to see one of the new variants described by Bob Will. (I have, however, been to a meeting where a patient thus affected was presented in detail).

Brain and Kelly used separately to collect unusual variants of thyroid disease – encephalopathies, and eye changes treated with iodine. One of the registrars, Ernest Jellinek, who worked for Reg Kelly, wrote a clinical M.D. on the neurological changes in thyroid disease, describing, inter alia, cerebellar ataxia in a patient with thyroid disease whom I clerked at a later stage. Ernest's father came over as a refugee to Oxford and was an expert on electric shock. Ernest wore a patch over one eye. As a German speaker, he had led a tank corps into a German town towards the end of the War, when a hand grenade was thrown at him. Another patient of Dr Kelly's I particularly remember was a coloured man from south Wales with Refsum's syndrome, due to an accumulation of phytanic acid in the blood. He had all the typical features of this disorder, retinal pigmentation, deafness, thickened nerves, ataxia, muscular atrophy and peripheral neuropathy. The slow degeneration which occurs over many years can be partially treated by a diet devoid of phytol, which is a derivative of chlorophyll. If you want to ensure that a condition has an eponymous name, call it something obscure as Refsum did – heredopathia atactica polyneuritiformis. It is a particularly rare syndrome, so much so that at John Hopkins Hospital, Baltimore they flew over two brothers from Northern Ireland in order to study the condition in depth.

I wish to discuss some of the neurological conditions which I have dealt with at practically every stage of my career, but which I associate to some extent initially with Maida Vale.

**Parkinson's Disease**
Parkinsonism or Parkinson's disease illustrates the fact that a common disease can, nonetheless, be fascinating. The shaking palsy was first described medically by James Parkinson in 1817 but dates from antiquity:-

> Remember your Creator in the flower of your age
> ere evil days come on,
> when the guards tremble in the house of life
> when its upholders bow,
> and even a walk has its terrors
> 
> (*Ecclesiastes* 12. Moffat Version)

Since then many varieties and causes of the condition have been described – idiopathic, familial, familial with depression, following encephalitis lethargica, carbon monoxide poisoning, drug or manganese induced, with electric shocks, dementia, motorneurone disease or Lewy body disease, etc. The basic pathology is now thought to be due to absence of dopamine in the substantia nigra – black bodies in the basal ganglia which become depigmented in the disorder – more so on the side opposite the more severe changes. It is essentially a parenchymatous disease with a triad of tremor rigidity and slowing (bradykinesia). In 1929 Macdonald Critchley described how the condition could be mimicked by arterio-sclerotic changes producing 'marche a petit pas'. This condition has been shrouded in controversy and he was forced, in deference to Melvin Yahr, to modify his title to arterio-sclerotic pseudo-parkinsonism. In the past year or two, the term arterio-sclerotic parkinsonism has regained acceptability and the condition has been reinstated by Andrew Lees in Europe and in the USA, with the nomenclature of lower limb parkinsonism.

Irving Cooper introduced stereotactic operations for parkinsonism to correct the tremor on the contralateral side. It had been noted that a stroke could abolish the tremor of parkinsonism, so that limited strokes were made surgically. On one occasion Irving Cooper had to stop the operation prematurely because of bleeding, but the tremor improved and he discovered that a small lesion made by an injection of alcohol into the basal ganglia could achieve the same result. This operation, by stereotaxis, could also be done with heat or freezing and for many years this was the standard treatment for parkinsonism. Tremor was reduced but other symptoms were not affected; thus a limb might appear to have returned to its normal state, but the patient would neglect its use. Bilateral operations, if not separated in time, could endanger breathing and weaken the voice. However, the major drawback to this operation, which was frequently performed at Maida Vale and at many other centres, was the risk of haemorrhage, especially in those with high blood pressure. The term arteriosclerotic parkinsonism very nearly became attached to those patients where vascular causes were a contra-indication to operation.

In 1962, Purdon Martin and Louis Hurwitz, described the negative features of parkinsonism based on post-encephalitic parkinsonian (PEP) patients from the Highlands Hospital in North London. Most of these patients had developed the condition in the years following the epidemic flu which came immediately after the 1st World War in 1919. Since then there have been a few patients following endemic (as opposed to epidemic) encephalitic illnesses, but PEP has since virtually disappeared. In these patients the key features were not of tremor, but of bradykinesia or even akinesia; so that they would stick or freeze in various postures. One minute they could be immobile, at another time of day they could move freely or even dance. In the event of a bell ringing or a fire, they might suddenly regain the ability to move, then freeze again. When walking, they might festinate, i.e. break into a run, unable to stop themselves except by crashing into a wall. On turning, they might find themselves taking a few steps backwards. There were other difficulties affecting speech, chewing and swallowing, posture, equilibrium and righting as well as locomotion. Many of these manifestations were the result of bilateral atrophy (shrinkage) of the pallidal structures in the basal ganglia.

Both Hurwitz and Martin came from Northern Ireland. As a Jew brought up in Belfast, Louis Hurwitz was asked whether he was a Prod Jew or a Catholic Jew. Purdon Martin, who died in his mid 90s, was originally a mathematician, qualified in Liverpool, and was recruited to Queen Square because of his knowledge of post-encephalitic parkinsonism. I used to see him walking across Hampstead Heath but had not met him until he visited Maida Vale to give a second opinion on a post-encephalitic parkinsonian patient. I had to unload large cushions from his car and, like a royal flunkey, process in with them behind him so that on the ward he could push and pull the patient in various directions without harm. Purdon Martin gave a demonstration of parkinsonism at Queen Square with a video of a man walking up to a railway line with considerable difficulty, but able to stride out with the visuo-spatial guide of the sleepers lying transversely across his path. So much so that he was able to walk along the top of the railway itself until he came to the end of the track, when he reverted to small awkward steps. Such visual cues can be helpful in getting parkinsonian patients started, moving through doors, or walking down a garden. A light from a torch shone in front of them can also provide the necessary stimulus.

Post-encephalitic parkinsonian patients had other problems. Such patients, and those following rauwolfia treatment, frequently experienced oculo-gyric crises when their eyes would fix, looking upwards for 20 or so minutes. One treatment used to be stramonium cigarettes, which took as long to smoke. They also had recurrent respiratory crises and disturbances of speech. Whereas in most parkinsonian patients, articulation becomes soft and limited, a few may exhibit a wide range of hyperkinetic disorders, including palilalia (auto-echolalia with compulsive repetition of the last word or two (or syllables) of a verbal statement), echolalial (the forced repetition of someone else's words again and again) and even coprolalia (the impulsive vocalization of vulgarities). Dystonic or dyskinetic movements may be associated with explosive utterances, crying out loud or shrieking (klaxaphonia) and talking in a far louder voice than usual (megaphonia). Other examples include tachyphemia (the tendency to rapid, stereotyped talk), logorrhoea and verbigeration.

Levodopa therapy was often poorly tolerated, with violent movements or dyskinesia. In 1970 Sacks and Kohl described 'incontinent nostalgia' in a 65 year-old female who had had post-encephalitic parkinsonism from the age of 18. L-dopa caused increased excitement (erethism) with coexistent memory release. She called for a tape recorder and over the next few days recalled the night-clubs and music halls of her youth. When the excitement became so bad that the dosage of laevodopa was reduced, she instantly 'forgot' all these early memories. Zutt, in 1932, had had a patient who complained of 'thousands of memories suddenly crowding on to his mind' during a memory surge occurring spontaneously whilst in an oculo-gyric crisis. It is just possible that my father's sleep singing of musical hall songs (see later) had a similar basis.

The last patient I had with post-encephalitic parkinsonism was 65 when I first met her, and had had parkinsonism from the age of 8 years. She was helped by atropinic drugs and by Amantadine, which had just come on the market, but lived a wheelchair existence. However, with bronchitis and urinary tract infections, the control of her involuntary movements was markedly reduced. She would fling her left arm about and tumble from her chair when not tied in. The violent dyskinesias were so gross that she had to be nursed at night on a mattress on the floor. Hyoscine injections could cause a temporary improvement, but with the ever-present danger of the skin breaking down. L-dopa only made matters worse. I tried numerous drugs – Valium, Lioresal, Nitoman, Priadel, Lorazepam, Sinequan, Cyclospasmol, and Melleril – over the next two and half years in a vain attempt to reduce the movements. She eventually had to be admitted to hospital as an emergency, with breathlessness and a high temperature (105°F). Her abdomen was bloated and she could not pass urine. Despite physiotherapy and antibiotics, she died after 5 days.

From the 19th c. until the late 1960s the only treatment for parkinsonism was belladonna and its derivatives. These have since been shown to affect cognition and nowadays are rarely used; but there was some earlier awareness that such drugs could have a deleterious effect on one's mental abilities. Thus Henry Head, a Neurologist who developed parkinsonism, preferred to go untreated rather than take artane. Hydrotherapy was being explored as a potent method of treatment of some patients, but was quickly superseded by the discovery of laevodopa by Hornykiewicz. Dopamine containing cell bodies is found in the zona compacta of the substantia nigra and at other sites such as the Corpus Luysii forming a dopaminergic pathway controlling tremor. Dopamine itself cannot cross the blood brain barrier but laevodopa can do so and then can be synthesized to dopamine. Laevodopa occurs naturally in the broad bean and velvet bean. Twenty-five grams of L-dopa can be extracted from 1 kilo of beans. However, from the 1920s, the only known action of L-dopa was as an emetic – it made people vomit. Furthermore, the isomeric form D-dopa, also present in the Fava bean, can cause haemolytic anaemia. Hornykiewicz gave L-dopa initially as an injection but Cotzias found that, started orally in low dosage, the emetic and anorexic effects could be overcome and therapeutic levels of L-dopa established after about 13 weeks therapy. This slow induction period was essential when the drug first became available, until a zinc-bound L-dopa was developed with reduced side effects. A further advance occurred with the addition of a decarboxylase inhibitor, which limited the breakdown of L-dopa in the intestines and blood, thereby allowing a smaller amount to be given to achieve adequate replacement of dopamine.

The marvellous results from laevodopa were trumpeted world-wide – literally so, as the jazz trumpeter, Maynard Ferguson, made a record 'L-Dopa'. People previously immobile could fell trees, play tennis, chase women, achieve heightened sexual arousal. And some paid the penalty with coronary heart disease or the unwanted effects of their sexual proclivity. They were given maximum dosages and dyskinetic movements soon replaced the previous rigidity. Perhaps some of these were amorphous movements from the disease, unmasked by the removal of rigidity, or overspill of dopamine to other brain cells. Dyskinetic movements could affect breathing, speech, cause unwanted and quasi-compulsive humming or whistling, lip-biting, or writhing movements alternating with episodic freezing (yo-yo effects). These side effects could be minimized or delayed if the aim was slight under-treatment and over-treatment was avoided.

I did not receive L-dopa until 1970 but was able, from the vast district I covered in North Lancashire, to treat 100 patients before any other centre in the U.K. My results received little attention but at the same time I gathered, and was able to analyse, 42 patients with Essential Tremor. Essential Tremor, recognized in the continental literature as various forms of minor tremor, had been overlooked in the English literature until a paper by Macdonald Critchley in 1949. Known as benign, familial hereditary or senile tremor, it assumed greater importance with the advent of laevodopa. Many G.P.s assumed that every tremor was parkinsonian and would respond to L-dopa, whilst missing those parkinsonian patients whose predominant disability is bradykinesia or paucity of movement. For some years people used two references for essential tremor: Critchley 1949; Critchley 1972. Despite failure to find an effective treatment – less harmful than the benign, but socially disconcerting, tremor – essential tremor has taken off. Just as there was a Nobel prize based on half a cranial nerve (Hallpike), and a professor of one peripheral nerve (Gilliatt), so there are specialists concentrating solely on essential tremor.

Although called hereditary tremor, 26 of the 42 patients were sporadic cases without an established genetic basis, 12 had a family history suggesting an autosomal dominant mode of transmission, and 4 were indeterminate. The tremor involved the upper extremities in 41 patients, the head in 25, lower limbs in 15 and the trunk in 2. Seven patients showed involvement of speech. Essential tremor appears to arise as an exaggeration of physiological tremor, with episodic increases in amplitude occurring against a background of tremor of the same frequency but of lower amplitude. As the malady worsens, there is much variation in the regularity of the wave form and in the severity and spread of the tremor; thus patients may present different types of tremor, either concurrently or in succession, as the disease progresses. It is this syndromic variation which makes the experimental simulation of essential tremor so fallible.

It is a socially disabling condition rather than a disease. Those with essential tremor may have difficulty staying still for a haircut. Eating in public may prove embarrassing. The tremor will almost certainly be worse when attending an interview or meeting people in the course of daily work. Some authors have regarded essential tremor as a monosymptomatic condition, but the more widely based series agree in that the presence of associated neurological signs in addition to tremor does not necessarily negate the diagnosis. These are clinical variants and occur in up to 25 % of established cases. Unfortunately there is no clear marker of the condition. Patients can be reassured that the condition is benign – it will not shorten life. Medication can be tried. Thus beta-blockers can be useful before an interview but their reaction must be tested beforehand. With longer term medication, the subject must weigh up the possibility of side effects from medication taken for a harmless condition against the possible benefit; and many prefer to avoid medication for this reason.

Differences between essential tremor and parkinsonism include titubation of the head sideways rather than the peri-oral tremors of parkinsonism, lack of rigidity and lack of bradykinesia. The handwriting is large and sprawly: that of parkinsonism small and cramped. Alcohol may improve some essential tremors, but patients often avoid alcohol altogether, possibly because other family members with the disorder have been accused of suffering from delirium tremens. In examining a patient with an extra-pyramidal tremor, one is advised to put them in a parkinsonian, semi-bent posture, observe any facial immobility, and check for frontal features with the glabella tap. Limitation of eye movements can occur in the elderly, but if grossly limited with marked rigidity elsewhere, it is probable that the parkinsonian patient has the progressive supranuclear palsy (Olszewski-Steele-Richardson) variant of the disorder. In testing for increased tone in parkinsonism (absent in essential tremor), passive movements of the neck and upper limbs are examined. Changes in tone are best observed over two joints, e.g. wrist and elbow, to minimize any voluntary activity, and minor changes can be brought out by synkinesis, i.e. asking the patient to make fists with the opposite hand. The patient can usually steady the end-point of an extrapyramidal tremor, as when touching the nose, but with the tremor of multiple sclerosis, achieving the end point results in a more violent movement.

To overcome the long induction period in the early days of L-dopa, potentiation with mono-oxidase inhibitors could be used but was not generally advised for fear of an allergic reaction with hypertension, intense headache and neck stiffness, which mimicked hypertensive encephalopathy. Once again from Hungary, Hornykiewicz developed a B form of monoamine oxidase inhibitor, namely selegiline, which potentiated L-dopa by about 20%. This was tried out by Gerald Stern and Donald Calne at University College Hospital, who received the substance as a powder. When they asked permission to do a double blind trial, they were told that the drug had been imported illegally. I had first met Donald Calne, one of the pioneers of L-dopa therapy and later of Dopamine agonists in the U.K., seeing membership patients when he worked at the London Chest Hospital, He developed many of these drugs at the Hammersmith Hospital with my colleague in Preston, Sarosh Vakil, before going firstly to the National Institutes of Health, Bethesda, Maryland, then to Vancouver, British Columbia. Selegiline next came to prominence when Langdon examined young drug addicts in California who had taken 'designer drugs' with the formula MPTP (1-methyl-4-phenyl-1,2,3,6-tetrahydropyridine), which is converted in the brain by monoamine oxidase B in glia into the toxic substance MPP+. Because selegiline could theoretically block this reaction, it was assumed that it could also delay the progression of parkinsonism. Two major multicentre trials were performed, the data-top study in North America and a multicentre study in the U.K. The data-top study was brought to a premature conclusion because the evidence in favour appeared initially to be overwhelming; that in the U.K. had a very different outcome. Analysed after 5 years, there was the unexplained suggestion that the mortality rate was higher in the selegiline arm of the trial. It is now thought that there is no convincing evidence of a delaying effect of the drug and that any early mortality might be explained by a blood pressure-lowering effect. If, without the intervention of drugs, the blood pressure falls precipitously, with changes in posture, disease involvement of the autonomic nervous system has occurred, resulting in the Shy-Drager syndrome or more universal A.N.S. failure as from multi-system atrophy.

Laevodopa replacement therapy remains the mainstay of treatment but does not prevent further deterioration or the development of dyskinetic and on-off side effects, which are initially dose-dependent. With progression of the disease, there is a gradual slowing of reflex responses and it may be difficult when to advise a patient to stop driving motor vehicles. The initial response over the first five years is usually good. Thereafter additional therapy, as with dopamine agonists, may need to be instituted. Claims have been made that the early institution of dopamine agonists can delay side effects, but with their use some side effects, such as hallucinations and depression, may be more prolonged and harder to control. The future lies with more selective forms of dopamine, the newer stereotactic operations and reversing the presumed degenerative causes of parkinsonism and trigger factors such as abnormalities of iron metabolism within the brain. An allied condition is that in which the genetic linkages are well established and in which there is the abnormal deposition of copper within the brain in Wilson's disease.

## Wilson's Disease

I first met Wilson's disease, or hepatolenticular degeneration, as a student in my uncle's clinic at King's. I remember it as a disease of rigidity, associated with dyskinetic grimacing, and it made me wonder in later years whether the rigidity of parkinsonism was to some extent a compensatory cloak for a whole range of underlying dyskinesias. King's was an appropriate setting, for S.A. Kinnear Wilson had been my uncle's predecessor at King's. Gower had called the condition tetanoid chorea and Westphal, pseudosclerosis, but Kinnear Wilson had recognized the association with degeneration of the liver and as a junior at the National Hospital for Nervous Diseases in Queen Square, had travelled to the south of France to recover the body of a patient in order to prove the association. It is said that Kinnear Wilson is turning in his grave from failure to recognize the brown granular pigmentation present in the cornea of the eyes – now known as the Kayser-Fleischer ring. In some patients it is obvious to the naked eye; in others a slit lamp examination is required. But it is the clue to the cause – an excess of copper in the body, damaging the liver and brain. Other aspects of the condition – the kidney and bone lesions, the low copper-carrying protein (caeruloplasmin) in the blood and amino-acids in the urine – have since been found.

From time to time the medical press contains papers suggesting that Wilson's disease is much more common than declared in hospital records. It is certainly more common in India and in countries where consanguinity increases the risk of recessively inherited disease. I have had only a handful of such patients under my care. The last such patient, in Preston, required treatment with a molybdenum preparation because penicillamine (the major drug used) did not work. One patient of mine, whom I followed for many years, had a successful pregnancy but developed contractures of her hands. Plastic surgery only made matters worse and was later repeated whilst she was given L-dopa to try to obtain some relaxation of her rigidity.

## Neurological Aspects of Tuberculosis

I cannot be certain whether I first came across tuberculous meningitis at Maida Vale or earlier, but certainly those patients I saw at Maida Vale with the condition stick in my mind. The management of all forms of meningitis has undergone considerable change over the years. Nowadays the diagnostic tests usually involve scanning before lumbar puncture, which is avoided in the young; newer, faster and more certain diagnostic tests have replaced reliance on gram and Ziehl-Neelsen stains, guinea pig inoculations, bromide tests and CSF chloride; and vastly improved treatment is started almost invariably before a firm diagnosis is reached. Only in the acute cases of tuberculous meningitis is the meningitic triad of photophobia, headache and neck stiffness present. In all forms of meningitis the triad may be absent at the extremes of life and with the subacute or slow onset of tuberculous meningitis, this may also be true in the adult cases. Furthermore, the temperature need not be raised and the initial spinal fluid may be unremarkable. Repeated lumbar puncture examinations, checking also for yeasts, were often required and the introduction of some air, causing a mild cellular reaction, could often help the pathologist, who would spend hours looking over Ziehl-Neelsen preparations to find acid-fast bacilli.

During the Second World War tuberculous meningitis was almost invariably fatal until the Hon. Honor V. Smith, working at Headington near Oxford, introduced a somewhat risky treatment using tuberculin, which saved some lives. The various anti-tuberculous antibiotics, used in combination, with streptomycin given intramuscularly and intra-thecally, dramatically altered the prognosis, though recovery was often prolonged with the persistence of cranial nerve problems such as deafness, vertigo and tinnitus. Even today relatives have to be forewarned of the seriousness of prognosis both as regards the risk to life and, with survival, the risk of complications including deafness and hemiplegia. A meningitis caused by yeasts was not only a primary differential diagnosis, but with the necessity for repeated lumbar puncture, diagnostically and to introduce streptomycin, yeasts could be introduced iatrogenically by repeated lumbar puncture. The lesson from Maida Vale, which has been repeated countless times since, is that the onset can be atypical, including tuberculous epidural abscesses, and the disease must be excluded where there is an unexplained pyrexia or cachexia.

One of the early questions was whether steroid therapy would help by aiding the entry of antibiotics to tuberculous lesions. This question is still extant but the answer, if the therapy is powerful enough and antibiotic resistance is not present, is yes it can help. Inadequately treated tuberculous can give rise to hydrocephalus by blocking the ventricular foramina or by causing an obstructive basal meningitis. There is thus the question: how long treatment should be continued: three months, six months, one year? Tuberculomas can form an icing sugar thickening over the surface of the brain or tumour-like collections, particularly in the posterior fossa. In the past it was necessary to operate, if only to confirm the diagnosis; but now, with CT scanning and antibiotic regimens, medical treatment monitored by serial scanning is the management of choice.

Endemic tuberculosis in the towns of Lancashire, particularly among the Pakistani population, was a continual problem, more probably related to pulmonary tuberculosis from cramped living conditions than from disease bought in from the Indian sub-continent. Most doctors were aware not only of the pulmonary forms of the disease but of neurological and other rarer forms. Professor David Graham, a distinguished neuro-pathologist from Glasgow, chose to talk in Preston on tuberculosis of the spine, prefacing his talk but explaining the rarity of such lesions nowadays, only to be told by the audience that they had all seen recent examples. My last case of tuberculous meningitis in fact involved a white lady from a town near Preston. Today we are seeing a recurrence of tuberculosis, including the avian form, among the immuno-compromized. I, along with most of the medical students who were my contemporaries at Oxford, was inoculated with the murine form – a live vaccine as opposed to the more common BCG.

**The Royal Free Hospital**
Working at a teaching hospital is as important to the study of neurology as within a specialized hospital. Referrals from allied disciplines, medicine, ophthalmology and orthopaedics, for example, can provide fascinating insights into the interplay of neurological and systemic conditions.

The predominant personality at the Royal Free was Professor Sheila Sherlock, who had advanced the treatment of liver disease as dramatically as laevodopa had advanced that of Parkinsonism. Although a neurological registrar, I was able to attend her grand rounds, where anyone present could be subjected to ferocious questioning. I remember a visiting Chest Physician being asked to explain 'what is dyspnoea'? I had to explain what was the active principle of Gower's mixture (tinct Gelsemium), the then treatment of trigeminal neuralgia. These rounds were my introduction to the neurological aspects of systemic disease, as for example hepatic encephalopathy. It was gratifying for a neurologist to learn that the most useful indicator of the severity of liver encephalopathy was the electro-encephalogram, with the development of pathognomic triple waves activity. The other indicator was the blood level of ammonia, quite a hazardous test for the biochemist, and one which I always asked for after talking specifically to the senior biochemist. The different presentations of Wilson's disease were illustrated by twins, one of whom had developed the neurological picture and the other liver disease.

At the Royal Free I had my first chance to learn some neurophysiology.

Campbell and Richardson would perform eight or more carpal tunnel tests in the same time that Prof Gilliatt at Queen Square would take to do one. I had had some experience of electro-encephalograms from Sam Nevin and Horace Townsend at Maida Vale, but now had regular sessions with Pampligione (Pep). Initially he had been a neuropathologist in Italy before coming to the U.K. to study EEGs, and became neurophysiologist to the Children's Hospital at Great Ormond Street and the Royal Free. His reports were always lengthy with well rounded sentences. His teaching methods were equally thorough. He had a particular interest in the evolution of childhood fevers – the exanthemata such as measles and rubella, and would load a heavy EEG machine on to his old Rolls Royce to take up to Melvin Ramsay's unit at Coppett's Wood Hospital. Rapidly progressing cancers were treated surgically by hypophysectomy and I was given the opportunity to study the EEG changes that resulted from removal of the pituitary gland.

Richardson, Ramsay, Pep and Dimsdale were all pre-eminent in the outbreak of Royal Free Disease shortly before I went there. This outbreak, like that at Akureyi in Iceland, had many similarities to the post-glandular fever syndrome or that following any viral or rickettsial disease, wherein symptoms, including depression and ready fatigue, persist for many months after the acute illness. By contrast, the diagnosis of chronic fatigue syndrome cannot accurately be made until at least 12 to 18 months have elapsed with continued symptoms,

Helen Dimsdale was joined by Professor Peter Kynaston Thomas, known as P.K. He had returned from Montreal, where he had been appointed, impatient for advancement in the U.K. The Royal Free was his main hospital but he also attended the Royal National Orthopaedic Hospital and Queen Square. P.K. was, and still is, the most hardworking and prolific of all the U.K. neurologists. On a Wednesday we would attend the lecture-demonstrations at Queen Square and afterwards have a game of squash followed by a curry in Drummond street before returning home. However, between 10 and 11 pm, he would head off to University College to complete his animal research. In those days he was a somewhat diffident lecturer and clinical presenter, but his writing has always been of the highest standard. His major research has been on peripheral neuropathies, culminating in the multi-volume *Peripheral Neuropathies*, written with Peter Dyck, which I once had to review. He was able to remove single nerve fibres for microscopic examination when performing peripheral nerve biopsies, and support his clinical judgment with refined electromyography and nerve conduction studies. At clinical meetings he inevitably carried a satchel of articles to examine and for years edited *Brain*, the *Journal of Anatomy* and several other journals. He fostered the development of Anita Harding, his second wife, as the leading neurogeneticist of the world until her untimely death. Their collaboration raised British neurology to new heights.

The accomplishment I am most proud of at the Royal Free was to meet and marry my wife, proposing to her during the interval of the *Magic Flute* at Glyndebourne.

**University College Hospital**
The neurological and neurosurgical beds at U.C.H. were situated in the old St Pancras Hospital. Also in St Pancras was the first geriatric department, presided over by Lord Almuree, noted for his red cloak and pervasive stutter. The third department was of Tropical Medicine and we shared with them a special unit – unique, even at that time – in keeping the malarial parasite for the treatment of tertiary neurosyphilis when other treatments had failed. Such fever treatment, it was claimed, could improve matters in one third of patients, stabilize another third, but fail to prevent progression in the rest. Tertiary neurosyphilis consists of two conditions which overlap: tabes dorsalis and general paralysis of the insane (GPI). The tabetic was unsteady, especially in the dark, had specific areas of sensory loss, and suffered from spontaneous visceral crises and neuralgic pains (often referred to as screws). The joints could be grossly deformed and unresponsive to painful stimuli. Those with GPI, classically would boastfully believe themselves to be very rich, throw money about in the street and make serious misjudgments. Today they are more likely to claim to have out-played Faldo at golf or out-shouted John McEnroe on the tennis court. Both Tabes and GPI have the pathognomic Argyll-Robertson pupils, named after a Scottish ophthalmologist. The pupils in an adult are small, irregular due to adhesions or synaechiae, and fail to react to light. The pupillary changes may be mimicked to a degree by Holmes-Adie pupils, which are regular but react poorly or not at all to light and accommodation. Both pupillary syndromes may be associated with loss of reflexes in the lower limbs. The Holmes-Adie syndrome is most commonly seen in middle-aged females and it caused some amusement to hear Dr Dimsdale explain to a virginal Hospital Matron that she did not have syphilis but had a benign unrelated condition.

Among the patients I admitted, I remember especially an artist with porphyria and Kartagener's syndrome. Kartagener's syndrome consists of absent frontal sinuses, bronchiectasis causing recurrent chest infections, and transposition of the viscera with dextrocardia. He also had ulceration of the shins and a history of intermittent neurological disease. Porphyria is an intermittent disorder, sometimes precipitated by drugs such as barbiturates, with acute abdominal pain, peripheral neuropathies, and cardio-respiratory crises. The urine during such episodes is darkened. A possible clue, taken with the history, to suggest Kartagener's syndrome is that he had an appendicectomy scar on the left side of the abdomen. I, along with a great many others, had had him as a patient in the membership examination. My interest, with the various hospital notes in front of me, was in the considerable time it had taken to establish the diagnosis in the first place.

Another rare condition, also giving rise to recurrent chest infections, is that of ataxia-telangiectasia due to deficiency of immunoglobulin A and occurring as an autosomal recessive genetic condition. It was first described by Madame Louis-Bar in 1941 but most descriptions of the disease rely on two hospitals in different parts of San Francisco often reporting the same 20 patients. The child is unsteady on its feet from infancy and unable to walk by about 10 years of age, the serum alpha-foeto-protein is raised and there is a substantial incidence of associated cancers. It has been mapped to chromosome 11q 22-23 with the suggestion that breakages of parts of the chromosome with realignment accounts for its occurrence. I was later to discuss all the syndromes of neurological disease with retinitis pigmentosa and suggest that similar fragmentations and reversal of chromosomal segments would account for their occurrence. The hereditary cerebellar syndromes always held a peculiar fascination for me. The best known one, though by no means the most common, had the delightful name which scans as an iambic pentameter: 'olivopontine cerebellar atrophy!' but is now only seen in its abbreviated form of OPCA. Similarly ataxia-telangiectasia has lost its hyphen, is never called the Louis-Bar syndrome, and is more commonly referred to as AT. The inherited ataxias are now talked of in terms of neurotransmitters, neuropeptides and second messenger systems.

We also had a patient who had been operated on for a tumour in the cervical spinal cord by Victor Horsley in 1913. The operation had been performed in two parts, an initial marsupialization of the tumour at the back of the neck and its subsequent removal. He presented to us with symptoms unrelated to this tumour.

Hypertensive encephalopathy is rarely seen nowadays. It can be mimicked by eclamptic conditions in pregnancy and these are treated with magnesium sulphate. But the full-blown picture has virtually disappeared. The blood pressure rises dramatically accompanied by loss of vision (amaurosis), a stiff neck, intense headache, even coma and focal neurological disturbances such as hemiplegia and convulsions. Other features may be papilloedema (increased pressure behind the eyes), loss of speech (aphasia) and nystagmus. The brain is oedematous with the risk of haemorrhages. In 1965 the mainstay of treatment was hexamethonium, a ganglion-blocking drug, which had to be injected and titrated very carefully lest the blood pressure fall precipitously.

Apart from ward and out-patient work, I continued seeing EEGs with Desmond Pond. Sir Desmond, as he soon became, was a foremost psychiatrist. His EEG reports were short and to the point, compared to the mellifluous reportage of Pep, and he was helpful also in discussion on the subject of dyslexia, which I began to study. I also visited Hallpike's department at Queen Square to learn his techniques for testing vertigo and started work on platelet stickiness under Professor Prankeard, as this test was in vogue for the assessment of multiple sclerosis. I felt, though I did the test at the senior consultant's request, that its usefulness had been overreached; but it was later to come in handy when I studied neuro-acanthocytosis. Soon after I arrived at U.C.H., Gerald Stern was appointed as the second Neurological Consultant. Once established, but after I left, he did tremendous work on parkinson's disease and set both Donald Calne and Andrew Lees on the same path. Even if I did not benefit from this aspect of his work, I appreciated his help and advice. I now turn to two subjects which occupied much of my time at U.C.H.

**Deafness and Hearing Children of Deaf Parents**
At this stage in my career I was planning my next steps, which included going to the United States to study neuro-paediatrics (Been To America [BTA] was a necessary requisite of one's C.V. in view of the difficulty in obtaining consultant posts) and I planned to write a book on *Speech Origins and Development*. I therefore decided to study the development of speech in deaf children and in the hearing children of deaf parents.

It is said that James I of England wanted to see the experiment tried of bringing up a couple of children without ever hearing the sound of a human voice. He conjectured that they would speak 'pure Hebrew'. In fact all the 'feral' children who have been studied have been considerably delayed in language acquisition and after a certain age fail to achieve. Very few deaf children fail to hear all sounds, but have great difficulty within the sound range of human speech. They may hear bells, the sound of thunder, or the clip-clop of horses' hooves. Even those with partial hearing, amplified by hearing aids, experience a number of distinctive difficulties which are not always appreciated.

A normal babe starts to babble. With no reflex encouragement – i.e. hearing their own babbling, – babbling dries up prematurely. Deaf babes have difficulty with syllables. Higher notes are distorted or not heard. Through lack of hearing, they develop a limited 'inner language' or vocabulary store. Concepts are inadequately understood; even such simple concepts as 'up, under, above, below', and this extends to other abstract words, 'mine, yours, his' and to ethical principles. Interests lack stimulus and new interests are acquired with difficulty. Because they cannot monitor their own speech, extraneous noises are not eliminated; and the speech may be offensive to others, harsh and monotonous. Sign language and finger spelling were frowned upon by educationalists for many years but by such means intelligent deaf people, especially among their own community, can achieve and build an adequate vocabulary. Often, however, on leaving school or a protected environment, they fall back because others are not prepared to listen and they must function in a speaking world. What then of lip-reading (or more correctly speech-reading)? Nine out of ten words must be guessed at and are only recognized if previously understood. I did however visit Pierre Gorman, Librarian at the Royal National Institute for the Deaf and himself deaf, and in the course of over an hour's conversation, he only required three words to be written down and they were names of people.

I started my study by taking a tape-recorder to listen to children born of deaf parents to see whether it was possible at an early stage to distinguish which children are likely to be deaf, or to be hearing, by recording their babbling. The Psychologist, Lenneberg, published a similar study in the same year as I did. There are other ways of testing hearing in babies such as the response to noises, and more recently by recording audio-acoustic potentials. Most of the families I studied in London appeared to be grouped around Heathrow airport! These studies were supported by an in-depth psychometric study of development in a few children and by following the social development of both deaf children and hearing children from deaf families.

Only about 12% of deaf children have deaf parents. For those with hearing parents in whom deafness has been present since birth, the stifling effect of the handicap is seen from the beginning. No parents ever expect a deaf child and the deafness may pass unnoticed and unattended to for months or years. The parents may be quite incapable of communicating with their deaf child. In addition, when the deafness is at last discovered and can no longer be ignored, feelings of guilt may result in family discord and the child is consequently shunned and neglected. Such neglect, resulting in lack of contact with the outside world, may affect the child's intellectual development.

The facility for speech is innate and the formative influences can be staged. Between 6 to 12 months the child shows readiness to listen and from

12-24 months readiness to speak. Even from as early as 8-9 months the vocalizations of a normal child will reflect the language sounds of its parents and one can distinguish between the babbling noises of a Japanese, French, American or German child. The child is a passive-receptive vehicle, receiving communication from the closeness of the mother and empathic emotional exchange. Thus the mother selects sounds from the vocalizations, reads meanings into the syllables – da, da; ma, ma; and constructs little situations to which the word is appropriate and the learning of speech begins. The child in fact constructs some meaning from the mother's facial expressions as well as her vocalizations. The result is that a speech or hearing defect may be first noticed only when the child moves away and begins to toddle. Alternatively, a severely deaf child will cease babbling at about 12 months and will then be left with no means of communication until instructed in speech when it reaches school.

With deaf parents, about one in nine of the offspring are also deaf. This may be anticipated if there is a clear genetic background. For a while babbling may appear to be reinforced by the mother's emotional expressions. The child's gestures will be treated as though they were signs and reinforced until true signing develops. Gesture may later be reinforced by finger spelling. Because through finger spelling and sign-language a start is made to vocabulary acquisition, a greater proportion of deaf children of deaf parents reach higher education (e.g. grammar schooling) than those from hearing parents.

Unlike Indian sign language, which was developed so that tribes with different oral languages might intercommunicate, deaf sign language needs to be reinforced by changes in facial expression. A deaf family discussing a topic may appear to the outsider as a highly charged emotional experience. Quite apart from lip-reading, where speech is attempted, if the person wears dark glasses or is facially hirsute, communication is impaired. The Scottish deaf community, in particular, will use finger spelling to a great extent, even spelling whole plays, but for most deaf people finger spelling is slow and laborious, and is reinforced by sign language. Sign language is essentially universal, has a grammar of its own but does not convey tenses, etc. It does require intelligence and may be very primitive in isolated deaf people. In Northern Ireland it is possible to tell whether a deaf person comes from a Protestant or Catholic background: those from a Protestant background will use the English bimanual method of finger spelling whereas the Catholics have adopted the American unimanual method.

Oral communication has been encouraged in the past and about 75% of deaf children will benefit from sound amplification. Older children may be upset with the distortion of noise created by the hearing-aid, especially as pain is common with high amplification of sound. Furthermore, the possibility exists that in the long run the effect of high amplification may simulate boilermaker's disease, with a further decrease in hearing. Children tend to use the hearing-aids in class but leave them off in the playground. The genetic argument, that by the use of hearing-aids deaf children will mix with non-deaf friends and not marry within the deaf community, is not true in practice. But for the partially hearing, hearing-aids may enable the child to hear the full speech range and receive education in a normal school.

The deaf remain segregated from society at large. There is also a clear-cut 'internal segregation', dependent upon the severity of deafness and the communication status of the deaf person And welfare services for the deaf assume that he is unable or unwilling to join in the activities of the non-deaf milieu. After leaving school, opportunities for work are limited and subtle difficulties of understanding, as overshades of meaning, affect the maintenance of deep life interests. They may be individually good at sports but fail to understand the necessity for team work. In childhood temper tantrums tend to persist for longer than with hearing children and as adults their seeming emotionality may not be acceptable to others. Because their harsh speech, often accompanied by extraneous noises which they have failed to eliminate, leads to awkward looks from hearing people as though suggesting that they are daft or cannot help it. They may speak less and less and lose much of their facility for speech. Thus regression and psychiatric reactions to their attempts to fit into a hearing world are commonplace.

In my study, I enquired into the question whether lack of understanding of social concepts leads to a diminished social responsibility. This is not a question sought in a vacuum, because many of those looking after deaf people are required to attend courts to act as interpreters for the deaf. Few deaf people receive any education in sex matters and fewer pass such information on to their hearing children. They may acquire their knowledge of sex at the wrong psychological age and in the wrong way. However, few sexual problems get as far as the courts. Accusations of loss of temper causing fights do occur and may reflect their emotional background. There are a few motor car offences. Motor vehicles are particularly popular among the deaf and form a frequent source of conversation. The most common offence arises when they are used as bookies' runners or are caught acting as lookouts for other children committing offences and seeking to delay discovery by placing a deaf person in the way of the police. The overall pattern one gets from visiting deaf families is that they are excessively careful not to cause trouble. They fear lest the T.V. is put on so loudly that it offends the neighbours. They keep the children well disciplined and they maintain their houses spotlessly. They represent a sober minority within society.

What becomes of the hearing children of deaf parents? This question is seldom addressed. Usually great care is taken that such children should not be disadvantaged. Concern is expressed by social workers, non-deaf relatives and by the deaf themselves. Should the child be brought up by non-deaf relatives? If so, when should the child leave home? Often the child does move to the home of a non-deaf relative; but people are then concerned at loss of maternal bonding. The pre-school child is liable to have a smaller vocabulary than others and to have some speech delay. When very deaf parents, who make little use of oral modes of communication within the home, have a non-deaf child, his development of speech sounds and language may not take place at the usual time in the manner observed in other non-deaf children because of the absence of a speaking environment. Television, cassettes and frequent contact with hearing people are advised. However, a common source of developmental failure occurs when a second hearing child is born and those who would otherwise express concern suppose that the second child will develop facility of speech easily from the first child.

Most deaf parents find that they can speak with their children without embarrassment. Their preference is for combining conventional signs with inexact finger spelling replete with abbreviations. Although the children do not necessarily become expert in finger spelling from an early age, many excel at spelling when young in advance of their vocabulary skills. Deaf parents take great pride in seeing their children read, but show little interest in what the child actually reads. As they possess little understanding of school examinations and opportunities and rarely communicate with the masters, the child's formal education can be rather haphazard. Decisions are usually made for the child without reference to their parents, who respect but do not understand authoritative persons.

The child begins to recognize that his parent is deaf in the first or second year. He finds that whereas noises often fail to attract attention, a gesture, or, better still, a touch, is almost always successful. The mothers are kindly and the child, quite unaware that they are in any way different from other mothers, suffers no psychological trauma. If the parents have some speech, the child may not be aware of any difference from other people until he starts school. However, once they start going to school, they can expect to be made aware that their parents are 'different'.

The first show of awareness of the difference in family background may be that they do not, or cannot, invite their friends to their home. The majority soon become fiercely protective of their parents Any hearing child of deaf parents will find himself called upon to act as interpreter and to make contacts for the rest of the family, answer the door or telephone, barter in shops, explain family ailments to the doctor, or increasingly aid in the discussion of business, income tax, insurance, hire-purchase, etc. From the age of 7 or 8, he may write all the family letters. If he becomes adept at these tasks, his services may be in demand beyond the family circle. Examples I collected included acting as interpreter for a deaf-blind man through a church service, writing to the Duke of Edinburgh when there was a threat to build houses on a children's playground, and telephoning the police because his younger sister had failed to return home from school at the usual hour. By contrast, deaf people, with their limited life experience, may not be able to anticipate the social situations which may arise with their teenage offspring.

Excessive responsibilities, as above, may not be evenly spread among the offspring and some escape responsibility altogether. In the USA Mr Yarborough of Texas, born of deaf parents, became both a Senator and a Judge. Those with lesser experience often gravitate to continuing social work with the deaf. Hearing girls of deaf parents who have taken on responsibilities from an early age may have difficulty adjusting to the conventional passive role of the female in most situations in modern society, but few are noticeably 'feminists' in their approach to life.

## Dyslexia and the Drift into Delinquency

My aim to study dyslexia took me once again to the Western part of London to a Remand Home and Assessment Centre for Juvenile Delinquents. Dyslexia is defined as failure to attain the language skills for reading, writing and spelling commensurate with that person's intellectual ability despite normal intelligence, intact senses, conventional instruction, adequate motivation and socio-cultural opportunity. The diagnostic label of 'developmental dyslexia' can be correctly applied to between 5-10% of children with reading problems. There may be a positive family history of reading difficulties or other evidence of slow speech development, comparative clumsiness or uncertain laterality; all of which may suggest a genetic or constitutional immaturity of the nervous system. The manifestations of dyslexia are far from uniform but may be explained nonetheless by such theories as delayed or defective myelination of nerve fibres to the association areas of the brain, minimal cerebral dysfunction or predisposed vulnerability. My chief in the States (David Clark) tried to correlate dyslexia with injury to the brainstem at birth, reducing neuronal activity and stimulation from that region to the developing bouton terminaux (the connecting nerve endings around other nerve cell bodies) in the association cortices of the cerebral hemispheres. More recent research suggests that the basic insult involves an abnormality of either chromosome 6 or chromosome 15.

I was interested in determining whether dyslexia was just a term applied to middle-class children to explain their school failure without arousing parental feelings of guilt, or whether other children could be found of normal intelligence who were specifically affected by this syndrome. By choosing to study children in a remand home, I was examining the suggestion that there might be a drift of such children from school failure into truancy and thence to delinquency. There was an added advantage in that these children had already been assessed medically to exclude eye and ear defects and their IQs had been determined by educational psychologists. It remained for me to take a history, assess them neurologically and then do specific tests involving laterality, speech, reading, writing and spelling skills to confirm the diagnosis.

The study of reading disability in criminals was pioneered by Dr Nathan Peyser in New York in the 1930s. School failure appeared to be more closely correlated with delinquency than were poverty, broken homes, physical and mental defects or psychopathic conditions. Reading disability came to be regarded as a measurable aspect of school failure. Those with a contented, apathetic disregard for their handicap and its results, or with a more generalized emotional blocking, were withdrawn and seldom delinquent; but those with a mild, paranoid reaction toward the teachers, or a more fully developed sense of inferiority, often responded with behavioural disorders in the school, truancy and depredation upon school property. Similar studies have been reported from Germany.

However, the majority of these children are undoubtedly of low intelligence or short attention span; but there have been examples of dyslexic children who have responded by similar aberrant behaviour. Credit for the specific association between dyslexia and criminality must go to a Danish Judge, Huno von Holstein. His treatise on *Ordblindhed og Kriminalitet* was published in 1951. He pleaded for the medico-legal recognition of the handicap of word-blindness, describing the martyrdom and frightful psychological trauma endured by the children concerned. Others have suggested by quotation from the numerous and bizarre spelling mistakes, made throughout their lives, that Joseph Sewell, the South London second-hand car dealer, and Lee Harvey Oswald (IQ 118) were dyslexic. At the Remand Home I came across the natural son of one of the Great Train Robbers, and, interested in the possible hereditary nature of the condition, wrote to Wandsworth Prison for permission to interview the father, only to learn that he had escaped. As Mrs Beaton would say, 'First catch your hare!'. No one would excuse a criminal on the grounds of dyslexia, but it is reasonable to question the possibility that the handicap may have been instrumental in setting him apart from society.

Overall, 60% of the children were retarded in reading by two years or more and 50% by over 3 years. Few children had disabilities of a general medical character but several had a positive family history, with performance and orientational impairments, diagnostic of developmental dyslexia. Left-handedness, crossed laterality and faulty pronunciation were found rather more frequently among the retarded readers than in the controls. What did surprise me was that many children showed uncertainty of handedness persisting to as late as 13 years of age.

The social hazards which a dyslexic adolescent or adult may encounter can lead them unwittingly into trouble as from signing forms without comprehending their meaning; taxation returns wrongly completed with numbers written back to front. Forced to cope with bookwork, their ineptitude may lead to accusations of 'swindling' or 'cooking the books'. He (4 males to every female) may also read traffic signs wrongly. As opposed to the older term 'word-blindness' or less crisp terms such as specific language retardation, I believe that the term 'dyslexia' has a value. The dyslexic can be helped, especially following early recognition, but may require individual tuition using innovative techniques. The value of the term – and, yes, its social acceptability – lies in the fact that it encourages early recognition, the seeking of advice, and the willingness of affected adults to seek instruction. It stops harmful labels, removes parental guilt and the emotional concomitants can be recognized as secondary manifestations. Thus it not only enables the achievement of his/her potential, but creates a social awareness of the social and community implications, and provisions which can be made in adjusting exam requirements. Finally, there are parallels with the acquired neurological condition of Alexia.

I was once ticked off by the editor of the *British Medical Journal* for describing someone as meticulous, quoting Partridge's *Usage and Abusage* – 'meticulous is erroneously used to mean careful of detail in a praiseworthy manner'; properly, it implies excess of care and an over-scrupulousness caused by timidity'. The term 'meticulous', not surprisingly, is often applied to neurologists: thus they make a sharp distinction between 'developmental dyslexia' and 'acquired alexia'. Acquired alexia is a condition I was to meet somewhat later, caused by a stroke, trauma or other pathological conditions most commonly affecting the Peri-Sylvian language zone of the brain.

Damage to the left angular gyrus down to the underlying white matter commonly results in alexia, with associated inability to write (agraphia) and inevitably some difficulty with speech (aphasia). Dependent on the site, other higher functions can be affected. By interrupting the fibres travelling in the white matter, disconnect or even isolation syndromes can develop. Thus a more posteriorly placed lesion may also cause impairment to part of the field of vision. If the lesion is posterior but sparing the left calcarine cortex, alexia may occur without agraphia or hemianopia. The identification of some of these syndromes, even separating semantic comprehension from phonological conversion, has proved helpful in differentiating specific pathways within the brain for encoding language, thereby providing a theoretical anatomy for reading.

I had my own theory relating to the learning of linguistic skills. Reversals or transpositions of letters, sounds, or words are seen in the initial stages of language acquisition and are related physiologically to the learning process. Such mistakes decrease with age and language experience but may occasionally persist. The orthodox hypotheses relate reversals in language to developmental defects of visuo-spatial or temporal orientation. For example, 'the mirror-like inversions of mirror speech and the "spoonerisms" of cluttered speech can thus be explained as arising as a problem which is a question of order or spacing in time'. My own theory placed greater emphasis upon the accuracy of stimulus perception and kinaesthetic feedback mechanisms.

To test this theory, I examined the output of school children learning to type for the first time and the errors made by typists taking part in the world speed championships. In the early 1920s, speed typists were carefully coached, notably at the Underwood Speed Training Group, and annual world championships were held in New York at the Old Madison Square Garden. The QWERTY typewriter, the lay-out of which was arrived at by chance to avoid the tendency for the keys on Sholes' early models to stick, is a left-handed instrument. Fifty-six percent (56%) of the strokes are made by the left hand and too much work is done by the weaker fingers. I found that in both the learning and expert groups, the proportion of the total errors which involved reversals or transposition of letters, was similar. The experts made far fewer errors than the trainees but the proportion of errors which could be said to involve visuo-spatial or temporal orientation did not change.

There is a tendency to make reversals during the learning process in learning to talk, read and write but even the most competent will continue to make or overlook errors of transposition in typing and proof-reading.

However, students learning to sing or to play musical instruments do not share this tendency. Only when tackling the reversed chromatic scale, when it is necessary for the two hands to move in opposite directions, can a student be tricked into such errors. The kinaesthetic feedback in music is dependent on auditory stimuli and is exceptionally pure. In contrast, the information feedback to the brain in touch-typing is probably crude and depends upon joint position, sensation and movement. Special concentration is necessary in order to avoid the tendency to overlook reversals when reading a proof. Thus, there appears to be a gradient of sophistication for the kinaesthetic mechanisms: those used in reading and writing are less precise than those involved in music but are more precise than those used for touch-typing or proof-reading. In speech, the tendency to make reversals is seen best in 2-4 year old children before auditory discrimination has fully developed.

## Bedford

Those who have looked critically at the appointments I have held will have noticed that apart from my Army service, I have had relatively little experience of general medicine. I therefore took the opportunity of three relatively free months before going to the USA to do a consultant locum in general medicine in Bedford, with an interest in gastroenterology. Dr Easton, the Consultant I took over from on his retirement, had the pleasing habit of prefacing his opinions with the phrase 'Methinks', always written as one word. The gastroenterology part of the job was made easy by the fact that the panacea at the time for all gastric and duodenal ulceration was liquorice, since discontinued because of unacceptable changes in potassium and other electrolytes within the body. An equally unusual character was that of David Lewis, who had been selected out of a hundred applicants to fill the cardiology post. He was experimenting with cardiographs (E.C.Gs.) Instead of using the expensive electrolyte paste to make contact between the skin and electrodes on the chest, he tried rubbing the skin to produce a vascular redness and the use of toothpaste or tomato ketchup as alternatives. He also believed that an ECG in the bed gave little information, whereas a remote ECG, with the patient mobile using a small radio-transmitter and asked to run up and down stairs, was of greater value.

Bedford was a necessary prelude whilst waiting to go to the USA. At that time 'B.T.A.' (been to America) was a necessary prerequisite to a consultant post in the U.K., providing an opportunity to widen one's experience and to initiate some research.

## America – Kentucky

On our arrival in New York, we were greeted with an internal airways strike and travelled on to Kentucky by greyhound bus. As we had a nine month-old child, we soon realized how convenient the buses were for travelling with children. Ours was fully air-conditioned and cool milk was also supplied. On reaching Lexington, we were met at the bus station by the chief himself, who immediately advised us to take half the clothing off our child because of the heat. David Barrett Clark appeared as a small to medium, slightly grisly looking man with a noticeable moustache – for an infant to try to touch that moustache was regarded by Dave Clark as a sign of intelligence – his hair was short cut and sparse. Unless he had a migraine, which we always knew from a pathognomic inequality of the pupils, his manner was friendly, often tinged with humour.

He was rightly considered the foremost American Neuro-paediatrician of his day, and was certainly the best clinician I ever worked for. He had left Johns Hopkins, where he had been head of Neuropaediatrics, because of shortage of in-patient beds for his speciality, and came to Kentucky to found a new Department of Neurology. Born in Chicago, he was a life-long anglophile, choosing to take his sabbaticals at Queen Square and setting aside a day each week to make himself an expert on the history of the Royal Navy from the library of the Greenwich Maritime Museum.

He had qualified as a vet but an interest in neuro-anatomy and pathology led to his taking up medicine. His early interests were never forgotten. On his ranch-like home he bred horses and Canada geese. He would teach without a note for two or more hours at a time, explaining, for example, the surface markings of the brain. His remarkable career as a clinician began when working for Dr Buchanan, the founder of paediatric neurology in North America. It is said that when he joined the Department, Dr Buchanan went on holiday leaving him to it for the first few weeks. On the one occasion I saw Dr Buchanan, I was amazed at the similarity of approach in getting the child he was examining to sit alongside him. From Chicago he transferred to Johns Hopkin's Hospital and for many years collaborated with Frank Ford, having a considerable in-put into Ford's *Textbook of Neuro-paediatrics*. Ford's textbook is a comprehensive but haphazard compendium and Dave Clark was expected to be responsible for further editions but could never reach agreement with the Trustees, and in particular with Ford's wife, about the need for extensive re-writing and compression of the text. I would also add that, though Clark's teaching and extempore presentations at clinical and histo-pathological conferences were superb, he would wrangle for months over written papers and consequently his literary output was small.

Even when not the attending physician, he would appear on a ward to see a difficult patient at any hour of the day, and then spend many hours doing a full round on all the rest. However he did not follow the usual 7 am start of many Departments, preferring what he described as the British practice of starting at 8 am. The Department was compact, with a pathology technician, Fran, and a social worker and departmental organiser, Mary Leonidakis, both of whom had come down with him from Johns Hopkins.

The Associate Professor was Mike McQuillen, a third-generation Irish Catholic, who always wore green even when the elbows came out of his sport's jacket. His father was in the same law firm as John Foster Dulles and he was even more staunchly Republican than David Clark. Despite his rather overt prejudices, he always appeared highly educated and compassionate, with a less earthy form of humour than Dave Clark. He loved nothing better than to spend hours in discussion, especially with his favourite priest, and today has given up neurology to become virtually a cleric – deeply concerned with medical ethics. His expertise lay in electro-myography and neuro-muscular disease. He was one of the first to show that steroids for the Guillain-Barre syndrome were unhelpful and could even be dangerous in those with the most severe (grades 3 and 4) forms of the disease, because of cardiac abnormalities resulting from electrolyte imbalance. He would take an extreme line on not performing thymectomy for myasthenia gravis, debating the issue vehemently at Neurological Congresses. He had joined Dave Clark from the Neurology Department at Johns Hopkins.

Doug Jamieson, the Assistant Professor, had been recruited from outside Dave Clark's normal ambit, from Wisconsin. His Christian beliefs were fundamentalist and he had a large family, reminiscent in appearance, and much else besides, of the early pilgrims. He looked after electro-encephalography. His methodical approach clinically and in EEG reporting was more rigid than that of the rest of the Department, but he was liked and respected and his early death was a shock to all. The departmental mix was completed by Harvey Cantor, extroverted and an orthodox Jew, and myself. Harvey was a remarkable neuro-paediatrician, later to go into private practice in his home town of St Louis. Whereas I was taught to allow a child to take one in first before starting to examine the child, he might enter a ward, pick the child up, throw it upwards, catch it and be on the best of terms. When asked, he explained that he had learnt this technique at Guy's hospital in London when an elective student.

American medicine is in many ways very different from English medicine. One must be prepared to see Departments based on strong Teutonic principles. Patients, though often with some insurance, have to negotiate admission. Students do not come on to a Department as a firm, but one or two will be present at any one time as electives. They will be expected to be around at all hours and this fact would appear to be more important than what they achieve. If they do not fit in, they can be damned by the report they receive. In out-patients one may see no more than 3 or 4 patients in an afternoon. If the student has seen them as well, the number may be even less. Patients expect a very full explanation of their symptoms, diagnosis and treatment. The strength of the American system is the residency programmes aimed at the Specialist Boards. This means in-built teaching sessions and a balanced experience of one's subject, including time set aside for the relevant pathology and radiology.

Kentucky sits like the fuselage of a jumbo jet, squashing below it a Tennessee pride sausage. To the north and west is the Ohio River. The largest town, Louisville, (pronounced Louerville) sits on the river. Covington is a suburb of Cincinnati on the opposite bank directly to the north of Lexington (mid-state). Other towns of diminishing size are Frankfurt (the capital), Paris, Versailles (pronounced nautically), Athens (pronounced (Ay-thens), London, Berea and others. All in all, Kentucky is a little bigger than England. I was to get to know the central part, the Bluegrass around Lexington, extending to the Appalachian mountains and Cumberland gap to the East, but no further than Lincoln's birthplace in Hardin County and the Mammoth Cave National Park to the west. The traditional South began below the Ohio River, Dixie rather than Yankie, southern cooking, southern Baptists, the Bible belt with the Bible College at Berea, ballads and folk music on the dulcimer and fiddle, but few blacks in my part of Kentucky except around Danville. The poor were white, the Scots-Irish, the inbred white people living along the 'creeks' or narrow river valleys, the Appalachian poor. Daniel Boone opened up the Cumberland gap crossing the Blue Ridge mountains to let them in. Forced to work on the plantations of Virginia to pay their passage to America, many chose to escape and live rough as frontiersmen. They found a creek with a bit of land, safe from other feuding wild men – the Hatfields and McCoys – married and produced offspring. The progeny moved further along the creek to poorer and poorer land, intermarrying with their own kith and kin. Genetic disease was rife, the youngest child of the family almost certainly the offspring of the eldest daughter, perhaps incestuously.

Their story is told in the literature of the region: *The Wilderness Road*, *Night Comes to the Cumberlands*, *Yesterday's People*, *New Perspectives of Poverty*, *Pissing in the Snow*, *Stinking Creek*, *South of Hell fer Sartin* and also in the beautiful tales of Jesse Stuart, whose books such as *God's Oddling* are written with a sense of language straight from Thomas Hardy. These were my patients. They came to the hospital. They sat in their swing porches. They scraped a living from the soil and opencast mining. They lived off welfare. My task was to open up regional clinics in the small towns, often called cities – the placard read City of Beativille, population 2,000. There was Pikeville – the All American City – Paintsville – where a panther came down the creek to lick salt; Hazard, Kentucky, Harlem, Kentucky. Because they lived off welfare, a judge had called them 'Happy-Pappies'. The name stuck. Because I did regional clinics there, I acquired the nick-name in the department of Dr Happy-Pappy. The name was transferred to my successor, Dr Paul Chuke from Nigeria.

One of my first tasks was to do an editorial on Achrondoplasia. I went for advice to John Hewitson, the neuroradiologist, who had just returned from England. Dave Clark decided that I should study adult reflexes in the newborn in the first four days of life. Roger Robinson was travelling the world with his reflex study relating to gestational age, and when I had finished, was able to advise on presentation. I found, for example, that the abdominal reflexes could nearly always be obtained if the test was done before otherwise disturbing the child. Flexor plantar reflexes were indicative of pathological abnormalities in two babes. My second son was number 380 of my series of 600 babes. I also studied retinal haemorrhages in the newborn. I had to examine over 300 babes before I could be certain of my interpretation. The haemorrhages were found in 13% but I felt that if I had used indirect ophthalmoscopy, which was later shown to me, the percentage would have been higher. There were relatively few patients with multiple sclerosis in Kentucky and mostly they had brainstem forms of the disease. I saw many more adolescents with subacute sclerosing pan-encephalitis, Dawson van Bogaert disease, than I had previously. Associated with the measles virus, it begins with little lapses of movement of the fingers and then elsewhere, with the patient falling into a comatose state and in nearly every instance it proves fatal.

Apart from the hospital work, I went about weekly to a regional clinic. We would hire a State limousine, seating at least six people and holding an EEG set, and travel down a state highway at about 90 mph (looking out for helicopters) to a National Park, where we would stay the night before an early start treating epilepsy, genetic diseases and other neurological disorders referred to us. Within the boundaries of Lexington was the Federal Narcotics Institute, where people came from all states to be dried out. Opiates were replaced with methadone, but more importantly, a test dose of a barbiturate was given to all comers. Barbiturate withdrawal can lead to life-threatening fits, which can only be controlled by more barbiturates, I was invited to help in a research project there, hooking rats on barbiturates to provide a research model for epilepsy, then examining the level of GABA (gamma amino butyric acid, which is an inter-neural inhibitor and the basis of some anticonvulsant drugs). The project was funded to the tune of $250,000 but a member of the team's wife died of cancer and another was moved elsewhere and the project folded up.

My next experience using the metabolic ward along with frequent visits to East Kentucky gave me the opportunity to examine a rare and fascinating condition in depth.

**Neuro-acanthocytosis**

I took Professor Jack Tizard, Clinical Psychologist at Great Ormond Street, out to Floyd County, firstly to see two siblings who exhibited mirror writing. It was likely that one had started to do so naturally and the other had copied to share in the acclaim. By the time we arrived, they had both stopped and reverted to normal writing. We then went on to see my prize patient. I will call him Terry, which is an alias. Jack Tizard was revolted at the appearance of the man, a lumbering, slightly bent figure, with numerous tics, bitten tongue and lips, saliva dribbling, to the ground and controlling himself as far as possible by a rag held to his mouth. In the vernacular 'jest a-settin and a-chawin the rag', which suggests that there have been other cases in the past.

Terry had presented to Abe Wikler, Professor of Psychiatry, Neurology and Pharmacy, who had attempted to try to control his movement disorder to no avail. Dave Clark was determined that he should be thoroughly investigated and the family studied and I was the man to do so. The tentative diagnosis had been Huntington's Chorea. A similar family had been studied in New England but there had been a number of false starts. One described hallucinations, schizophrenia and a movement disorder; another presumed that there was hypolipoproteinaemia with steatorrhoea. It was some time before acanthocytes were observed in the peripheral blood with normolipoproteinaemia. There was a suggestion of a myopathy, questionable fasciculations, and a tendency to shoulder dislocations.

Acanthocytes are misshapen red blood corpuscles with thorn-like projections. The number seen is less than in the allied syndrome of abetalipoproteinaemia but their presence is diagnostic.

Terry was a 29 year-old white male. When first seen at the age of 26, he exhibited involuntary movements and had a grossly swollen, raw, bitten tongue. He had had 15-20 similar episodes of tongue, lip and cheek biting, which often occurred at night. The episodes started six years earlier on a background of increasing generalized weakness, nervousness, 'fits and jerks', and had increased in frequency and severity. The involuntary movements included finger-snapping, grimacing, dystonic and choreiform movements, hyperextension of the trunk, twisting movements of his shoulders, sucking noises, plosive sounds, and drooling. Coprolalia, seen in the Gilles de la Tourette syndromes was not evident. There had been times when he could not speak plainly: 'the inside of his mouth would draw', he would 'snap at his lips, and his stomach would stick'. When he ate, his tongue would involuntarily push his food out on to his plate. For four years he had preferred to retire to a separate room to eat.

He showed no psychotic or hallucinatory behaviour, but on his later admissions, appeared somewhat disinhibited sexually. Over two years he had two episodes of 'passing out' preceded by abnormal noises and shaking or tremor of the abdomen and outstretched extremities, 'drawing up of the legs'. These episodes, which lasted for 30 minutes, were followed by confusion and a 'wild look' which persisted for approximately one hour. On admission in 1967, his involuntary movements were so intense that he could not walk without assistance. He was alert, well-orientated, had no gross memory defects, and was disturbed by his own repulsive appearance. He slurred and stuttered when talking, was often indistinct and had occasional inappropriate laughter. Despite the involuntary movements, there was no ataxia and co-ordination tests were intact. He had generalized hypotonia, flexor plantar responses, and loss of deep tendon reflexes. There was a suspicion of thinning with coarse twitching of the calves. His IQ was 72 (WAIS), verbal 81, and performance 61. All neurological tests were non-contributory. These included repeated electromyographic tests.

He was the 10th child. The eldest died of seizures, bit her tongue and had involuntary limb movements. She became forgetful, emaciated and bedfast with violent shaking of her limbs. Two others also died about the age of 26. The fourth child had an illness of two years duration, with passing out spells and rejection of food from the mouth. The fifth gave birth to an unaffected child and soon afterwards became bedfast and emaciated. The ninth remained healthy till aged 31, before developing choreic movements and grand mal fits. She has always refused admission to hospital but did permit an examination on herself and her normal 17-month child. I witnessed what appeared to be an attack of hystero-epilepsy with partial loss of consciousness, opisthotonous (bending the back in hyperextension) and drawing and grasping movements of all four limbs. Speech and swallowing were normal but she showed facial grimacings and distal choreic movements. The deep tendon reflexes were absent and the diagnosis of acanthocytosis confirmed.

The niece, aged 27, daughter of the presumably-affected eldest sibling, we will refer to as Tralee. She had a pleasant demeanour and was investigated in depth. She had a neurological disorder resembling Friedreich's ataxia with extensive myocardial involvement but no involuntary movements. There were only a few cells resembling acanthocytes in the blood, and it is possible that the association is fortuitous; but it is tempting to regard her clinical state as linking the Bassen-Kornzweig (see below) and normoliproteinaemic syndromes.

She weighed 4.1 kg at birth, walked late at 17 months and had weak legs before the onset of 'rheumatic fever' when aged seven years. Her joints and hearing were affected. At about 11 years of age she found that she had to hold on to the furniture when moving about the house and needed assistance out of doors. She became overtly ataxic aged 13 and has not walked, even with support, since her 20th year. She needed a hearing aid, has become dysarthric and clumsy and shown subtle changes in mentation. She has never had steatorrhoea, fits, or involuntary movements. Her vocabulary was surprisingly good in view of a limited formal education. There was no evidence of retinitis pigmentosa, the discs were pale with moderate constriction of the visual fields and intermittent spontaneous nystagmus (jerky eye movements).

She needed to be tied into her wheel chair. The joints were lax and hypotonic and there was a mild curvature of the back. Legs and arms were tapered, with club feet and equinovarus deformity. She could not support her outstretched arms for more than two minutes. Besides cerebellar signs, there was glove and stocking sensory loss and defective joint position sensibility.

Thirty years later I refereed a Japanese paper suggesting a new syndrome. They quoted my original paper but clearly had not read it. The similarity to that of Tralee was striking.

I screened, with the help of a haematologist, 34 other members of the family for acanthocytosis and neurological signs. Many of the younger members had pale fundi and a minor degree of clumsiness. Only one boy aged 16 had a significant acanthocytosis but no neurological illness. However his tendon reflexes were uniformly absent. From the history, it is possible that two others were similarly affected: a paternal nephew, married with nine normal children, who died aged 43 after a three-year illness and subject to fits, slurring of speech and bad nerves; and a maternal nephew aged 43, married with 10 normal children, but subject to fits. However in the latter case the fits appear to be alcohol-related, but while drinking or sobering up, he 'draws, jerks, and slobbers at the mouth'. He also holds on to things or pulls things.

**The Second Family**
Within a year of my return to England, a 30 year-old patient was referred to me. Her parents were unrelated and until her marriage in 1965, her medical history had been unremarkable. She held a semi-skilled job assembling electronic valves. However, her husband had noticed during their courtship that her walk was ungainly and had avoided drinking with her in company because of her tendency to slobber. After the birth of her first child in 1967, she became forgetful and unreliable and was twice accused of neglecting her child. At times she would have difficulty in co-ordinating movements and would bump into objects, or, when sitting quietly, suddenly fall to the floor. Her husband became increasingly irritated by grunting noises, of which at first she was unaware. During her second pregnancy she gave birth prematurely after 7 months gestation When examined at 4.5 years, the child appeared healthy but small and blood films showed a few acanthocytes.

After the birth of her second child, she became tense and depressed with crying episodes. Her mother-in-law accused her of being mental. She started to lose weight and thought she had leukaemia. On her own volition she attended the ENT and Psychiatric clinics, complaining of intermittent difficulty in swallowing and a tightness in the throat. At that time her speech was noticed to be slurred and the psychiatrist made a provisional diagnosis of multiple sclerosis. There was no history suggestive of steatorrhoea.

When I first examined her she was thin with high arched feet, 5ft 4in in height and weighing only 125 pounds. She was alert and oriented, yet appeared unkempt and dishevelled. Many of her symptoms distressed her but there were others of which she was apparently unaware until her attention had been directed to them Most disturbing were the wide variety of oro-facial tics. At times these appeared compulsive or even hysterical. They were continually present during waking hours, though fluctuating in severity from day to day and partially improved by benzhexol and diazepam. Her speech was dysarthric, partly broken by involuntary movements. She would also grunt, suck, cluck, make repetitive sounds, bite her tongue and lower lip, or struggle to control the pooling of saliva.

The involuntary limb movements were sometimes dystonic and choreiform, with hyperextension and flexion of her trunk and throwing out of an arm or leg. Her gait was variable with a tendency to drag her leg. She performed purposive movements fairly well despite an apparent loss of manual and finger dexterity. There was no nystamus or ocular abnormality,

The reflexes were just present and sensation was intact. Her blood pressure was 160/100. The full scale IQ (WAIS) was 86, verbal 91 and performance 81. All tests, including the electromyographic ones, were normal. To confirm the diagnosis, I referred her to David Weatherall in Liverpool but she was then sent by her G.P. to Professor Gilliatt at Queen Square, who had nothing new to offer. Over a two-year period she remained much the same and her movements became more distressing and failed to respond to medication. Cinematographic studies of her swallowing confirmed the difficulty in initiating deglutition and showed lack of co-ordination, weakness and flaccidity involving the soft palate and hypopharynx. She left her husband and the neighbourhood, maintaining an uneasy relationship with her mother and brother. In March 1971 she took her own life, drowning in her bath. A coroner's postmortem was cursorily performed and with difficulty a small section of brain was recovered to be examined by our neuropathologist., Really the portion was insufficient for any diagnosis but was sent on to Professor Cummings to look for phospholipid and sphingolipid patterns. These were normal.

Since that time there have been many other families, examined by Aminoff and Anita Harding in the U.K., across America and in Japan. The Japanese refer to the syndrome as the Levine-Critchley syndrome, a name which pleased my son in Liverpool, whose best friend was also called Levine.

Of considerable scientific interest is why or how patients with normal lipids can have misshapen red blood cells. The problem has yet to be solved. They differed from the red cells of the other syndrome, where there is lack of beta-lipoprotein (abetalipoproteinaemia) in three essentials. Clumping (rouleaux formation) can occur, the sedimentation rate is normal and not reduced, and there are fewer acanthocytes. They were described by Dr Worth Estes, who studied the first New England family: '... the spines of the acanthocytes are equally distributed over the cells, are perpendicular to the cell and often have terminal bud-like swellings'. Under the electron microscope at 4,900 to 12,800 times magnification they cannot be distinguished from those of abetalipoproteinaemia. All other manifestations of abnormalities of the blood were absent. In Preston I was able to arrange some experimental investigation of the red blood corpuscles with Professors Betts and Nicholson at the then Harris College. These experiments were designed to study whether the unique morphology of the acanthocytic red cell can be attributed to abnormal lipid structures in the red cell membrane and the influence of adsorbed plasma components on the red cells and platelets. In essence the cells were washed, subjected to different chemicals and enzymes and studied in electrokinetic fields. Even with these tests, we were unable to find a difference from normal red blood cells.

**Abetalipoproteinaemia and related syndromes**
Oxford University, after considerable delay, would only accept a thesis if I included other acanthocytic syndromes. In this respect I had some examples from Kentucky and in Lancashire was able to see patients under the paediatrician (Gordon Hesling) in Preston and Ted Holmes (gastro-enterologist) in Manchester. I was later to inherit Gordon Heslings' patient as he outgrew the Paediatric Department. There would appear to be three clear syndromes: that of abetalipoprotein (the Bassen-Kornzweig syndrome), Familial hypobetalipoproteinaemia, and secondary hypobetalipoproteinaemia with acanthocytosis.

Bassen and Kornzweig in New York first presented the case of an 18 year-old Jewish girl exhibiting the association of atypical retinitis pigmentosa with malformation of erythrocytes. The parents were second cousins. Her sister was similarly affected. They were ataxic with arreflexia, slender, weak, but not atrophic, legs, and restriction of the visual fields. Such a combination was well known but the addition of crenated red cells was something new.

The condition can present in one of three ways, neurologically, with failure to thrive or as a disorder dependent on malabsorption. The earliest presentation is of fatty stools (steatorrhoea), in the first year of life before coeliac disease normally occurs. Unsurprisingly, the child fails to gain weight and the tummy may be distended. The child may outgrow this stage and by five years the steatorrhoea becomes less troublesome. The stools remain bulky and they are dwarfed in stature. Treatment is necessarily symptomatic but can be very effective. Adequate nutrition is essential, with a low fat diet, given preferably in the form of low chain triglyerides. The fat soluble vitamins have to be replaced, in particular vitamins A (delaying any deterioration in the retinitis pigmentosa), and E. The neurological picture resembles Friedreich's ataxia. The first signs of this may be noticed, incidentally, with a tendency to stumble. Later there is loss of manual dexterity, thick speech – with a broken and monotonous timbre, the gait is broad-based, balance poor. The subject may shake and display nystagmus. The distinctive combination of ataxia, absent tendon reflexes and extensor plantar reflexes in a young person is equally suggestive of Friedreich's ataxia and abetalipoproteinaemia. The differentiation comes from the examination of plasma lipids and the examination of the blood with both phase contrast (wet) and Wright stain (dry) preparations.

One patient whom I eventually took over from Gordon Hesling and Professor (now Dame) June Lloyd, presented with failure to thrive at 8 months, worsening over the next year. The tendon reflexes could not be elicited but there was no other neurological abnormality. He sat at 9 months, stood at 14 and walked at 19 months. At 20 months he weighed only 9.75 kilograms (height 81 inches), ate well, appeared lively, but passed bulky, foul-smelling, often greasy stools, once or twice daily. Investigated when aged 2 in December 1965, the serum cholestoerol was 50mg%, betalipoprotein was absent on basic testing and 90% of the circulating erythrocytes were acanthocytes (as opposed to 30-40 in those with normolipoproteinaemic acanthocytosis). At nine years of age his symptoms remained satisfactorily controlled on a low fat diet with iron and vitamin supplementation. The deep tendon reflexes could not be elicited and apart from an obvious choroidal pattern, the fundi were normal. His height was still between the 25th and 50th percentile. Throughout his 20s he was well, of reasonable height and he had run at least one marathon race.

With the second personal patient, the first symptoms followed a change from half cream to full cream milk at 2 weeks of age. She was investigated for continuing ill health at 7 months and the diagnosis made. A third, aged 17 when first seen, had an early feeding problem with weight loss and early loose, pale bulky motions. She developed spontaneous bruising and loss of blood until 4.5 months old. She was treated with vitamin K and put on a low fat diet. Intellectual development has been normal. Following gastro-enteritis on a caravan holiday, she was found to be anaemic and menorrhagic but recovered. Her height at 17 years of age was 4 ft 11.5 in and she weighed 40.8 K. She was thin with a poor texture to her skin, with small musculature but no discrete wasting. Her feet were high arched, vision normal and limbs mildly hypotonic. Tendon reflexes could not be elicited. Movements of her limbs were clumsy, with noticeable truncal ataxia. She was being investigated at the age of 17 because her parents were concerned by her failure to grow and gain weight.

Most of the cases of transient acanthocysois have followed severe malnutrition or diarrhoeal disorders from infancy or with intercurrent infection leading to hypoalbuminaemia and hypobetalipoproteinaemia. The patient I saw with this syndrome was the 5 year-old sister of one of the abetalipoproteinaemia patients She was initially well, though passing somewhat bulky stools. Vitamin and lipid levels were all normal and on several occasions in early life, but not thereafter, transient acanthocytosis was noted.

In conclusion, the syndrome of abetalipoproteinaemia is of considerable interest to practically every branch of internal medicine That of normolipoproteinemia acanthocytois further adds fascination to the scientific puzzle.

## Back to Kentucky

Herpes simplex encephalitis can be a devastating illness with a high fatality rate. Usually the onset is sudden, with a urinary tract infection, and the encephalitis develops within 6 weeks; but the onset can be delayed. There was a judge in Kentucky, noted for his harsh judgments, but over 3 to 6 months they became unrealistically harsh before he succumbed to herpes simplex encephalitis. The EEG pattern is characteristic, with periodic complexes, but the condition, if not thought of, may be mistaken for a tumour, Even on angiography, or with modern scanning methods, parts of the brain such as the temporal lobe may appear swollen. The possible misinterpretation is increased by the finding of a more than usual number of red blood cells in the spinal fluid as the result of vascular cuffing by the infection allowing some leakage or seepage of blood.

As stated, those doing residencies in neurology were expected to learn some radiology. To do an air-encephalogram, using air to show the outlines of the ventricles of the brain, we had a machine which swung the patient through 360 degrees, head over heels. Even without this procedure, patients used to get intense headaches afterwards, unless they were demented, when they often did not turn a hair. In Preston, the late neurosurgeon had an alternative procedure, prior to operation, done under a general anaesthetic, whereby a few drops of myodil fluid were introduced via a needle into the 3rd or 4th ventricle. Either procedure was needed to establish the diagnosis of benign intracranial hypertension. Today both have been replaced by non-invasive CT (computerized tomography), or MR (magnetic resonance) scanning. We were also taught how to do angiographs, often with direct puncture of a brachial artery and the use of a pump Even till the 1980s direct-puncture angiography was used for carotid and vertebral angiography. The risks were higher and bleeding into the neck could occur, but radiologists were able to perform 6 such procedures in the time now taken to do two catheter studies.

One aspect of the work of the Department in which I took only a peripheral interest was the electrodiagnostic nerve and muscle studies performed by Mike McQuillen. Lexington is situated at the centre of the Blue Grass, surrounded by horse farms. Even I knew the names of some of the horses at stud. But there was trouble on the farms. Each year some of the best foals were dying prematurely of 'shaker foal disease'. Shortly after weaning they would become ill, reject food, develop wobbliness and fail to stand. Death would follow quickly or after one to two weeks. Mike McQuillen and Harvey Cantor performed EMGs on one or two foals, finding a presynaptic block akin to botulism. These observations were noted but not published and the diagnosis remained unestablished.

## Johns Hopkins Hospital

I was sent for a month to Johns Hopkins Hospital in Baltimore, Maryland to Victor McKusick's Department of Medical Genetics. I had spent my last two terms at school awaiting entrance to University, learning the then basics of genetics. At Johns Hopkins I would spend much time laboriously cutting out and matching chromosomes by shape and size – an inaccurate technique no longer required. Dave Clark had told me to contact his old chief, Frank Ford, and this I did.

I spent a day with him and we visited a mental home south of Baltimore. One of the patients we saw had the Lesch-Nyhan syndrome, which links up well with the normolipoproteinaemic acanthocytic syndrome just discussed. Catel and Schmidt (1959) first described severe choreoathetosis and spasticity in children with hyperuricaemia, and in 1964 Lesch and Nyhan (a medical student) defined the unusual neurological characteristics of this rare X-linked disorder, which is thus confined to males. Nyhan witnessed very similar disturbances in the Lesch-Nyhan syndrome:

> These children have a compulsive behaviour which they obviously do not like at all. As soon as restraints are removed, he generally appears quite terrified. The hand goes directly to the mouth and he begins tearing at his flesh, screaming all the time, as if in pain.

The mothers also have raised blood levels of uric acid but are of high intelligence, the children retarded. In both conditions, the Lesch-Nyhan and NLA acanthocytosis, self-mutilation is a characteristic, though not an invariable accompaniment, in association with involuntary and compulsive movements. In the L-N syndrome the biochemical disorder results from hypoxanthine guanine phosphoribozyl transferase (HG-PRTase) deficiency and is inherited. The children are normal at birth but towards the end of the first year, developmental and mental retardation become apparent with choreo-athetosis and spastic cerebral palsy. The IQ is usually less than 50 and the children are unable to walk or crawl. They experience difficulties with swallowing and are dysarthric. Aggressive and compulsive behaviour may begin as early as 2 years but more commonly starts at 6-8 years, with convulsions in one third of patients. These behavioural abnormalities reflect the level of uric acid and fluctuate with it.

Compulsive behaviour at conscious level – compulsive eating, anorexia, nail-biting, narcolepsy, appear to be sited at hypothalamic or basal ganglia level. Much earlier I referred to quasi-compulsive whistling, humming and lip-biting in Parkinsonian patients overdosed on laevodopa. As with the noises, tics and coprolalia of the Gilles de la Tourette syndrome, these features can be controlled for a short period but only at the distress of the patient. Control comes if the dosage of laevodopa can be lowered, or a non-suppressive form of treatment for the G-d-l-T syndrome given. Self-mutilation also occurs in the syndrome of congenital indifference to pain. Experimentally, in rats self-mutilation has been induced by feeding caffeine or theophylline. Caffeine, laevodopa, uric acid all possess a rather unusual common electronic structure with electron-donor properties. The site of action is believed to be the anterior hypothalamus but no histological confirmation has been shown.

The other patient I was shown was a tall eunuchoid male with mental retardation and aggressive tendencies. There are several forms of chromosome reduplication such as the Kinefelter syndrome of XXY, with XXXY and XXXXY variants. This patient exhibited the XYY syndrome, present in a significant proportion of tall, subnormal, psychopaths with 'dangerous, violent or criminal propensities'. I was to return to this Mental Institution with McKusicks' team who had gone on ahead to present more than 20 syndromic forms of retardation.

Victor McKusick was one of a pair of megancephalic* twins: both he and his brother, a lawyer, are extremely bright. His career mirrors what one might expect of an RMO (Residential Medical Officer) at a London Teaching Hospital. He had an echo-cardiograph which he took round everyone's patients. He was given a chronic diseases clinic, mainly involving neuro-syphilis. He introduced patients with Marfan's disease (the presumed explanation of Abraham Lincoln's stature) to the clinic. Then in 1962 he held a symposium on the X chromosome in man and henceforth became an internationally renowned geneticist, backed up by his *Mendelian Inheritance in Man*, the first book to be kept up to date by computer. He attracted people worldwide to his department – Alan Johnston (RMO when I was at UCH, later to become consultant in Aberdeen, while his brother was a headmaster

---

*Megancephaly = enlargement of the brain. This may be an incidental feature along with other malformations, or may be related to an overgrowth of the supporting cells of the brain or associated with otherwise normal development and cyto-architecture. At birth the head may be large, though not as a rule large enough to attract notice, with large fontanelles and wide sutures. The skull soon begins to enlarge disproportionately and assume a hydrocephalic-like shape, with the fontanelles and sutures remaining open but differs from that of hydrocephalus in having less pronounced parietal eminences. It may often be associated with outstanding intellect as with Thackeray, Turgeniev 2,012 Grams; Bismark 1,790 Grams, Byron 1,807 Grams. Among Neurologists, Kinear Wilson was megancephalic.

locally), Ferguson-Smith, Renwick, Alan Emery, David Weatherall, and Brian Walker – in short all major British geneticists will have been there. Having said this, his Department hangs out in a corridor split up into small cubicles by bookcases.

Only one person has ever scored over Victor McKusick. Professor Dent came out to deliver his lecture on homocysteinuria. By that afternoon McKusick had gathered six examples from his collection of patients with Marfan's syndrome. He had several stratagems for collecting genetic data. One was to help organize conferences of 'The Little People of America'. They would meet, pass resolutions that the height of telephones in booths should be lowered, etc. and he would take the opportunity to put his Department into action interviewing and, with their support, examining, those with a possible genetic basis. Next year he would repeat the procedure with the 'Tall People of America'. Fragile bones, albinos, people from the islands of Chesapeake Bay, might be invited. Cardiovascular diseases which could be inherited were gathered. I remember his journal clubs looking at reports from elsewhere and grand rounds where the presenting doctor, showing someone with Marfan's, might describe the patient as 'non-competitive' – the sport of basket ball is very much to the advantage of someone who is exceptionally tall. Perhaps his single greatest source of genetic information was from the Old Order Amish. He even recruited doctors from the wider Amish community to advance his work.

I made two trips to Intercourse, Lancaster county, Pennsylvania: once on a special trip driven by Prof McKusick with Ingrid Gamstrop[*], the Swedish neuro-geneticist, and once with his team.

Because of their unusual socio-religious tenets and practices, the Old Order Amish are well-known in North America. They eschew personal adornment and follow closely prescribed habits of dress. They resist technological advances, specifically using the horse and buggy for transport and horse-drawn agricultural equipment. Their homes are devoid of electricity and telephones. Most Amish are farmers. In Lancaster county most are prosperous and a few fairly wealthy. Private enterprise with mutual assistance characterises the Amish economic system. And inter-community magazines, gossipy about family illnesses, connecting the 80% who live in

---

[*] I associate Ingrid Gamstrop with a condition she described called adynamia episodica hereditaria. There are various forms of periodic paralysis, all of which can be difficult to treat, wherein paralysis can occur after physical exertion, large carbohydrate meals, with thyrotoxicosis or with sweating. I had a patient who developed paralysis from sunbathing with loss of sodium and potassium in the sweat. They may respond to potassium, sodium or calcium infusions. Correction with the wrong salt can be fatal. Gamstrop's form could be induced by eating ice-cream, temporarily paralysing the swallowing mechanism.

Pennsylvania, Ohio and Indiana with scattered groups elsewhere, serve as a source of data from which to start genetic investigations.

The Amish sect originated in the Canton of Berne, Switzerland, in 1693, when Jacob Amman led a split from the older and more extensive Mennonite church. Converts were acquired in Alsace, Lorraine, the Palatine, and neighbouring areas of southern Germany and eastern France. Many of these converts were Swiss, who had moved to these areas in the preceding century. Migration to eastern Pennsylvania began about 1720 and continued until 1770. Most present-day Lancaster County Amish are descendants of pre-revolutionary immigrants, who probably totalled no more than 200 persons. Waves of Amish immigration continued until about 1850, with these later immigrants moving on to Ohio and Indiana. The migration patterns account for the peculiarities of distribution of family names and certain genes within the United States and Canada.

Known also as Pennsylvania Dutch, some Amish are trilingual and all bilingual (not speaking English). Religious services, conducted in German and 'Dutch' (for Deutsch, the south German dialect of the Palatine), are held in several homes or barns in rotation. (There is now a separate, breakaway community called Church Amish who use churches). Their beliefs are based on literal interpretations of the old German Bible. A strong system of sanctions, including excommunication and shunning (Meidung), helps maintain the group. They oppose infant baptism. Reception into church membership by baptism is practiced at an age of decision, usually the late teens. Footwashing is a characteristic part of the service twice yearly and no formally educated clergy exist, but bishops, preachers and deacons, chosen from the laity, are responsible for almost all aspects of religious and community life. Resistance to consolidated schools and to education beyond the legal minimum, absolute pacifism, and in general separateness from the world are other cardinal features. Contact with other children is not so much shunned as the corruption of their children from the teaching of science, gymnastic activities and the wearing of non-Amish school uniforms. They frequently court trouble through failure to satisfy the minimum requirements for schooling, to make social security payments and by not electrifying their dairy barns. Despite appreciable loss through persons leaving the faith and therefore the community, its numbers have increased many times faster than the average for the United States, though with no new source of diluting genetic material, the genes of the original 200 or so ancestors form the basis for the whole community of Lancaster County.

Perhaps the most striking example of the genetic concentration of disease among the Old Order Amish is dwarfism of Ellis-van Creveld type. The features of chondro-ectodermal dysplasia are lack of hair, poor dentition, extra fingers, chondro-dysplasia and congenital heart malformations. The nails are small, deformed and with ridges. Peripheral bones are shortened and 50% die in infancy of respiratory insufficiency. McIntosh described one case in 1933, Ellis and van Creveld another in 1940. Metrakos and Fraser assembled 7 reported cases and added 5 of their own in 1954, enabling the condition to be established as an autosomal recessive. In 1969, McKusick's team identified 61 from Lancaster county.

With huge, complex charts of interbreeding and second-cousin marriages, other genetic syndromes have been described in profusion. Dwarfism with cartilage hair hypoplasia, from Lancaster County; pyruvate kinase deficiency haemolytic anaemia from Mifflin County Pennsylvania; limb-girdle muscular dystrophy from Adams and Allen Counties, Indiana; haemophilia B in Ohio.

From the many populations in the United States and even elsewhere, McKusick has studied Ashkenazic Jews, Sephardic Jews, Africans (most American Negroes have 40% European genes), Korean, Mexican, Inuit, Hawaiians (Polynesian), American Indian and other ethnic groups. The syndromes associated with deafness were reclassified and extended. Radiologists, Biochemics, Cardiologists abounded to help with the task. Often the most unique contribution can come from a Dentist.

## Charcot's Hysteria Renaissant

Whilst at Johns Hopkins, I made good use of the library to look at Charcot's original descriptions of hysteria. The Medical Library at the University of Kentucky Medical Center was excellent. The Librarian had been given several million dollars to travel Europe to obtain back editions of important textbooks etc., but the Library at Johns Hopkins was superb.

Conversion hysteria, i.e. psychologically induced physical illness, can affect anyone, even those of high intelligence: as for example a medical secretary who believed she had carcinoma of the pancreas. However, it is mostly associated with low intelligence and a failure of understanding between patient and doctor, doctor and patient. Within our department there was a consensus that hysteria was rife throughout Kentucky and there were many discussions as to how we should catalogue its frequent presentation. Classical forms such as 'running fits' had been seen for many years in patients from Kentucky's Appalachian counties. Confirmation of its high incidence came from several other Departments of the Medical Center, and in particular from the Departments of Psychiatry and Community Medicine, substantiated by sociological surveys from the University's Department of Sociology. The literature of the region: *The Southern Appalachian Region – a*

*Survey*; *Health and Demography in Kentucky*; *Night Comes to the Cumberlands*; *They Shall take up Serpents*; *Yesterday's People* – is strewn with references to hysterical neuroses and behaviour.

In an early attempt to write up our findings, I propounded a hypothesis:-

> The sex and age distribution of conversion hysteria in Eastern Kentucky does not conform to accepted hypotheses. The high incidence of hysterical reactions among males cannot be explained by direct comparison with those circumstances in which hysteria predominantly occurs among males; in particular the aspect of secondary gain, as normally understood, is not a prominent factor. The majority of individuals studied came from the lowest social strata and sought obscurity in their environment. The hypothesis is presented that conversion hysteria may represent one kind, one form, of social maladaptive behaviour by the least guided, non-verbal, members of society in response to repeated adversity. In developing this hypothesis, attention is paid to the social history and ecology of Eastern Kentucky; the full meaning engendered in the term 'non-verbal'; and the spectrum of events whereby a 'depressed' society attempts to voice its grievances as a 'protesting' society, and finally succeeds in achieving its political goals.

David Clark was extremely worried about the potential backlash which any description of hysteria as particularly prevalent in Eastern Kentucky might have in jeopardizing the Medical Center and grants to the Neurology department. It was only some years later that Harvey Cantor and I were able to publish a description of Charcot's original observations, with parallel cases from Kentucky, complete with their neuro-radiological and neuro-physiological findings and subsequent interpretation. Let us preface this report with two observations:

a) the diagnosis of hysteria even in its most florid forms must be made with caution;

b) the physician has the added duty of understanding why the patient has taken to express himself, or herself, subconsciously in this manner.

One of the most startling forms of hysteria which Charcot described was 'La Grande Hysterie', otherwise called hysteria major or hystero-epilepsy, with distinctive crises. He presented 10 patients (both men and women) with this condition and described La Grande Hysterie as consisting of four phases:

(1) the epileptoid,
(2) that of violent movements,
(3) that of attitudes passionnelles (the hallucinatory phase),
(4) that of the concluding delirium.

According to Charcot, all the various forms of an hysterical attack (which as a matter of fact are more frequently observed than the full grande attaque) are derived from a shortening, lengthening, omission or isolation of these separate phases.

He described the first two phases as follows:

> Attacks either start spontaneously or may be provoked by stimulation of part of the body. There follows a well defined painful aura arising from the stomach to the throat, producing a feeling of constriction and throbbing pain in the head. Then the patient loses consciousness and the epileptoid stage starts. The limbs stretch out. The wrists flex and become twisted in a position of exaggerated pronation. The arms contort, with extremely violent movements of salutation and disorderly gestures owing to convulsive contractions of the pectoral muscles. The patient breaks and tears apart everything on which he can lay his hands. From time to time the contortions stop for a moment and give way to the characteristic attitude of an 'arc en cercle', with opisthotonus and forward or lateral curvature of the spine.

Our parallel example was a 33 year-old patient, in whom we witnessed several attacks, filming one. Another occurred in a lecture room before an audience. She had had seizures from age 10, but latterly they had become more severe and for 10 days before admission had been almost continuous without relief from phenytoin 100 mg three times daily. Her first seizure had occurred when she was 10 in a school playground and was almost certainly epileptic. She recalls nothing of it except that she fainted and woke some time later, sleepy and confused, with the teacher washing dirt from her face. From puberty her seizures occurred premenstrually. They were accompanied by an aura of flushing and a feeling of warmth over her face. She then felt that she had to sit down lest she should fall. She never bit her tongue, never foamed at the mouth, never fell hurting herself, never had a seizure when on her own, and when pregnant on four occasions, never had a fit after the first month of gestation.

Her present dramatic attacks could be provoked by entering into a discussion with her husband and obtaining from him a description of the course of events. She would then complain of a feeling of warmth, and as he began to show how she wrings her hands at the start of an attack, she would proceed to do likewise, falling back in a state of tonic rigidity. She would enter into a stage of agitation: drawing her hands upward in an apparently purposeful and strong movement and exclaiming in a clear voice, 'I will bite, I will bite', at which her husband would hasten to place a rolled handkerchief in her mouth. The next stage consisted of a series of tonic and usually symmetric posturings accompanied by moaning. She would often raise herself on her head and heels in a state of opisthotonus (arc of a circle). Some tonic posturings would occur for several minutes after the opsithotonus, but at this stage her husband claimed to be able to break the fit by rubbing the sides of her neck.

The results of clinical examination and investigation were normal. The cerebro-spinal fluid contained 2 white cells and a protein concentration of

6 g/l. The electroencephalogram, including a sleeping and waking record, was within normal limits.

It was felt that these attacks closely simulated Charcot's original description. Charcot was well aware that hysterical and epileptic attacks may be seen together in the same patient. Two other points need to be made. Although the blood levels of phenytoin were within the normal range for treatment, toxic levels can be associated with an increase in the number of fits and they can simulate hysterical attacks. Secondly patients are at times able to avert an attack, usually in the initial stages by various means, such as fist clenching or rubbing an affected area of the body.

The next example concerns the hallucinatory phase of La Grande Hysterie.

> Then comes the third stage, called the period of passionate attitudes, during which he utters words and cries in keeping with his gloomy delirium, and the terrifying visions which persecute him. At length he regains consciousness, recognizes and names people round him, but the delirium and hallucinations persist yet awhile; he seeks around him and under the bed for the dark beasts which threaten him; he examines his arms, expecting to find the bites of animals which he thinks he felt. Then he comes to himself, the attack is finished, but very often only to begin again a few seconds later, until, after 3 or 4 successive attacks, the patient regains his normal condition.'

Our patient was a 30 year-old male admitted for investigation of epilepsy. He was said to have rolled 200 feet down a railroad embankment. He had periods of disorientation as to place and if approached at such times was often belligerent. One afternoon he disappeared from the ward and was not found for several minutes. He was located in a washroom lying against the wall with his eyes closed. When aroused, he was communicative, explaining that we were in the woods hunting snakes with our hands. He was placed in a wheelchair and taken back to his room, where he slid out of the chair, grasping the side rail of the bed with a powerful, unrelenting grip and asked for pliers to remove the snake's teeth. All the while he stared straight ahead. When asked, he would explain what he was doing, but if touched he became belligerent. He remained on the floor for another 10 minutes, then got up quite unaware of where he was or how he got there.

He showed focal abnormalities on the EEG including delta activity from the left temporal region. On x-ray there was a patch of calcification at the left temporal tip. Bilateral carotid angiograms and an air-encephalogram were normal. He undoubtedly had temporal lobe epilepsy and this could have been accompanied by either a schizo-affective state or ocular hallucinations.

Most certainly there was a severe personality disorder accompanying the focal disturbance, thus making hystero-epilepsy the most probable diagnosis.

Hysterical Hemianaesthesia is yet another form which may accompany hysteria major. Charcot described a young girl with hemianaesthesia of hysteria in a form that is altogether characteristic. On the left side there is insensibility to pricking, cold and other forms of stimuli. This loss of general sensibility is found in the upper extremity, the lower extremity, half of the trunk and the head. This girl bears the most intense faradization without suffering the slightest inconvenience and the anaesthesia occupies not only the skin, but even the deeper parts, the muscles and nerve trunks. In most cases, when there is insensibility of one side of the body and of the face, a more or less pronounced disturbance of vision is also manifest in the corresponding eye, a sort of amblyopia which rarely amounts to amaurosis.

We presented two examples of this condition. Firstly, a 53 year-old male who had had two prolonged periods of unconsciousness in the previous 8 months. When he recovered from the second episode, he noted a numbness over the right side of his face and complained of headache over the right half of the head. He had several episodes of sudden and generalized right-sided weakness occurring about every three days and lasting two days. These were unaccompanied by any alteration of his level of consciousness. Further examination showed bilateral tunnel vision and right ear deafness. In other respects his sensory loss was total over the right half of his body and face. Sensation to light touch, pin prick, joint position testing, vibration and temperature were absent up to the midline. There was no difference in the reflexes or in the corneal responses from either side. Skull and chest x-rays, blood serology, glucose determinations ECG and EEG were all normal before he took his own discharge. It is just possible that he had hemiplegic migraine, which can be associated with prolonged episodes of loss of consciousness, but objective tests such as sensation over the corneae, and reflexes bilaterally similar, suggest hysteria. Despite his 'sensory loss' he was still able to identify objects in either hand by feel and touch.

Our second patient had a dense, unselective, sensory neuropathy with normal deep tendon reflexes. A pin could be stuck into his tongue without evoking pain. These symptoms followed the finding of silicosis affecting both lungs. Over 6 weeks a feeling of numbness and heaviness spread over his whole body. Even so, there was no alteration in muscle tone or strength and he could stand on either foot with his eyes closed. With antituberculous therapy and psychiatric treatment all his symptoms cleared within six weeks.

Rather than continue with yet further parallel descriptions of Charcot's, including monoplegia, and hysterical gaits, I will describe a highly cultured man from West Africa who came to see me with loss of voice. The physiotherapy department were able to treat him with direct laryngeal stimulation, but it transpired that he was a financial adviser to a government in the region and monetary problems had arisen. The most dramatic recovery from an hysterical paralysis I have witnessed was a 45 year-old man, a former rugby player, whom I had inherited from academic departments at two separate neurological centres. He was bloated as the result of repeated courses of steroid therapy, could not move his legs and could barely move his arms. I was called to see him as he had been transferred to a Cheshire Home. I entered the ward office to be greeted by a tall thin individual, who recognized me and whom I in turn thought I knew but could not place. This was the patient. Apparently his wife had left him and he had made a startling recovery. There are recorded instances of several patients with hysterical paraplegia who have been admitted to renowned paraplegic units before the nature of their diagnosis has been recognized.

It is not enough to relate case-histories of patients with conversion symptoms. Hysteria asks questions of neurology, psychiatry, and re-emphasizes the fact that we know so little of the workings of the mind. As a diagnosis, it is generally considered a problem for psychiatry yet the historical and contemporary associations are largely neurological. It is amazing how often, with a question of a legal nature, the physician is regarded as being at fault if he has not asked for the opinion of a psychiatrist, and yet that same court will ignore the psychiatrist's prognostications, preferring the 'common sense approach' of the physician. There is always a certain 'tortuosity' to definitions of hysteria. Thus the World Health Organisation definition reads: 'a mental disorder in which motives, of which the patient seems unaware, produce either a restriction of the field of consciousness or disturbance of motor and sensory function which may seem to have psychological advantage or symbolic value'. Other statements suggest a disparity between neurological signs and symptoms thus being medically inexplicable, 'a temporal relationship between symptom onset and some external event or psychological conflict, or the symptom allows the individual to avoid unpleasant activity or the symptom provides the opportunity for support which may not have been otherwise available.' The alternative concept, introduced by Pilowsky in 1975, is of Abnormal Illness Behaviour – the persistence of an inappropriate mode of perceiving, evaluating, acting in relation to one's state of health, despite the fact that a doctor has offered a reasonably lucid explanation of the nature of the illness, and the appropriate course of management to be followed, based on a thorough medical examination.

These factors come much to the fore in discussing hysterical fugue states in which there is overlap with aspects of self-recognition and esteem, psychotic illness and recognition of familiarity. Thus hysterical fugues are but one form of a spectrum of dissociated reactions. They are usually more clearly so than other forms of hysteria, recognizable as a direct response to severe or overwhelming stress. Shorter trance states, also with dissociation of the personality, may occur, as in the scene in Shakespeare's play where Lady Macbeth is tormented by the guilt of Duncan's murder. In hysterical fugues, a wife, suddenly reacting to her husband's infidelity, may leave home without notice and is discovered wandering aimlessly in a state of dissociated or restricted consciousness for days or even for weeks. Similarly, a businessman may suddenly quit when faced with failure of his firm or an undiscovered fraud. On recovery from the fugue, there is usually no recollection of the events of the fugue. The patient may appear dazed, confused and with loss of identity. Alternatively, he may have apparently settled down to another life as a normal individual, carrying out an occupation and exhibiting a mode of life and behaviour different from his previous one. The patient has no access to the memories of his usual personality and, on recovery, no recollection of the events of his fugue.

Variants of this theme include: hysterical amnesia – thus, as in the Podola case, a prisoner may be unable to plead in respect of a crime; the Ganser syndrome of hysterical pseudo-dementia (straw in his hair, etc.), where failure of memory is accompanied by bizarre behaviour aping madness; or the much rarer syndrome of multiple personality, as exemplified by R.L. Stevenson's novel *The Strange Case of Dr Jekyll and Mr Hyde*. The fugue individual may take on a distinctly different personality than the premorbid personality – and usually a rasher, less conventional behaviour pattern emerges. The two personalities can interchange but remain unaware of the other half of the 'split'. Where two or more subsidiary personalities emerge, these may be aware of, and make disparaging remarks about, the original timid, conforming personality but still remain unaware of one another, and the original personality remains unaware of them. The emergence of the alter ego is ushered in by a fugue and the new personality builds up an entirely new life, acquiring a new job, a new circle of friends in different communities, but can occasionally alternate in the same setting. As with other hysterical phenomena, it thrives on the fascination it engenders, and a direct link with a suggestive stimulus is usually discernible.

Hysterical fugues are met with rarely, and unfortunately are so clearly related to the patient that reproduction without describing the patient whereby he and his illness can be recognized, is rarely possible. However, I have outlined the fugue state because so many neurological conditions abut on to it and require differentiation from it.

**Kentucky Again**
Like Stephen Foster, let me sing of my old Kentucky home, or rather three such homes. We were able to stay in the houses of members of the University who had left on sabbaticals. Our first, with elegant cherry-wood furniture, was the home of the widow of an expert on the Marquis de Sade! This lay at the end of a long avenue of pin-oaks. Our next move was to the house next door, ostensibly in another road. It belonged to an engineer and his young family. Every house had a basement, with laundry facilities and a pump because the water level was so high. The story goes that one lady, listening to a radio commentary whilst washing, put on her son's baseball hat so that the hung clothes would not drip onto her hair, and at the last minute decided to throw in her smalls to complete the wash, leaving herself naked. Just then the meter reader arrived and seeing her thus, the football commentary dominating the room, exclaimed: 'May your team win!' and fled. Our third house was covered in paintings by the owner, even in the toilet, and filling a junk room. My wife was able to work for much of the time, firstly in anaesthetics then doing ventilation/perfusion studies on the lungs. We had – almost a record – the same negro lass to look after our children when Mair was at work. She was excellent and her name was Dovey. She would arrive each morning along with other negro workers by bus, dubbed the slave wagon by certain of our non-traditional friends.

We were fortunate that besides the medical friends, who in themselves were very hospitable, we met up with two of my parent's friends from Ethiopia. Rozanne was a social worker and her husband Bob a professor of law. They were Jewish from New York and unlikely people for conservative Kentucky. He would fight civil liberty cases (race and women's lib) from the county courts all the way to the Supreme Court, and was, in effect, drummed out of Kentucky at a later stage. Our other friends were neighbours who befriended Mair when she was at home with the young babe. One, an ENT surgeon in town, would check his cholesterol level twice weekly to determine what he should eat. His family came from East Kentucky and there had been several State Governors among them. The gathering of the Coombs clan was an international event with over 3,000 attenders.

Mair was taken, with great protests of sadness that she was not American, to the League of Women Voters. They were thinking of putting up a candidate for jailer as they protested at the prisoners being led through the streets in chains. Travelling through the countryside, one saw not only posters for governor but graffiti on stones – so-and-so for jailer. In addition, on the outside of the town jails there would be notices not to talk to the prisoners through the bars. Kentucky politics were strange affairs. Everything was voted for with balanced town-country lists which never worked out because cross-party voting would ensure that the country got all the posts. A man standing for Attorney General had, as his policy platform, that if elected he would investigate the people investigating his income tax. And the advice most listened to came from 'A'dolph Rupp, coach of the Kentucky basketball team.

The association with the League of Women Voters was not quite as bizarre as that of Dave Clark's daughters being invited to join the Daughters of the American Revolution. Dr Clark was able to reply that, yes, their ancestors were in the States at the time of the American War of Independence, but they fought on the other side. That apparently did not matter; the fact was that they were in America then.

Towards the end of my two years in America, I flew to Manchester for an interview from which I obtained a Consultant Post in the U.K. based on Preston. The Neurosurgeon clearly wanted to dominate, questioning why I had also asked to meet the senior physician!

Just before I left, I had done a regional clinic in Manchester, Kentucky. There were the jumping Sizemores, suffering from lack of ability to sweat, so in hot weather they used to cool by bathing in the creek. There was also an example of a porcupine man: small headed, with fits and scaley skin (icthyosis). I drew up a genetic table of the families under the title of ectodermal dysplasia, but it is likely that the Sizemores had the Christ-Siemens syndrome of anhidrotic ectodermal dysplasia, which is a sex-linked recessive, with partial or complete absence of sweat glands, a thin flattened skin, some disturbance of the underlying collagen and elastic fibres, and icthyosis more apparent than real. The female carriers can also be recognized by dental defects, sparse hair, reduced sweating and dermatoglyphic changes. Among other patients seen that day was the son of the local sheriff and of the local bootlegger. Parts of Kentucky, and even parts of Bourbon County, are dry, with an illicit trade in Moonshine. Apparently the Sheriff had frisked down the bootlegger before he went in to see me! Another family with six retarded children, one of whom was especially interesting, also attended. The Health Visitor explained that the father, in this case, had been an ex-miner injured in the mine shaft and had drawn for years (drawn welfare), but only the other day someone had drawn on him and shot him dead. Now the problem was to transfer the welfare money into the wife's name. On the subject of Drawin' and Shootin' dead, there is, in Appalachian Kentucky, a subtle distinction made between shootin', killin' and murder. A shootin' in the course of an argument is a shootin', the outcome of a minor fracas after whisky or when an outsider annoys you on your land. A killin' is more deliberate; it is necessary to lie in wait and shoot deliberately in pursuit of a feud or a family affair. Murder is murder, but it rarely is murder and usually a lenient view is taken anyway.

Kentucky is part of the Bible Belt and as such is the home of many revivalist and fanatical sects. Baptism by total immersion is commonly practiced. So too is the gift of tongues to the apostles, reinacted in 'talking in tongues' similar to the Welsh *hwyl* of the beginning of this century. Ira Jay Martin, professor of Bible and Religion, has written on glossolalia in the Apostolic Church and many of the books on Kentucky vouch for its regular practice. In the Jesse Stuart Harvest, a short story, 'Snake Teeth', describes Unknown Tongues revivals going on to the more spectacular event, which is the cause of one or two deaths each year in various parts of Kentucky – the Snake Handling Ceremonies. I had seen the film made by Sir William Sargeant, Consultant Psychiatrist at St Thomas's, London, who was shown the Ethiopian equivalent by my parents in Addis Ababa. And in the last few weeks before leaving I was on stand-by to attend a clandestine snake-handling ceremony. These ceremonies are justified by a quotation from St Mark's gospel, and 'they shall take up serpents'. The idea being that to handle deadly vipers displayed one's faith and to die by such means guaranteed a path to heaven.

If I failed to attend a snake-handling service, I was able to attend a very pleasing little event before leaving Kentucky. Prof. Abe Wikler gave a dinner party for those leaving Kentucky and arranged that a violinist should visit each table playing a tune from whence they came, and another, rather more light-hearted, to whence they would depart. At our table he played Greensleeves, followed by Col. Bogey from the Bridge over the River Kwai. I was able to explain gently to him the slightly inappropriate words which commonly went with the tune.

**Early American English**

I do not wish to leave Kentucky without describing another of our quests to understand more of the people of this deprived part of the opulent USA. The peoples of East Kentucky have had a new lease of life with the need to search for fossil fuels including shale. Consequently there has been a revival of their fortunes bringing in new resources to Appalachia. They will never be on a par with the rest of the USA, but relative prosperity has occurred.

My interest was aroused when an educational psychologist reported that she had found school children who spoke a kind of idioglossia – they could understand each other but could not be understood by outsiders. We therefore telephoned one of the schools. 'Yes, they had a few such children, but our inquiries would be more fruitful if we rang the school further up the creek.' The answer from the principal of the second school was different, with perhaps a hint of paranoia: 'Children who speak funnily? – No, unless you think we all do, but then we speak the oldest English going.'

The school was in Magoffin county. The county had been one of the more isolated in Kentucky until the mountain parkway had been completed three years earlier, linking the Blue Grass of central Kentucky with the eastern townships of Paintsville, Pikeville and Prestonsbury. The parkway led through Powell and Estill Counties in a maze of geological splendour; to the left, the Red River Gorge, to the right, one hundred natural arches and the Natural Bridge State Park. At the end of 120 miles of fast road, there remained only 11 further miles of desultory, broken black-top to reach the town of Fredville, formed by the intersection of a single-track railroad, the mainstreet and the banks of the Licking River. The school lay two miles beyond, set against a hill in apparent isolation.

My wife and I made the first exploratory trip to the school to interview the School Principal in his study. A spitoon lay to his right and he chewed and spat tobacco blissfully as we chatted. He came 'from the soil here, born and bred in this section'. He had actually left the State to learn his profession. Back home, he had no wish to move. He hunted a pack of hounds, knew the neighbourhood, and was himself someone in the community. He had declined many offers of better paid work elsewhere. In co-operating with us, he was as good as his word.

Once assured of the opportunity to study the local dialect, I sought out the most professional help possible. The University Calendar showed that Lexington boasted a Professor of Phonetics, Dr Gifford Blyton. It took very little persuasion to obtain his help in the venture. Because we were each to depart at the conclusion of the academic term, there was some haste in preparation, but after further advice from Dr Cratis Williams, an acknowledged expert on Kentucky dialects, we devised questionnnaires and sought to record with a tape-recorder as much conversation as possible. Dr Blyton had previously attempted to study dialect in another part of Kentucky, leaving the tape-recorder in a village store, and with the help of the store-keeper obtained some valuable material – only to lose it when someone borrowed the tapes.

The advice we were given in sampling folk speech at its uninhibited best is to induce people to speak freely about their experiences. An old gentleman 'hosting' his guests on his front porch likes to give narrative accounts of floods, droughts, murders, strange occurrences, hunting experiences, the peculiar behaviour of outsiders. His speech will be more nearly true when he is swept into his account. Your admiration is of his tale, not his speech. If you admire his accent and want to tape it, he will become even more excited if he is not too mike-shy. It is then that his metaphors, strong preterites, elisions, and archaic expressions, flow. Women tend to preserve the traditional more faithfully than men but 'mountain' women are more likely to be inhibited than 'mountain' men.

Where do we look for the oldest dialects? It is rarely in the cities or where there is contact with other languages, but where a group of people, often inbred, have sheltered from change. Norman French is preserved in Jervaisse – the language of Jersey, and old French in the French-owned islands off New Foundland. In Orkney and Shetland, old words are preserved but their origins are obscure – they could as certainly be of Norse origin as of old English. In America, in the islands of Chesapeake bay – Smith and Tangier islands – in the Ozark country of Kansas, in the creeks of Kentucky, where there is inbreeding but little in-migration, old forms are preserved but it is probably best to go to completely isolated colonies, such as were on the island of Tristan Da Cunha, to find the oldest forms.

What did we seek? We sought those characteristics which render an old dialect most interesting – terms from ancient languages which fit most closely to Elizabethan English. Thus there is a proliferation of package phrases, replete with redundancies, answers which repeat the same stereotyped, clumsy, almost rhetorical phraseology, preterites which are used more frequently than in present-day English, etc. As Cratis Williams declares, 'Writers of fiction have been most impressed with those verbs which retain either the strong preterites of Middle English or variant preterites of the English dialects. It is perhaps these verbs that most readily attract the attention of outsiders to the peculiarities of mountain usage. Not unusual in English dialects, they are impressive solely because of their frequency.'

Suffixes and prefixes, too, attract attention. Many are frequently Chaucerian, some Shakespearean. En-, un-, a-, dis-, be-, mis- take on a new lease of life: unthoughted, apast, pears for appears, anent, disfurnish, dismission, misput, that's what's be-giving off. The exchange of civilities, metaphor, the 'r' and 'th' sounds especially, the rhythm and prosody of speech, pleonasms e.g. hound-dog, spade-shovel, the stress placed on final syllables, and prepositions all add spice to our enjoyment of dialect. Diphthongs are used differently, vowels lengthened, 'n' rather than 'ng'. Soured milk is 'clabbered'. Children are 'raised'.

We are left with generalizations:-

Inbreeding and rural depopulation lead to the ossification of the local vernacular,

Rules of grammar with archaisms tend to be preserved.

Primary languages, uninfluenced by other trends, tend to have large, often redundant vocabularies and a complex syntax.

I am left with the thought that the study of the fast-disappearing old forms of English would be a worthwhile hobby when time permits.

PART II

# NEUROLOGICAL CONSULTANT

**Preston and the Surrounding Area**

THE SUB-REGIONAL neurological centre based on Preston served a population of 1.8 million, to whom I was the sole neurologist. The area covered all Lancashire outside Greater Manchester and Merseyside, and included Furness and south Cumbria. Apart from my weekly clinic in Preston, I did fortnightly clinics in Blackpool, Blackburn, Burnley, and Lancaster, with patients from Barrow and Cumbria coming to Lancaster. I also attended the Epileptic Colony (later to be called Centre) at Langho on a weekly basis and in all visited 60 different hospitals at one time or another. I had charge of neurophysiology, reporting all EEGs and doing my own electromyography and nerve conduction studies as necessary.

The centre had been set up by Ken Tutton five years previously. He had been first assistant to Sir Jeffrey Jefferson in Manchester. Sir Jeffrey was renowned for his seminal monograph outlining the detailed anatomy of the cavernous sinus at the base of the brain, transversed by arteries and nerves. His sons, Anthony, a neurosurgeon and Michael, a neurologist, were highly regarded. Tutton's senior position in Manchester was not in doubt. He had spent a year in North America. His M.Ch thesis had been on cerebral abscess formation. At this stage he went to Sheffield as a locum Consultant Neurosurgeon, only to find that Anthony Jefferson was appointed to the permanent post. This was to cause deep acrimony and whilst Sir Jeffrey was away, Mr Tutton approached the Regional Board, explaining that one third of all Neurosurgery came to Manchester from further north and that it would be logical to start a centre at Preston. He succeeded in his endeavour breaking completely from Sir Jeffrey Jefferson.

He began work in Preston with no assigned beds. He encouraged both the General Pathologist and General Radiologist to develop the necessary expertise to cover neuro-surgery. He would see patients and even operate at any major hospital in the area, and in addition to Preston, set up a small unit at Lancaster Moor, where, with the help of a psychiatrist with an interest in EEGs and electro-corticography, he performed temporal lobectomies and even leucotomies. A ward was built for him at the Infirmary, with a recovery ward in an old EMS hospital devoid of facilities half a mile away. After a gap of a few years, he was joined by Dr Neil Gordon, who travelled from Manchester each week to do a neurological clinic in Preston and the same afternoon would travel to Lancaster to do an additional clinic. About this time, a second neurosurgeon was appointed. Two years before I came, Dr Gordon became a full-time Neuro-Paediatrician in Manchester and Susan Woodcock was appointed Neurologist to Preston, only to leave in December 1967 to get married.

Tutton and his colleague, Alex Daws, were technically able and good clinical opinions but extremely difficult to work with. Ken Tutton's retirement dinner was marred by an altercation with Alex Daws, unbefitting such an occasion. Tutton claimed to have adopted Sir Jeffrey's time-keeping, 'if you arrive early or on time for something, clearly you have not spent sufficient time at the previous engagement'. He could be exasperating one minute and then, by taking over a case urgently, could be most helpful. His abiding interest was golf. A steady player, not given to great hits, he became President of the Royal Lytham and St Annes Golf Club. He was more supportive of his golfing mates than of his colleagues, given at times to indiscretions and to damning comments in case-notes.

Relationships with neuro-surgeons are vitally important. There are considerable disadvantages in the practice of neurology away from a neuro-surgical centre. Discussion with them, and with the neuro-radiologists, disputing where necessary, is very much in the best interests of all concerned and particularly of the patient. But they can be prickly and awkward creatures. Alexander Pope must have met them. 'Wrapt in a Gown, for Sickness, and for Show'. Time and seniority in neurology enable one to curb their excesses. However, over the years, I have found the newer neuro-surgeons more accommodating and easier to deal with. All nevertheless deserve praise for their skills and abilities.

The neurological situation was far from ideal; but this was only one of two neurological posts vacant that year in the U.K. My part of the unit consisted of a senior house officer, a clinical assistant (a good local G.P.) in outpatients, a secretary and an EEG technician. My beds were all in Deepdale Hospital, the EMS hospital half a mile from the infirmary – with no direct access to intensive care facilities. For any investigation – straightforward x-rays, EEGs, myelograms, angiograms and air-encephalograms, some needing anaesthetics – the patient had to be transported by ambulance to the Infirmary and returned to Deepdale. It was over ten years before my beds were transferred to the Infirmary.

Although I reported EEGs, my approach was far more sceptical than that of Mr Tutton, who had used EEGs with unusual electrode placements to localize abscesses in his M.Ch thesis. Localised delta (slow wave) activity could indicate a tumour or abscess. Phase reversal with sharp outlines pointing upwards in one set of leads and downwards in another could provide further localization, and one may see an area of electrical silence. Dead cells have no electrical activity, damaged cells produce abnormal electrical activity. Even using these criteria, my confidence limits were less than his in this respect. We waited about 5 years for isotope scanning to be installed. By being able to swing regional policy, we obtained a CT scan (originally called an EMI scan until they lost the franchise, then CAT scanning, only later to be shortened to CT) as soon as they were generally available throughout the U.K. There was some value in seeing all the EEGs. I could monitor the general scene and predict what was likely to come my way. I continued to report EEGs for over 24 years, until a neurophysiologist was appointed.

The sensitivity of EEG machines has increased over the years and I was always careful to select the most advanced machine in order to attract technicians to Preston. A common practice used to be to remove anticonvulsant drugs prior to an EEG so as to increase the likelihood of abnormal EEG findings. There were dangers inherent in this procedure in that fits and even status epilepticus could be precipitated as the result of drug withdrawal. We also used activation techniques with sphenoidal needles inserted to lie beneath the temporal lobes to gather information not available to electrodes situated over the surface of the skull. Thin wire electrodes replaced larger sphenoidal needles, and the methodology could be enhanced by short-acting barbiturate anaesthesia. These techniques have been mostly set aside. A routine or a sleep EEG, can provide the necessary information. In the routine EEG hyperventilation will blow off carbon dioxide, altering the blood gases, and stroboscopic stimulation (flicker) at various rates can display any photosensitivity. It is regular practice also to compare the EEG with ECG leads for any underlying vascular abnormality and to monitor blood glucose or blood calcium if a metabolic cause for the EEG abnormality is seen.

The value of EEG departments has often been disputed. Small, single-technician departments in which the technician is responsible for the clinical report are generally inadequate. Not every doctor who does reports has the necessary expertise. I feel that every neurologist should be able to report on EEGs but that advance in the subject, if it is to occur, can only come from dedicated neurophysiologists – and these can be a rare breed. We were able, within a few years, to open up a neurophysiology hut with two or more technicians. Our technicians, over the years, proved to be of high calibre and subject to in-house training within the region. The other major criticism levelled at EEG departments is that clinical opinions based on the EEG report often rely on inadequate referral information presented on tiny slips of paper. There are several sources of referral and by speaking to people and interchanging information, we achieved a reasonable standard of referral. 40% were from our own Department, 27% from physicians including geriatricians, 12% from paediatricians, 11% from psychiatrists and 7% from neurosurgeons.

The commonest cause of referral is the possibility of epilepsy. Always the best evidence of epileptic attacks is obtained from a careful history and from eye-witnesses to the attacks. Even so, a high proportion of adults and approximately 3 out of every 10 children are not, in fact, epileptic. The differential diagnosis of epilepsy includes syncopal attacks (faints), psychogenic seizures, cardiac arrhythmias, narcolepsy (falling asleep), vertigo and basilar migraine. I once wrote that

> ... it is both courteous and wise to substantiate an opinion contrary to that of the referring physician by obtaining an EEG; thus, although a non-specific or a normal EEG does not exclude the possibility of epilepsy, it may be the only way to convince a general practitioner than a man of 50, presenting with episodes of confusion, does not have petit mal.

The essential role of the EEG in the study of epilepsy is the detection of sources of seizure discharge. An unstable EEG with a definite pattern seen between attacks (inter-ictal) can suggest a particular type of epilepsy. Evidence of focal abnormalities or instabilities may help also in the prescription of the most specific anticonvulsants for that person's condition. Other evidence may be required as to the cause of the epilepsy, e.g. a tumour or vascular malformation. Even early on in the development of scanning the sensitivity of the EEG in the diagnosis of space-taking lesions compared unfavourably with scanning techniques. Nonetheless, the EEG remains the only major non-invasive physiological technique for the assessment of cerebral function; only recently rivalled in special centres by the use of single photon emission tomography (SPECT) or positron emission tomography (PET), which give information of blood flow or metabolism.

Careful study of discharges picked up by the electro-encephalogram does not facilitate easy interpretation. The propagation of a discharge from one site to another may occur whether or not the fit is overt or subclinical. Many of the discharges represent inhibitory mechanisms; thus mirror foci (found on the contra-lateral – the other – cerebral hemisphere) are predominantly seen in the non-epileptic group. During temporal lobe epilepsy, the EEG may be flattened, slowed or suppressed, with release or spread after the event, possibly coinciding with automatic behaviours (automatisms).

There are many uses of the electro-encephalogram. One patient under a Mental Health order by reason of alcoholism was referred from another hospital and used the occasion, whilst awaiting the EEG, to get on the telephone to plead successfully that, because he was a member of the House of Lords, he could not be declared insane. Was he aware that one member of the British flora, Arum maculatum, known as 'Lords and Ladies', is also called 'cuckoopint'?

Although interpretation may be difficult, the EEG can be highly sensitive to metabolic changes, e.g. a low blood sugar; to encephalitis; to vascular insufficiency, and there are certain conditions for which the EEG may be pathognomonic:- subacute sclerosing panencephalitis (Dawson-van Bogaert disease); Creutzfeld-Jakob disease (excepting those due to pituitary tissue or to the more recent variant likened to BSE); to hepatic (liver) failure and herpes simplex encephalitis. In coma it may distinguish between drug intoxication, post-ictal states (i.e. after convulsions), and metabolic disturbances. It may distinguish between primary pituitary failure and myxoedema from an underactive thyroid. And, lastly, the presence of bifrontal slow activity may serve as a reminder that neurosyphilis has not entirely disappeared and should be excluded. In intensive care units, especially abroad, an EEG is often run routinely with the ECG to alert the therapist to any cerebral events.

The diagnosis of brain death now depends on showing that brain-stem function has been destroyed. This is achieved by repeated testing of brainstem responses, once drug and metabolic stability has been achieved. However, before these criteria were established, evidence of an isoelectric EEG as a result of loss of electrical activity over the cortex was considered to be an essential requirement before brain death could be considered. Thus for several years, like many other neurologists, I was called upon to attend every intensive care unit to monitor the EEGs before death could be declared. Although I reported EEGs for 24 years or more, I was less happy to provide other aspects of a neurophysiology service. When, after five years in Preston, my first colleague was appointed, I was pleased to hand over electro-myography to him, thence to his wife, then to a G.P. who later became a Consultant Neurophysiologist, and eventually to accredited experts in the field.

I will continue with the practice I have adopted hitherto of taking one topic at a time and following it through regardless of chronology. My service commitment on arrival in Preston was heavy and included many patients with epilepsy, parkinsonism once laevodopa became available, migraine, multiple sclerosis, stroke, investigation of tumours, and the unusual second family with neuro-acanthocytosis.

**Epilepsy**
Our ideas of epilepsy are based on an uneasy medley of keenly observed clinical events and ill-understood physiological concepts. As a result, no definition is wholly satisfactory. In practice, even when visiting an Epileptic Centre, it is rare to witness a true fit from beginning to end. Dr Tim Betts, a psychiatrist with a particular interest in epilepsy, begins any talk to sufferers from the disorder by saying that anyone who has a fit during his talk is probably having a pseudo-seizure. It is quite amazing how the number of fits, when talking to a group belonging, say, to the British Epilepsy Association, decreases from 5 or 6 to nil if one begins with Betts' statement.

Most textbook definitions define epilepsy as a paroxysmal and transitory disturbance of the functions of the brain which develop suddenly, cease spontaneously, and exhibit a conspicuous tendency to recur. There are, of course, many other paroxysmal phenomena of cerebral origin. Pathological phenomena include migraine, transient ischaemic attacks, narcolepsy, cataplexy, drop attacks and myoclonus. There are behavioural phenomena – sneezing, grimacing, yawning, startle responses, weeping, coughing, vomiting, hiccough. And lastly we should add urination, defaecation and copulation.

A good, though complex, definition of epilepsy is that of Neil Gordon: 'A disturbance of cerebral function resulting in localized involuntary movements or spontaneous sensations or in loss or alteration of consciousness, with or without generalized convulsions'. Any part of this sequence of events can constitute a fit. There may be a warning, an aura, this may be triggered – 'reflex epilepsy'. The aura can take the form of a sensation arising from the stomach, momentary dizziness, visual, olfactory or auditory hallucinations, or a sensation of fear. Objects may appear different in size or colour. There may be a Jacksonian march from one part of the body to another over a matter of seconds, e.g. from the thumb to the arm to the face and leg, before consciousness is lost; this may be of sensory changes or motor disturbances. And there may be adversive attacks with head turning: quickly turning the person through a circle before falling if the supplementary motor area is the site of irritation; slowly with head turning as if staring if the origin lies in the temporal lobe. An aura is always an indication of the part of the cortex initiating the fit. Unfortunately many patients are amnesic immediately after recovery and cannot recall the initial occurrence.

A minor fit may be associated with staring, day-dreaming, disruption of concentration or flickering of the eyelids. A minor attack may be devastating if, with akinetic or myoclonic epilepsy, the patient falls heavily against an object such as the corner of a table, damaging, for example, an eye. Such patients are advised to wear crash helmets if their fits cannot be completely controlled. Minor fits with an EEG pattern of 3 per second spike and wave activity are due to petit mal and may give rise to major attacks in adult life in approximately half those affected in childhood. Alternatively, minor attacks can be due to partial seizures of temporal lobe origin or even from the mesial frontal cortex. In either case there is usually some partial loss of consciousness. In grand mal epilepsy – I prefer the American term 'major-motor' seizures – there is an early tonic phase with muscle contraction, followed by a clonic phase of contraction and relaxation, during which the patient may yell, bite his tongue, foam at the mouth, roll up his eyes, urinate or defaecate. Afterwards patients commonly go into a state of deep sleep before recovery. The late phase may be associated with automatic behaviour, confusion, amnesia with or without loss of speech or headache – both of which may have a localizing value concerning the major focus of the attack. Patients commonly feel rough for some time (minutes or days) afterwards. Actual paralysis (named after Richard Bentley Todd) may also occur. Todd's paralysis was felt to be an inhibitory phase following the seizure in children and lasting at most some 20 minutes. In adults it is often indicative of underlying pathology such as a tumour, but is being increasingly recognized as an inhibitory phenomenon in the elderly. Continuous epilepsy activity can be confined to one part of the anatomy, e.g. to twitching of the thumb. This is referred to as epilepsia partialis continua and is more commonly seen with localised atrophy of the cortex (i.e. loss of cortical substance) than with a tumour.

The aura and nature of the attack help to define the locus from which it arose. Even petit mal cannot occur without some functioning cortex. Frontal lobe fits may present as a series of fits. Status epilepticus can develop with the risk of brain damage from lack of oxygen (anoxia) when one convulsion follows another within 20 minutes. The usual cause for status epilepticus, giving a dramatic series of frontal lobe fits, is either an open head injury or a 'butterfly' glioblastoma involving both hemispheres. The other setting in which status epilepticus occurs is one of sudden drug withdrawal, as when a teenager gets fed up with taking medication and stops suddenly. Lesser forms of frontal lobe seizure may be very difficult to interpret. There may be sudden vocalisations or speech arrest, forced thinking, amnesia, stereotyped behaviour or laughing epilepsy. Consciousness may be partially lost, the patient may fall without warning, and adversive attacks start with rapid head

turning. Many such attacks are misdiagnosed as pseudo-seizures. Over the motor cortex or sensory cortex, a fit may present with twitching of a thumb or of the flank or numbness at a similar site. The visual cortex will give rise to lights or more formed visions. The auditory cortex to noises or to formed words. In the adjoining association cortex more complex phenomena may arise such as the re-enactment of a battle scene with sounds, smells and visions. Disorders of the temporal lobe may bring together several sensory modalities, for instance sensations of taste, smell or touch, and visual (particularly from the non-dominant hemisphere) and auditory hallucinations in the form of continuous scenes recalling previous experiences. Alternatively, the sensory imagery may show a characteristic distortion, for example dysmegalopsia (alteration in the size of an object) macro-acusis, acoustic quick motion, and alterations in familiarity (déjà vu or jamais vu) or in personalization (autoscopy). Thus a patient of mine with temporal lobe epilepsy complained of:
1. A repetitive sound as of a tap dripping or echoing footsteps which lasted for 40 minutes at a time,
2. Déjà vu phenomena in which she could almost feel that she knew what was coming round the next corner although she had never been there before,
3. A sensation that someone was walking past her window; she would go to the door to meet them,
4. A feeling of re-living situations many times,
5. A robot-like attraction to certain noises,
6. Thought fixation on her grandfather, who had died some years earlier.

This patient's attacks were considerably helped by surgery, but many years later she had problems with memory, particularly involving facial recognition.

Epilepsy should always be thought of as a symptom, not a disease. This requires that we always consider and investigate for a cause – either from the blood supply to the brain with lack of oxygen or a low blood sugar; or from an irritative lesion affecting the brain itself. A small proportion of epilepsy is related to hereditary disease in defined syndromes, but infection, trauma, tumours and disease underlie the development of epilepsy in most cases.

One of my interests is in less usual forms of epilepsy. Kinnear Wilson in 1928 said that a faint, a cry, a laugh can be a fit and no rigid semilogical framework can embrace all its phenomena. I have been interested in the basis of emotional expression, which has been of prime scientific interest since Darwin's 1872 book on *The Expression of the Emotions* in man and animals. He felt that facial expression of emotions had evolved as an adaptive, serviceable habit to communicate information about probable future behaviour. There are in all physiological expressions a higher centre component, the facial expression itself, and a visceral component. Many believe that the facial expression in turn provides an important feedback reinforcing the emotional response. Pathological laughter, often as epilepsy, was the subject of a key-note lecture from one of my chiefs at Maida Vale. Redvers Ironside was a bachelor neurologist of the old school who happened to live in the same mews as Dr Ward of Profumo, Keller, Rice-Davies notoriety. He was one of a number of neurologists — Purdon Martin (1950), Kinnear Wilson (1924) among them — who collected evidence over a number of years that one could die of laughter.

The first description of laughter associated with epilepsy is possibly that of Erastus in 1581, who described a girl, '. . . if left to herself, she laughed, talked to strange things, and after the paroxysm had no memory of it'. Laughter can arise from several levels of the nervous system. Patients with bulbar palsy or pseudo-bulbar palsy affecting the brainstem may be afflicted with bursts of inappropriate laughing or crying. With frontal lobe lesions the word 'witzelsucht' is applied to inappropriate behaviour, laughing or punning. A patient with vascular lesions (infarction) of the temporal lobe may have released involuntary laughter. Above the temporal lobe lies the Sylvian sulcus, passing upwards to the top of the brain and dividing the motor and sensory areas. Here chuckling or glugging seizures accompanied by EEG spiking may occur. But inappropriate laughter is most commonly associated with the hypothalamus. All such attacks of pathological laughter occur without appropriate emotional feeling, as if a spark fired the magazine and the consequences are not commensurate with the cause. The term 'sham mirth' is often used.

The most dramatic examples of laughter epilepsy come from the early days of neurosurgery, when major operations were performed on the brain (which is itself insensitive to handling) under local anaesthesia. In 1933 Foerster and Gagel described several such patients. One patient had been lying quietly until removal of a craniopharyngioma was attempted in the region of the hypothalamus. He than began to talk incessantly, made jokes, witty remarks, gesticulated and laughed. After the operation, he remained confused and died of hyperpyrexia. Another patient started joking and whistling when blood was swabbed from the third ventricle overlying the hypothalamus. This type of response seemed to be obtained by touching the infundibular region. Percival Bailey, in 1948, described attacks of laughing and weeping in a boy during the recovery phase of removal of a third ventricular tumour.

The term 'gelastic epilepsy' (Yelos = mirth) is used in a wider connotation to include both a subjective feeling of merriment or complex co-ordinated movements with grinning, giggling or joyful weeping. Involuntary smiling can occur with petit mal or with partial seizures from the temporal lobe. The most quoted example comes from Dostoyevski's *The Idiot*, almost certainly based on the author's personal experience.

> There are moments, and it is only a matter of five or six seconds, when you feel the presence of the eternal harmony... a terrible thing is the frightful clearness with which it manifests itself and the rapture with which it fills you. If this state were to last more than five seconds, the soul could not endure it and would have to disappear. During these five seconds I live a whole human existence and for that I would give my whole life and not think that I was paying it too dearly... remember Mohammed's water jug: for the space of time it took to empty it, the prophet was rapt into paradise. Your five seconds are the jar... Paradise is your harmony... and Mohammed was epileptic!

Pleasurable sensations accompanying epilepsy can include intermittent sexual activity or sensations. The pleasure can be momentary, the after-feelings catastrophic and embarrassing. Running epilepsy, with an episodic alteration of awareness associated with running, was a form of epilepsy examined along with pseudo-seizures. One of the earliest papers on epilepsia cursiva (the syndrome of running fits) came from Louisville, Kentucky, suggesting that they were surveying a similar population to those whom we had examined but there are reports from elsewhere, and one of our Kentucky patients nearly knocked his head through a wall during a running fit. One paper from Lucknow describes a patient with gelastic, cursive and quiritarian (screaming) epilepsy. As with temporal lobe epilepsy, which can be associated with schizo-affective behaviour, there are always possible psychological factors tied up with epilepsy, not amounting to pseudo-seizures. Thus Frank Elliott in New York has examined dyscontrol seizures in which a person will repeatedly ram a car against a tree.

Another intriguing form of epilepsy is 'reflex epilepsy', in which an external factor brings about a seizure. Seizures can be triggered by emotion – excitement, a quarrel, hyperventilation during a fight, sorrow, etc. They can even be triggered by an unusual emotion – a sense of awe during a church service. The various forms of reflex epilepsy due to an external cause have been dismissed as neurological exotica, yet they can affect 1-6% of people with epilepsy.

The most common modality of sensory precipitation is visual: 20-40% of epileptics show abnormal EEG responses to flickering lights and in 2-4% seizures can be induced by the laboratory stroboscope or – more importantly

– in the course of daily activities. Flicker may be induced by swimming underwater with one's eyes open and the sun shining on the surface, or by driving along an avenue of trees through which the sun's rays shine. Black and white television sets with coarse dots used to induce attacks. They are less frequent with colour television. Those susceptible are advised to sit at least two yards from the set and have another source of lighting in the room. If they have to adjust the set, they should cover or close one eye. Attacks may occur in discotheques. Photochromic glasses are not enough. One eye can be covered or a prism used, but avoidance is the best solution. Some children induce petit mal attacks by quasi-compulsive hand movements, flickering the light shining on their faces. Less commonly there may be reading epilepsy. Reading is accompanied by patterned visual and proprioceptive stimuli which could act as triggers, and some patients with reading epilepsy are photosensitive. Others, however, are affected only by interesting, difficult, or emotionally charged material.

The next most common form of reflex epilepsy is musicogenic. A Russian music critic had to stop work because listening to Beethoven could induce attacks. More commonly it is 'musack' as in supermarkets which is responsible for causing an attack. The first example in Britain occurred at Queen Square. My uncle was giving out anticonvulsants to members of the staff with epilepsy when one cleaner said, 'it's music what sends me, Doctor'. They then set up an experiment with the subject on a couch and a gramophone played behind a curtain. The first record caused no response. 'It has to be classy.' They searched for something more classical and came up with Valse de Fleurs. Sure enough she had an attack.

Other examples of reflex epilepsy have been recorded with mathematical calculation and sequential decision-making under stress. Prolonged hot baths can induce fits, as reported from Newcastle, but hot water epilepsy is more commonly described in India, where people take showers using buckets of hot water. Many intriguing case histories have been published and the precise conditions necessary for seizure induction have been investigated with great ingenuity. The findings suggest that the apparent distinction between external and internal precipitants cannot be maintained. For instance, a simple and highly specific sensory stimulus, such as touching a particular part of the body, may prove ineffective unless combined with an element of surprise. Sometimes the possibility of conditioning arises, e.g. with a safety pin fetishist.

For twelve years, until they ran into financial difficulties and limited their operations, I was on the medical advisory panel of the British Epilepsy Association. I was also part of a team headed by Maurice Parsonage,

Consultant Neurologist in Leeds, who used to lecture to teachers and lay groups about epilepsy. Our main aim was to remove the prejudice against epilepsy, often thought of in Biblical terms, and to obtain its wider recognition and help. The secretary of the British Epilepsy Association at that time, who would talk on the social implications of epilepsy, was George Burden. I had first come across him when, as a medical student, I attended Dr Denis Hill's psychiatric clinics. He was Dr Hill's principal social worker and also ran Camberwell Borough Council. George Burden explained to me that it took him some time to realize that epilepsy presented to other Departments besides psychiatry. There are many psychiatric and psychological overtones to epilepsy. As mentioned, schizo-affective states can occur with temporal lobe epilepsy and the more dramatic automatisms, such as undressing in the street, usually indicate psychiatric problems. These automatisms, which may follow a fit, can take several forms: amnesia, dreamy states, stereotyped sensations of fear, smell, etc., chewing, lip-smacking, drooling, swallowing and choking, apathy, or purposeless behaviour with fighting, running, laughter or incoherent speech. Just occasionally someone may go and do the washing up after a fit without realizing what they are doing.

The tenor of our talks would begin by explaining that epileptics are not a race apart. Anyone can have a fit given the appropriate circumstances. Examples include following spree drinking, blood loss following the trauma of a stillborn child, or, if everyone gave a pint of blood, some might faint and some even twitch. Next we would explain that a fit need not be a recurrent event, lasts for only a few seconds or minutes of one's life, and should not prejudice the rest of one's existence. How is a patient treated during an attack? If possible their head is protected by a cushion. Unless they are fighting when disturbed, they should be turned on to their left side so that if they vomit the vomitus does not enter the lungs. Nothing should be placed in the mouth and no attempt should be made to remove false teeth during an attack. The best way to prevent the tongue falling back in the mouth is to bring the lower jaw forward by placing one's fingers behind the angles of the jaw and drawing them forward. Drugs can help. They must be taken regularly. But in overdosage they can dull the person and lead to more, rather than to fewer, fits. Certain situations such as employment and driving are then discussed, explaining the regulations in force. By and large people with epilepsy make conscientious workers, tend to fall backwards if they were to have a fit, and rarely have fits when actively engaged. Fits mostly occur when relaxing, drifting off to sleep or waking from sleep.

We also stressed that many of the causes of epilepsy were preventable.

Counselling could help with a few with hereditary epileptic tendencies, but the major concern was with improved obstetric care, avoiding toxaemia of pregnancy, bleeding during pregnancy, risks with the first child or multiple births, and small-for-dates children. Infections could also be avoided or treated early. Some of these were intra-uterine, including cytomegalovirus infections, toxoplasmosis and syphilis. Meningitis in the first year of life was a problem. Diseases such as phenylketonuria could be screened for and treated with the appropriate diets and the safety of immunizations improved over the years. Febrile convulsions can be inherited, and if poorly treated, can give rise to temporal lobe epilepsy in later life. Their correct treatment is obviously important. Finally one can add trauma from road accidents, from accidents within the home, from glue sniffing and drug habits.

Apart from hospital work involving epilepsy, I also attended Langho Epileptic Colony, a large institution which in its heyday had over 500 patients. The North West had other sizeable epileptic centres based on similar German institutions, at Maghull north of Liverpool and the David Lewis centre south of Manchester. Langho was unique in that it was run by Manchester Corporation. In the Ribble Valley where Langho was situated were other large institutions – Brockhall and Calderstones, initially for the mentally subnormal; the Whittingham, a psychiatric hospital of 2,000 beds and its own rail link with Preston station; and – added for the sake of completeness – Stonyhurst, the famous Catholic public school.

When I first attended Langho, it was run by Dr George Thompson, the Medical Superintendent. The male and female homes were kept well apart. There was even a dividing line which they were not to cross. When dances were held, no one could have more than two dances with a particular partner. George Thompson soon retired. It was the time of the Reid report on *People with Epilepsy* in 1969, and Harry Hayward, the Chief Nurse, took over. He immediately introduced many reforms. Several evening classes were offered. Patients, now called residents, could mix. The colony became a centre. Those wishing to marry and eventually moving out into the community were provided with a flat where they could learn the rudiments of looking after themselves. With the Reid Report, the policy changed to movement of as many as possible into the community and eventually, after nearly 20 years, the centre closed completely. Many of the original residents had come in for inadequate reasons such as having fits in public places. Most of the later residents had either very poorly controlled fits or additional multiple handicaps.

There is an interesting side light on the fact that unwanted pregnancies did not occur. A pathologist did a survey with us of folic acid levels and trichomonas infection. People on long-term anticonvulsants have low levels of folic acid. In fact we often tried to correct their responsiveness to anticonvulsants by giving a neocytamen injection followed by folic acid. Folic acid is a vitamin and when lacking, trichomonas infections occur more readily. The combination of factors reduces fertility.

Besides giving medical advice on treatment and as necessary on investigation, Langho provided Dr Vakil and myself with a population of severe epileptics who could be studied in depth. We obtained a grant from the DHSS which enabled us to employ a research nurse, Vivian Owen, who had previously been sister on the ward in Liverpool where the early studies of rhesus incompatibility were performed. We were able to document all the patients to examine the aetiological factors responsible for their epilepsy. With the help of an ophthalmologist and examination of the blood sera of all the residents, we were able to examine the possible effect of infection by two dissimilar parasitic organisms, Toxoplasma and Toxocara, both of which have been incriminated as a cause of epilepsy.

Toxoplasma gondii has a wide distribution in the tissues of animals and birds, and infection can follow the ingestion of uncooked meat. However, the cat is the definitive host, and cysts, pseudocysts, and oocysts secreted into the intestine can contaminate soil with subsequent human infection. Congenital transmission following maternal infection in pregnancy may produce a tetrad of hydrocephalus, choroido-retinitis, convulsions and intracranial calcification. Congenital infection can run a protracted clinical course, sometimes followed by sequelae becoming obvious at a later date. Acute illness acquired in childhood or early adult life can be predominantly lymphatic, exanthematous, or cerebro-spinal. All will produce changes in the sera.

Toxocara canis or Toxocara cati, the common roundworms of dogs or cats, may produce a syndrome due to larvae migrating through the body with an immune reaction and eosinophilic changes in the blood. They may also cross the sinusoids of the liver and disperse to the brain and eyes. Involvement of the eye may lead to blindness or granulomatous and tumour-like formations within the eye. Involvement of the brain can cause a severe illness with encephalopathy and convulsions.

With both Toxoplasma and Toxocara, screening tests of the blood were followed by more exact test procedures. Of 204 residents, 60 were positive for Toxoplasma antibody tests, 24 for Toxocara and 10 reacted to both tests; thus leaving 110 people who were negative. Less than 5 residents overall showed eye changes or calcification within the brain, which might suggest clinical infection with one or other of the organisms. There was no difference in the age of each group. We were then able to analyse each group by age and by the extent to which we had an alternative explanation of the cause of their epilepsy.

Looking at those with positive antibodies to Toxoplasma. Their incidence was only slightly more than that found in an adult non-epileptic population. In half the group another clear explanation of their fits was possible; but this 50% were in no other way different from the 50% in which the cause of convulsions remained unclear. Fifty-eight percent of the fits started in childhood, but there was a wide scatter of age of onset. The proportion of focal to non-focal EEG abnormalities was not diagnostically significant, nor could we find physical signs which might suggest a syndromic connection with Toxoplasma antibodies.

By contrast, the incidence of positive Toxocara antibodies was three times greater than that recorded in non-epileptic populations and more than twice that observed elsewhere among epileptic children. In 40% the aetiology was not otherwise explained. Again most fits started in childhood, with a wide scatter of age of onset. The ratio of focal to non-focal EEGs was not significant, but there was a possible association between locomotor defects – hemiplegia, spasticity and ataxia – and Toxocara. What emerged most clearly from the studies of both Toxocara and Toxoplasma was that the incidence of positive antibodies increased with age, from which we concluded uncertainty of the significance of the parasites in causing epilepsy, but among epileptic persons the more they bit the dust, as it were, during attacks, the more liable they were to acquire immune responses to parasitic infections found in the soil.

Prolonged treatment with anticonvulsants can produce a variety of side effects. Liver functions are mildly altered as anticonvulsants induct or slow the action of enzymes produced by the liver with faster or slower turnover of drugs, contraceptive pills, etc. through liver metabolism. Calcium can be lost from bones. The cerebellum can be damaged with some loss of steadiness of gait. And a subclinical peripheral neuropathy – rarely causing noticeable trouble – has been frequently reported using neurophysiological techniques. A side effect which came to the fore as the result of our survey was that of tissue thickening at certain sites, namely Dupuytren's disease or contractures. Bands of thickening of the palms of the hands extending into the fingers are seen far more frequently than in the general population. In fact they were recorded in 56% of our epileptics. In addition to contractions, knuckle pads, palmar and plantar nodules (Lederhose disease), were observed. More rarely other thickenings of subcutaneous fascia have been reported, including for example, under the skin of the penis, but this was not a feature of our sample population. Naturally we tried to find causal factors. Some of the residents had large hands and we checked their growth factors – hormones produced by the pituitary gland which increase height before adult life and can lead to acromegaly later. The growth hormone levels were not raised. Nor was there any difference between the type and cause of the epilepsy. But there was an increase in the duration of epilepsy which led us to examine the relationship to anticonvulsants.

The majority of the residents with epilepsy took several different types of anticonvulsants and had done so for years. Where possible we tried to simplify treatment so that they took a few drugs in adequate doses. Almost invariably we failed to take them off what were euphemistically known as 'working medicines', used to treat constipation. Of the anticonvulsants, 41 took only one drug, 69 two different drugs, 100 three drugs and 76 four or more anticonvulsants. Those most commonly used at the time were phenobarbitone, phenytoin and primidone (which breaks down to phenobarbitone plus another anticonvulsant). Further analysis suggested that phenobarbitone was the drug most directly connected with the raised incidence of Dupuytren's disease. I presented our findings at a joint meeting with the Danish Neurological Association, as they had done much of the early work on the subject. When I returned to my seat, I sat down next to Sir Charles Symonds, a venerated neurologist, who showed me his hand with a Dupuytren's contracture and explained that he had taken barbiturates at night for years.

Our major interest within the centre was to try out new anticonvulsants to see whether they could improve fit control, but it was also necessary to establish what counts as a fit and to obtain an accurate assessment of the number of fits each resident had. Nocturnal fits were most difficult to establish. Several of the residents had persistent bed-wetting at night (average age 51 years) and a few actually defaecated in their sleep (encopresis). Were these fits? This sub-group had sustained epilepsy following head injury, invariably with complications such as alcoholism, blood clots (extradural haematomata), raised blood pressure, uraemia or diabetes, or were progressing into dementia. Unfortunately attention to their anticonvulsant medication rarely influenced the frequency of enuresis or encopresis.

Over the years we examined the effects of giving all the anticonvulsants as a single daily dose, e.g. at night, and seeing whether sodium valproate (Epilim), Clonazepam, and later Clobazam, could improve epileptic control. My colleague, Dr Vakil, had had experience of high-powered drug trials, mainly for Parkinson's disease, whilst working at the Hammersmith Hospital. We had a biochemist, Seymour Cocks, who was very bright but congenitally deaf, doing the blood level studies. In every case, even though research ethical committees had not been established, we explained to each resident what we would like to do and obtained their permission (which could be withheld) to participate. We simplified the anticonvulsant regime for each one to two standard drugs and waited till we had established a stable baseline incidence of fits on the two-drug regimen before introducing the new drug on a double-blind cross-over procedure with a wash-out period separating drug and placebo. Our concerns were with the consequent reduction in fits, any rebound in the number of fits after reducing and stopping the new drug, the effect of adding the new drug to the blood levels of other anticonvulsants, and any biochemical or other side effects.

Clobazam (Frisium) may not be a particularly well-known drug. It was introduced as an anxietolytic drug, but Professor Gastaut in Marseilles found that it was helpful in epileptic children. Archie Martin, a psychiatrist in Lancaster, who was a friend of Gastaut's, learnt of this fact and tried it on children attending Sedgwick House School for Epilepsy. Around that time I took over from Manchester neuro-paediatricians in visiting that school twice a term to advise on treatment. Children in that school, which has since closed, not only had epilepsy but other multiple handicaps. However they were encouraged to lead an active life, even doing rock climbing under careful supervision. Undoubtedly in the short run clobazam reduced the number of fits they had, but after a while many lost tolerance to the drug and were no better off. It did, nonetheless, provide an interval in which their potential could be assessed and enabled an alternative anticonvulsant regimen to be established. We established its worth by a double blind cross-over trial at Langho and it is still used where people are subject to fits only in relation to period times or in children where a temporary improvement in control has to be established rapidly, so that other assessment can be made and if necessary a later switch to clonazepam is made to maintain control.

One of the old school of neurologists from Glasgow used to have a standard letter on all people with epilepsy, pointing out that reduction of fits may not mean improvement; it can occur with progression of an underlying tumour hitherto responsible for the fits. Much of our time in treating people with epilepsy is understanding why their fit frequency has varied. Has some psychological trauma overwhelmed any damping down of the fits by drugs? Is there an underlying tumour or other cause? Is someone safe to drive? Can he/she come off drugs having been fit-free for a period? And there are yet newer drugs which need assessment. With the closure of large institutions and more neurologists to deal with epilepsy, progress nowadays depends especially on multi-centre trials, which require considerable pre-arrangement and cooperation. Modern drugs are, by and large, kinder. They may have different side effects and require initiation in different ways. Even so, relatively smaller fixed doses of some of the older drugs are more effective, and should not be disregarded. The subject continues to hold our interest.

## Pain

I cannot recall how I first came into contact with Dr Robert Maher, general physician in Rochdale. Most probably I had one or two patients with multiple sclerosis and marked spasticity so that they were unable to straighten their legs, and I wished to learn his methods for their treatment. Dr Maher was one of the characters of medicine, grizzly, potentially difficult and argumentative, awkward, even cantankerous and idiosyncratic in his opinions. He was also one of the few people who had had not just one, but two, original ideas in his life-time. He had pioneered the use of intra-thecal phenol for pain and intra-thecal chlorocresol for spasticity. He had started the development of pain clinics (and stood with Mr Steptoe of Oldham, who developed in-vitro fertilization and John Charnley of Wrightington who started hip-replacement) as one of those in the North West outside the teaching hospital ambit who had altered the practice of medicine in this century. He was often in demand to lecture abroad; but unlike the goolis from the establishment, with their fellowships, his degrees read M.D., M.R.C.P. and he was constantly asked why that was so. He therefore wrote to the Registrar of the College of Physicians to ask what he had to do to become a fellow. The answer he received was brief: 'You are canvassing'. He replied, 'If I cannot ask you, who can I ask?' He received the same reply 'You are canvassing'. His Irish background and Jesuit education took command and he duly returned his membership to the college.

Dupuytren, whose name has been attached to contractures, wrote in 1840 that 'pain kills like haemorrhage', and others have stated that of all the ills man is subject to, pain seems the most urgently requiring treatment. Dr Maher addressed the issue of cancer pain, dividing the pains into continuous – the remorseless fixed pain which continues day and night till death occurs, mediated by the small 'c' pain fibres – and incident pain caused by events such as a fracture, activated by the larger 'a' fibres. Incident pain can be treated by immobilization. Continuous pain requires analgesics, thymoleptics and specific measures of relief. He took over a small hospital at Ramsbottom in order to treat patients who continued to complain of pain whatever the nature of the underlying lesion. It was later to be a Sikh temple.

Pain hurts. It is an unpleasant experience which we primarily associate with tissue damage. We presume it to be a defence of the body against harm or potential danger, and indeed, those without pain sensation, with congenital analgesia, asymbolia or universal indifference to pain, invariably show evidence of damage which they cannot prevent. Aristotle called pain 'a passion of the soul', and Leriche described it 'as a sinister gift which diminishes man, which makes him sicker than he would be without it'. It is an imprecise symptom that achieves recognition as a percept within the mind. The central appreciation of pain involves the cerebral cortex, and probably also the lower end of the thalamus and upper end of the midbrain. There is both an organic component – often described in terms relating to injury – and a psychological component, as interpretation takes place only in the mind. So that the information recorded there is entirely personal, a private matter that cannot be shared by anyone else or described in terms that mean the same thing to another person.

However, we can accurately describe the provoking stimuli as NOXAE and use the word 'pain' to apply to the whole complex of events forming the subjective experience. Thus the appreciation of pain is dependent upon the integrity of the nervous system, previous experience, the state of consciousness, fatigue, fear, anxiety, tension, knowledge and understanding, attention and distraction, and whether associated with pleasurable emotion, suggestion, religious or hysterical overtones. Many talk of the modulation of pain or modulation of the nociceptive response. The skin and membranes of the body, like any other sense organ (hearing, sight, smell), only react to certain predetermined stimuli. The skin cannot appreciate magnetism or ultraviolet light until a burn actually occurs. Acupuncture and Tiger Balm act by counter-irritation to dampen the pain. There are many instances when pain passes unrecognized because vigilance is directed elsewhere. A rugby player may not realize his injury until after the match The person hit by a stray bullet may be aware of blood on his clothes before complaining of pain. The Marquis of Anglesea, Henry William Paget, had his horse shot from under him at Waterloo and afterwards realized that he had also lost a leg. Pain signals reaching the spinal cord are 'gated', some passing through, some building up before recognition. The gate control theory of Melzack and Wall is accepted as a working hypothesis of the modulation of pain, though other experts, such as Peter Nathan and P.K. Thomas, have questioned certain aspects of the 'gate'. I have spoken of P.K. Thomas. Peter Nathan, a millionaire when such matters counted, who preferred to work at Queen Square, did research into pain mechanisms over many years. He wisely concluded his critique of the gate control theory with the statement, 'ideas need to be fruitful; they do not have to be right'. Melzack and Wall's theory has enshrined a major concept and it has had a powerful impact on research, theory and treatment. Yet we still have to label the precise mechanisms, and the duality of function necessary for triggering the hypothetical gate remains far from proven. Within the spinal cord other influences combine:- chemical, hormonal, electrical, inputs from elsewhere, and descending impulses from higher up the nervous system. Eventually modulated signals ascend to the brain and mind participating in a 'central matrix'. There may be an immediate reflex reaction such as avoidance or kicking out; but the conscious, and indeed subconscious, response is centrally determined.

I return to the work of Robert Maher. The main innovation was the use of spinal injections. Pain at a limited site such as a leg can be treated by cordotomy — cutting fibre tracts as they ascend the spinal cord. The operation can be done as an open procedure with the insertion of a knife to cut an arc of fibres within the cord, or even, though with less certainty, by using a needle penetrating the tissues under x-ray control, then moved through a similar arc. Such operations cannot safely be done to both sides of the body without risk of affecting respiration, and they cannot prevent the spread of disease which might cause a return of similar symptoms from another site. Thus cordotomy is not a suitable treatment with the spread of cancer. By contrast, spinal injections can be repeated with ease. They can also be performed at home without moving the patient or having the necessity to admit to hospital. Five percent phenol in glycerin is injected around the nerve roots below the termination of the spinal cord and followed immediately by positioning the patient on one side so that particular nerve roots can be destroyed. The procedure is limited in that neighbouring nerve roots may not entirely escape destruction. Thus, if the patient is not already incontinent, some impairment of bladder and bowel control may occur. This treatment has largely been superseded in recent years by the use of TENS machines, giving electrical stimulation to the spinal cord, or by intra-thecal baclophen.

Dr Maher would also use nerve blocks. Blockade of nerves using local anaesthetic agents had been available for some time but his use of phenol could provide a more permanent amelioration. Phenol was injected by a needle below the zygoma, missing the temporo-mandibular joint and passing into the trigeminal ganglion in order to alleviate the pain of trigeminal neuralgia (tic douloureux); or around the sacrum to treat coxalgia; or extra-durally, spreading in a honey-comb fashion, to relieve pain at the back of the neck. If the pain was not helped by the use of phenol, chlorocresol often provided a useful alternative.

Painful spasticity can be a feature of multiple sclerosis. The legs may be drawn up in spasm, causing contractures, so that they cannot be straightened, thereby making nursing difficult and ambulation impossible. Tenotomies can relieve spasm in a limited number of muscles, but for more general relief intrathecal treatment is required. I never understood why multiple sclerosis, which causes demyelination of nerves within the spinal cord and brain, should be associated with more resistant than usual peripheral nerves as they emerge from the spinal cord. Why they require stronger injections than are needed to lighten spasticity in other disease states. Chlorocresol is effective in the relief of spasticity associated with multiple sclerosis but carries a comparable risk of further impairment of bowel and bladder control as does intra-thecal phenol. Most of Dr Maher's procedures have now been supplanted and constitute the industrial archaeology of pain relief, but their originality cannot be denied and Robert Maher can justly claim to have been the father of pain clinics world-wide.

I moved away from pain relief work for two main reasons. Anaesthetists had taken up the challenge and started pain clinics and I felt that unless I was performing these potentially dangerous procedures on a regular basis, accidents could happen. However, I was grateful to Robert Maher and the experience I gained, and there are many aspects of pain which abut on the practice of neurology.

Pains, particularly those arising within the body, may be bizarrely localized. Their area of referral more closely depends on the embryonic site of the organ or viscus involved than on its present situation. Cardiac pain gives rise to angina — from the word for strangling or choking — as it is transmitted up the neck to the jaw; and it may also pass down the left arm as far as the wrist. Pain from the spleen may be felt at the shoulder tip. These pains enter and mingle in the same sensory pools as do nociceptive stimuli from the muscles and skin. These sensory pools (and I am purposely using an imprecise term) at various levels of the nervous system from the thalamus to parts of the spinal cord can give rise, if damaged, to persistent or spontaneous pains. Many theories explain their occurrence: reverberating cycles undampened by inhibitory impulses; rogue firing by isolated nerve fibres; nerve damage disrupting the normal firing sequences; accumulation of pain-sensitive chemicals. Melzack suggests that excessive or otherwise abnormal stimulation may bring about a prolonged bias of the 'gate' mechanism.

A demoralizing pain, usually felt at the end of a limb and accompanied by vascular changes and atrophy of the surrounding tissues, was first described by Weir Mitchell during the American Civil War. Causalgia often has a burning quality notoriously resistant to treatment and can arise after seemingly minor trauma such as a crush injury, fracture or even sprain. Blockade of the sympathetic nerves has been tried time and time again but Schott has demonstrated that it is not the sympathetic nerves which are responsible for the release of harmful neuropeptides but visceral afferents related to the blood vessels which travel with the autonomic nerves. Incomplete injury to larger nerves with spontaneous firing gives rise to neuralgic pains, usually unresponsive to analgesia. Cutting the nerve or other forms of direct treatment may leave an unacceptable numbness. Relief of the anxiety occasioned by the pain may prove more successful than dampening the pain by soporific analgesics.

Phantom limbs was yet another term coined by Weir Mitchell in order to describe the persistent sensation of the missing limb as an almost invariable consequence of amputation. Further experience over the years has confirmed his original observations that phantoms are almost invariable in adults following trauma. They are rare in mutilating diseases such as leprosy or gangrene, or in children before reaching four years of age. Thus children borne with phocomelia (absent limbs) do not get phantom sensations. A phantom may last for years, and even when lost may return under stress. A phantom is an illusory awareness of the missing part. With time the phantom tends to weaken in intensity and the limb appears to telescope in towards the stump until the fingers or toes of the phantom merge into its substance. A painful phantom is less likely to shrink in size with the passage of time and may remain, continuing to cripple and oppress. Thus 5-10% of patients continue to describe disagreeable sensations, variously described as cramp, shooting, burning and crushing. The pain following amputation may closely resemble the quality and localization of pain prior to amputation, and if the limb had been stressed in an awkward posture, that sensation may also be preserved. Pain emanates from pressure on specially sensitive areas such as the stump. Trigger zones, initially confined to the injured part, can gradually spread to other areas of the body which are healthy and unrelated to the injury; so much so that urination, defaecation and ejaculation may be accompanied by a burning sensation in both the phantom and the stump end.

In normal subjects, phantom-limb-like sensations can be generated by local anaesthesia of peripheral nerves, loss of sensation in a limb numbed by post-infective neuritis (e.g. the Guillain-Barre syndrome), or by avulsion of the brachial plexus as in a road traffic accident. This fact would appear to indicate that the phantom can be generated centrally within the nervous system in the absence of neural impulses from affected dermatomes (parts of the body).

Phantom phenomena affecting other organs have been described – after castration, enucleation of an eye, tooth extraction, facial mutilation and mastectomy – but such phantom pains and non-painful phantom sensations rarely affect more than 20-30% at other sites. However the incidence of phantoms varies. Such feelings are rare after removal of a breast or an ear, but common after enucleation of an eye, excision of the rectum, or removal of the larynx. Most curious is the fact that phantom phenomena of paraplegics differ from those of amputees. Whereas the vividness of the phantoms are obvious from discussion with any amputee, a similar complaint may be hard to elicit from a paraplegic. Telescoping does not occur and painful phenomena are absent. Patients with paraplegia and an amputated arm will complain of phantom pains in their arm but not elsewhere.

The term 'synaesthesia', a phenomenon whereby a stimulus presented in one mode seems to call up a sensation of a different type, has a special and distinctive application with respect to spinal injury or amputation of limbs. Abnormal spread of sensation can occur and the term synchiria, is applied when a stimulus such as a pin-prick applied to the unaffected side produces an unpleasant sensation bilaterally. When this occurs unilaterally – affecting the mirror point on the opposite side of the body – it is known as allochiria. Stimulation of an anaesthetic zone of a successful cordotomy may produce a sensation of pain either on the same side just above the level of the cordotomy or else on the opposite side. Other terms used include allaesthesia and synaesthesialgia.

Each sense organ produces its own specific sensations but occasionally a splashing over of sensations from one sensory modality to another can occur. Artists, composers, and writers have sought to evoke additional imagery – usually between sound and colour – in the course of their works, harmonizing the senses. Psychedelic drugs may have a similar effect. Certain groups of people, defined by Cytowic as 'synesthetes' are particularly sensitive to such phenomena. The level of the nervous system at which such a mingling of the senses can occur is subject to much dispute. I have explored three possibilities:-

a cross-talk or interaction between nerve fibres as they ascend together and possibly anastomose in the course of stimulus modulation from sense organ to central transmission, recognition and perception;

as release phenomena akin to hallucinations, illusions, central pain syndromes and even delusions;

and as an interplay between higher cerebral functions combining emotion, perception, memory and language.

All three mechanisms are recognized anatomical and physiological occurrences and, at a subconscious level, it is not yet possible to declare dogmatically that one mechanism predominates or that other mechanisms do not interact.

## Speech
What is the origin of speech: the second divine creation?

> ...Philosophers who chase
> A panting syllable through time and space,
> Start it at home, and hunt it in the dark
> To Gaul, to Greece and into Noah's Ark.

There is a power in language, a mystical property, which has perplexed man throughout the ages. He remains in awe of his own ability to speak and use language. Wise words have averted mortal conflict, injudicious words have produced disaster.

Words have never seemed to be earthly. They belong to the spirit or soul, and rest uneasily on the body. They depart with the breath of life. They are man's link with the supernatural. In more regions than not, it has been supposed that language is the direct gift of the immortals to their chosen creation – to mankind at large.

The early gods were gruesome. The words they spake were terrifying and mighty. Man was subjugated by language. He faltered when he came to reply. He strove for a greater share of the secret of language, and even today the mystique remains; for ability to harness the full power of language for the benefit of man eludes us still.

The Greek gods were kinder. They were almost human and shared the gossip, the depravity and the tittle-tattle of humans. But the tradition that language came from the gods continued. In Christendom a similar assumption was held. God made Adam to speak. The first language may therefore be termed the lingua adamaica. In the beginning was the word, and the word was with God, and the word was God. The original language was supposed to be perfect: its successors degenerate. Would Adam have further opportunity to be entrusted with the naming of the animals? There is no more enthralling scene in the Old Testament than that in the Garden of Eden when God brought every beast of the field and every fowl of the air before Adam to see what he would call them. With his invisible breath he devised unheard-of names, substantial enough to be freighted with deep thoughts and mobile enough to waft their precious cargo down the ages. God had created the earth, and Adam had festooned it with a web of words.

The theories of the Darwinian evolutionists led naturally to a consideration of man's position in relation to the animals. It was reasonable for them to conclude that man is not the only animal that can express what is passing in his mind and can understand, more or less, what is so expressed by another. For them human communication had its origins in animal communication. Wallace's theories in particular anticipated the recognition of prolonged foetalisation, enabling a development of the brain permitting speech as an instrument developed in advance of the needs of its possessor. A science of language, a *Sprachwissenschaft*, was developed. The showman, philologist and lecturer, Max Muller, took the theories of the day; damned each and threw them together. The onomatopoeic theory that language is made up through imitation of natural sounds, he dubbed the 'bow-wow' hypothesis. He supposed a mysterious or psychological harmony between sound and sense in language, which in turn was dubbed the 'ding-dong' hypothesis. Interjections of pain or delight became the 'pooh-pooh' hypothesis, of automatic activity of the laryngeal sphincter the 'colly-wobble' theory, involuntary sounds accompanying bodily effort the 'yo-heave-ho' theory, gesture with speech the 'ta-ta' theory, and that accompanying eating the 'yum-yum' hypothesis. Gesture, bodily movement and involuntary noises were harnessed together by Donovan into the festal origin of speech – the 'tarara-boom-de-ay' hypothesis. A more serious philologist, Jespersen, noted how early literature was structurally more rigid, relying on prosody and alliteration, closely allied to, and often enhanced by, music. Primitive language, he declared, was musical and passionate.

Wallace himself felt that language evolved from gesture, mouth and lip pointing. These gestures would be used for hunting, to elaborate the action of the group. The use of mimicry of animal sounds to lure their prey into the trap, gesture as the trap closes, but hunting would most probably take place at twilight and the arms engaged in throwing and hurling stones and weapons, so that as the battle proceeds, sounds would be increasingly required to direct the efforts of the tribe and to frighten the animal, rendering it more defenceless.

At what stage primitive man developed speech is unclear. Very little of what we say is replete with conceptual thought. Much conversation aims to establish an empathic relationship and is full of intimacy clauses. As the hostage John McCarthy describes: 'I desperately missed conversation. In the past I'd talked a lot of nonsense, playing with words, using humour to get to know people. It may have been frivolous, but it was contact, an intimate bond with others.' Primitive man may not have used much propositional speech but shouted and sang along with others as part of the bonding of the tribe. How large a brain was needed is unclear. Whether the larynx was situated high in the neck, permitting only grunts or in a lower position, allowing distinct speech sounds, may not have been important in the initiation of the evolution of speech. Excitement exists in the way language has evolved. As Polanyi describes:-

> The natural laws governing the formation of guttural laryngeal sounds and mouth clicks do not account for the combination of sounds into words

controlled by a vocabulary. Similarly the rules regulating the development of vocabulary do not presuppose the formation of sentences controlled by syntax and grammar. At each stage the principles governing the isolated particulars of a lower level leave indeterminate conditions to be controlled by a higher principle. Consequently, the operation of a higher level cannot be accounted for by the laws governing its particulars on the next lower level.

Vocabulary is not derived automatically from phonetics, nor grammar from vocabulary; a correct use of grammar does not anticipate style or content as in the prose and poetry of Shakespeare or Milton. Speech did not inevitably lead to writing or the written word to the advanced audio-visual devices of today.

My justification for starting with the origin of speech is to allow me to discuss an aspect of speech which has received scant attention elsewhere, namely the humoral influences on human speech. I searched for a quotation contrasting the monosyllabic noises of the average teenage male with the chatty loquaciousness of his female counterpart, and was forced through want of a suitable quote to devise my own doggerel:-

> Hamstrung – He,
> Incessant – She
> Swift, high and flowing.
> He, with a groan, replies.

Humoral secretions from the neuroendocrine system are believed to provide a chemical trigger for animal vocalization. Birds and some mammals, such as deer, produce distinctive calls during the reproductive season but at no other time. That courtship song is dependent upon endocrine change has been shown by its artificial production in zebra finches treated after hatching with oestradiol, then testosterone. In animals, with the exception of homo sapiens and the great apes, stimulation of the neocortex does not result in vocalization; but electrically evoked vocalizations can be obtained by implanted depth electrodes in cats, sea-gulls, pigeons, squirrel monkeys and rhesus monkeys.

The corollary is that animal vocalization utilizes mechanisms separate from the neocortical control needed for human speech. There could be a segregation of speech mechanisms into a phylogenetically older starting mechanism involving the cingulate gyrus and central grey matter, and a newer laryngeal system which includes pulvinar and posterior cerebral cortex; and in humans these two mechanisms could possibly function in parallel, producing a dual control of social communication. In fact there is considerable evidence that this is so. Patients with non-fluent aphasia may display selective preservation of vulgar or profane speech under emotional stress, reflexly releasing a stereotyped utterance under threat. Also, during states of hallucinatory excitement, previously aphasic, schizophrenic patients may exhibit considerable verbal fluency. States of mutism localized to the frontal lobes and deeper structures of the brain away from the normal speech areas can occur in otherwise alert patients.

Stuttering provides further evidence of the influence of the vegetative nervous system. A patient may stutter at length without getting out a single statement until he becomes impatient and rattles forth with perfect fluency the exclamation, 'Blast it, today is worse than ever'. A peculiar meterotropism is also noticeable in many stutterers. They are said to be aware of approaching weather changes through increased verbal and general insecurity, displaying on these occasions a deterioration in speaking ability. The possibility that stuttering may be influenced biochemically is suggested by reported observations that diabetics almost never stutter. Stimulation by laevodopa of the dopamine system can influence the speech of parkinsonian patients; and articulation worsened if anticholinergic drugs are stopped suddenly. The Gilles de la Tourette syndrome could presumably arise from hormonal dysregulation. Speech becomes slow and hoarse in hypothyroidism. In thyrotoxicosis the singing voice is often tremulous, with a tendency to fatigue and a broken pot timbre.

Changes occur in the voice as a result of the secondary action of sex hormones. At puberty the voice 'breaks' in males to a deeper adult tone. During menstruation females may experience a slight decrease in the quality of their singing voice, affecting particularly the notes in the highest register. With menopause the entire vocal range for speaking and singing may be lowered; and, with senescence, increasing virilism of voice may occur. At all ages and in both sexes, the rate, clarity and fluency of speech appear to be under endocrine control.

My other major concern is that most textbooks of neurology refer to the aphasic syndromes as sharply localized and immutable; and most of my colleagues have permitted such inaccuracy to be carried from one textbook to the next. Hughlings Jackson wrote that to locate the damage which destroys speech and to locate speech are two different things. We can equate an holistic view of speech with acknowledgement that conduction disorders can disrupt the pathways for speech to produce distinctive syndromes. However even with such localization, backed up by modern scanning, few aphasic disorders remain static when viewed longitudinally. It is possible for a lesion in the same part of the brain to cause a different type of aphasia, each related to the age of onset of the aphasia. Plasticity of the central nervous system is well-recognised in childhood and does not entirely disappear with ageing. I would separate from the other aphasic syndromes Wernicke's aphasia with its circumlocutions, disinhibition of verbal output, and a tendency to ramble. Wernicke's aphasia occurs, on average, 10 years later than other aphasic syndromes, and could be linked to vascular changes, dementia and even to the hormonal changes of senescence.

There have been several generations of neurologists, very few of whom have had any interest in speech or, indeed, in the higher functions of the nervous system. They have been happy to hand over aphasia to psychologists without so much as a backward glance. And psychologists in their turn have sought to devise pathways through the brain connecting the presumed sites of differing functions without recourse to any anatomical linkages. I am therefore unashamedly going to trumpet an holistic view of language and speech to blast them out of their stupor.

Memory, the initiation of propositional thought, mental feelings, and much else besides are psychically amalgamated in preparation for speech. They collate as inner language, groomed as recognizable concepts and clothed in syntax grammar, to be launched with prosody and emphasis. Several writers have tried to describe the intermediate stage between thought and speech: with such terms as 'Vorgestalt', 'schema' or 'preverbitum'. Impairment may have a tangible effect on personality but more directly leave that person lame in thought and void of ideas. Any organic process which gravely impairs speech also disturbs other functions not usually classed with the use of language. Changes in intelligence must be anticipated. Nor can aphasia be divided sharply into motor and sensory components, for the more carefully the patient with aphasia is examined, the certainty with which his disorder corresponds with any preconceived category diminishes expedientially.

Everyone acknowledges the pre-eminence of the peri-Sylvian language zone, which may vary in its unilateral or bilateral representation according to handedness or the presence of early brain damage. The majority of polyglots recovering from aphasia do not show any differences in the rate of recovery for different languages, and when a second language is acquired at an early age, the normal rules of cerebral dominance tend to be followed. But the study of the minority with a differential recovery has led to the supposition that there may be anatomically different centres for certain languages, depending upon such acquisition parameters as handedness, age, gender, and the manner and modality of second language acquisition:- in effect that the language organization of the average bilingual may be more ambilateral than that for the monolingual.

One of my patients sustained a subarachnoid haemorrhage when aged 57, with a left thalamic haematoma, right hemiplegia and aphasia. She later became dysphasic with an extreme degree of jargon speech, but over the next five years her aphasia improved with only occasional word-finding difficulties. However, six years after the initial event, she complained of repeated episodes of numbness of the left arm and leg, a persisting feeling of unsteadiness, and the onset of uncontrollable inner speech vocalizations that she described as a 'nattering inside her'. These internal vocalizations would commence at a particular time of day – the timing varying from week to week, but often beginning mid-morning – and would then persist throughout the day. They would only stop when she was talking, listening to others or reading. There was no suggestion of any psychiatric disorder, dementia, epilepsy or incipient deafness. She explained that the 'natterings' had always been her own voice talking. The content was often a mixture of prayers, hymns, and fragments of the Latin Mass, which she had learnt by heart as a girl when she sang in the school choir. The natterings were not coherent nor did they 'speak to her'. Their only quasi-compulsive aspect was that she sometimes felt the urge to change words in phrases or sentences that were making up the content of the natterings at the time. Unfortunately she was unable to supply anything like a transcript of the natterings. She complained that they were too fast and too fragmentary to be externalized There may also have been an element of reluctance relating to the embarrassment she felt at experiencing these vocalizations.

If we examine the right non-dominant hemisphere further, we can identify the fact that reading and writing are less unilaterally displayed than normal speech. Prosody of speech most certainly involves the right hemisphere, gesture is bilateral, and certain higher-level linguistic functions show a right-hemisphere emphasis. These include verbal humour, metaphor interpretation, spatial reasoning, abstract concepts, word-finding, problem-solving, creative literature, punch-line selection, and story recall. Mann (1898) showed that there can be a centre for music – a mirror focus of Broca's area – on the non-dominant half of the brain. Blood flow studies, even with propositional speech, show very little asymmetry. According to Ross (1981) this finding can be totally explained in terms of the prosody of speech; a supposition which has to be approached with caution.

There are three types of prosody: the intrinsic standard prosodic patterns inherent in language; stress used to express various subtle shades of meaning; and the added changes in tone and rhythm conveying emotion. All these are used by the native speaker, whose alterations in volume, pitch and tempo reflect his mood. But the violent, often loud, diction of the unsure foreigner may be wildly misinterpreted. With ageing, dialects, presumed lost, may return and deepen. Patients with cerebral lesions may occasionally appear to assume a foreign accent. An echo or delayed feedback may impede the self-monitoring and flow of speech. A similar distortion of feedback mechanisms may account for loss of prosody with right-hemisphere damage. Even so, it is not possible to claim that prosody is an entirely right hemisphere function. We must remain cautious of such interpretations. A conundrum has been asked of the extreme localizers: 'If we talk with our major hemisphere and sing with our minor, by what cerebral legerdemain do we continue to cope with those intermediate vocalizations such as chanting and recitative?'

Psychiatrists have entered the speech domain left by neurologists, analysing the speech deficiencies of patients with schizophrenia, mania, depression and dementia, and exploring the role of the frontal lobe in the regulation, intentionality, programming and execution of sequential actions such as speech. These are the growth points of medical linguistics. Some localization of frontal lobe functions has been suggested. Impairment of the left dorsolateral region may show as difficulty in processing verbal messages, facilitating verbal instructions and behavioural tasks. Sentences may be shortened with a tendency to perseveration. A similar lesion in the left orbito-frontal region will affect ongoing activity, with failure to monitor interference and consequent digression or confabulation. Right frontal lesions may influence the final implementation of verbal tasks with dyspraxia, misarticulation, displacement or misinterpretation.

In learning how to perform complex tasks, speech is used to reinforce the sequence of actions. A normal or bright child performing the task gives himself/herself the commands aloud and later plans actions through inner speech. This ability to use the regulatory role of verbal instruction is effected in most children between the ages of 5 or 6, when the frontal lobes attain the first stage of their myelination.

Another approach used by psychiatrists and paediatricians has been essentially theoretical, analysing speech development or disintegration, in terms of linguistics as developed by Noam Chomsky. In order to try to understand Chomsky's transformational grammar, I attended courses at Lancaster University Department of English for a number of years and took advantage of their library. Linguistics can be mocked:-

> How frightful is the self-inflicted fate
> Of learned men who cleverly create
> Strange forks that, prongless, fail to bifurcate.
> (Botha, 1989)

For linguistics to be meaningful in a psychiatric context, it is not enough to analyse the grammatical or propositional context. It is also necessary to establish the act accomplished by an utterance, the relevance of the discourse, and the resulting social interaction between speaker and listener. We should not enter too hastily upon an analysis of schizophrenic speech without taking note of the culture of the patients and the languages they use: isolating languages which depend on word order; inflecting languages where suffixes alter the meaning of words; or polysyllabic and agglutinating languages with words built from long sequences of units (e.g. anti-dis-establish-ment-arian-ism). The same applies to aphasia, which can depend on the underlying syntactic structure. Thus so-called agrammatic speech disorders feature more prominently in German papers on aphasia than in English.

There is much evidence, which at first sight is surprising, that the structure of a language is of greater help to those who are least bright. The language of primitive communities has to be grammatically correct. Foreigners are liable to be misunderstood if their pronunciation is inexact or they fail to use the proper portmanteau phrase. Italian is a more structured and inflected language than English. Yet Italian children with developmental language impairment made fewer morphological errors during the learning process than did their English counterparts.

Psycholinguistics, in particular cohesion analysis – 'mapping grammar on to the mind' – and discourse analysis – examining the socio-cultural context of communication – have provided major advances in understanding the accessory requirements of speech. Conversation requires the integration of communicative, social and emotional skills, the use of social signals and interactive strategies, for example encouragement and partial withdrawal, as in bargaining. Speech strategies include an appreciation of the listener's needs in following speech, a flexible plan of action sequences, and ability to inhibit or defer a response to a more appropriate time. The flexibility of normal conversation among reasonably bright people, often at the expense of syntax, reaches its apotheosis in the mutual repair of speech errors during rapid, abbreviated exchanges. Using similar principles, the disorganized speech of schizophrenics can be seen as a multi-level disturbance involving a true thought disorder, a pragmatic language disturbance, and faulty social cognition. And it may be that these disturbances – including perseveration and the abnormal behaviours associated with them – arise from dysfunctions, as yet unanalysed, within the frontal lobes.

## Hallucinations

I challenge any clinician to deny that they derive pleasure from taking a history of hallucinations. To all not prone to hallucinations themselves, hallucinations appear fascinating, their unexpected arrival is tantalising, their nature extraordinary. There are caveats galore. The patient may be worried and embarrassed by the thought that the hallucination could be a sign of insanity. Localization of the site of hallucinations, though sometimes possible, may be fraught with danger. Furthermore, the degree of insight by the patient as to the nature of the hallucination may be difficult to determine.

The Latin hallucinatio or alucinatio means to dream, to talk idly, or to wander mentally. Imagery forms part of everyone's mental processes, providing thought-vehicles for reasoning, for memory, and for taking in sensory data, as in rapid reading. The quality of visual imagery varies from person to person, with every inflexion from achromatic silhouettes to the vivid recollection of colours and hues. Graham Reed, in the *Psychology of Anomalous Experience*, believes that 'imagery' can be construed as an experience which revives or copies a previous perceptual experience in the absence of the original sensory stimulation – in other words that it is quasi-perceptual. Knowing is a pre-requisite to seeing and strongly determines what we see. In effect, we perceive only what we can conceive and any rigid distinction between imagery and perception becomes artificial.

Let us put to one side a quite different visual impression which has nothing to do with hallucinations. Galton coined the term 'eidetic imagery' to describe visile thoughts but the term is nowadays specifically applied to exteriorized imagery seen in great detail. Every now and again the media turn up a child, not necessarily intelligent, sometimes far from intelligent, with the ability to repeat, draw or paint a complex scene from memory. A strong visualizer with eidetic or crystal imagery may see the image in front of his eyes, as might an artist painting a portrait from memory. With true eidetism, the thought-object is seen in actuality and cannot be processed from visual to auditory memory. So-called photographic memories are different in that they can be reinforced by additional associations such as sounds, the emotional content, or the descriptions of others. Eidetic images are most often seen in childhood. They have features in common with after-images but are usually richer in detail, evoked more readily and persist for longer.

Berrios, a brilliant Peruvian psychiatrist working in Cambridge (U.K.), provides a modern definition of hallucinations as 'verbal reports of "sensory" experiences, with or without insight, not vouchsafed by a relevant stimulus.' But reliance is still placed upon that of Esquirol (1817), who defined hallucinations as perceptions without an object. Esquirol failed to clarify the unusual nature of the experience as distinct from special kinds of mental imagery which are perceived but evaluated as fictitious (pseudohallucinations); but succeeded in providing a continuity with delusions – false beliefs impervious to reason – and with illusions – misinterpretations of the form of external stimuli.

My first foray into the nature of hallucinations was in a commentary on the neurological localization of visual hallucinations based on an analysis of personal case-reports by Alwyn Davies-Jones. Organic hallucinations, not arising from the psychological mechanisms of thought, originate from instability of cortical cells. Visual hallucinations are a relatively infrequent accompaniment of damage to the occipital and calcarine (visual) cortices, yet may also occur as a false localizing symptom of frontal or subtentorial lesions. Considerable overlap had been previously observed in the types of recorded hallucinations by Ritchie Russell and Whitty when tabulating the varied complexity of visual hallucinations found in soldiers with localized head wounds. But there are theoretical reasons, amplified by direct stimulation of the cortex, which suggest a degree of localization. At the occipital pole stimulation produces static lights and stars. With more anterior lesions the light appears at the periphery and moves towards the centre. Further out in the parastriate area (18) luminous sensation may be obtained of coloured flashes or rings, or alternatively, stimulation may produce negative phenomena described as a grey or black fog similar to the scotomata of migraine. From parastriate area 19 and over the parietal cortex, the hallucinations become more stereotyped, with an emphasis on objects, people, and animals. These bizarre apparitions are one degree more complex than the flashes, zigzags, and whorls of colour obtained from the primary receptive cortex. Visual hallucinations over a large area of the non-dominant temporal lobe may be combined with auditory hallucinations with distortions in size or brightness, or with changes in the sense of familiarity or depersonalization. Similar 'focal' hallucinations, ranging from simple bangs and clicks to musical sounds, words or complex thoughts allied to vision, can occur over the temporal auditory areas and the parieto-temporal association areas.

Other phenomena from the visual association areas may occur alongside visual hallucinations. There may be perseveration of the image in time (palinopsia), in space (visual illusory spread – as in some of Matisse's paintings of Madame Matisse), defective perceptions of colours with errors in naming them (achromatopsia and anomia) or defective visual localization.

The list given so far does not exhaust the types of visual hallucinations seen. Many hallucinations arise because we are not fully alert. Even when fully conscious, we guess, we anticipate, we assume, we fear, we suppose. We use a far quicker, more superficial strategy with those with whom we are familiar, gauging their presence or reaction from the voice, from vibes, from glimpses rather than carefully reading their expressions. As Shakespeare says, 'Love looks not with the eyes, but with the mind'*. This may be part of the explanation behind the wish-fulfilment hallucinations of the bereaved. They anticipate the presence of their loved one, they half assume, and then they realize. To the psychiatrist this is just a pseudo-hallucination. He is not required. End of story. Impaired cerebration is an essential causal factor underlying the hallucinations in dementia, in arteriosclerosis, with toxic states, from hallucinogenic drugs — or from disturbances of sleep or consciousness due to 'dissociation' of the reticular activating system in the brainstem which cyclically alerts or dampens cortical activity.

In the *Neurology of Familiarity* (*Behavioural Neurology* 1989 2. 195-200) I said the phenomenon of familiarity affects our perception of ourselves and of others to whom we are emotionally or psychodynamically linked in the world around us; familiarity intrudes upon the means whereby we recognize others, often defying accepted forms of perception.

Anthony Storr, in the *Dynamics of Creation* 1972, states:

> We all know that our subjective involvement with a person interferes with our capacity to describe him. If we want to give a friend a convincing portrait of a favourite child, or of someone with whom we are in love, we find it difficult to do so, and we describe the difficulty by saying that we are 'too close' to the person we are trying to portray. We cannot view a loved person as objectively as we would like because we cannot separate ourselves from those we love, and cannot therefore stand back and see them in perspective. Detachment from the object or 'psychical distance' as it has been called, is a necessary precursor not only of science but also of art.

With sensory deprivation, the trigger for an hallucination may be a little glimmer of light, moistening of the skin, a faint scratch, a change of temperature. Most anomalous experiences related to sensory deprivation come into the realm of pseudo-hallucinations and some are clearly illusional and dependent on the few remaining stimuli. Accidents and errors by long-distance night truck drivers (highway hypnosis), jet pilots and radar sentinels become more understandable when it is realized that they are caused by perceptual distortions and impaired sensory stimulation. Other factors may be present such as stress, anxiety or sleep deprivation. After cataract

---
**Midsummer Night's Dream* 1, i 234
Love looks not with the eyes, but with the mind;
And therefore is wing'd Cupid painted blind.

extraction, black patch delirium in the elderly probably results from sensory deprivation in the presence of mild senile brain changes, and is more frequent when hearing is also impaired. Captain Joshua Slocum, a solitary navigator through a storm at night, imagined that the pilot of Columbus's ship the Pinta had taken over the helm. Before setting sail from the Azores, he took aboard a quantity of over-ripe plums which could have caused additional intoxication. Admiral Richard Byrd, isolated for six months in a small hut in Antarctica, developed psychotic obsessions and hallucinations until he realised that they were triggered by carbon monoxide poisoning from the tunnel vent of his shelter. In the *Neurological Boundaries of Reality*, I was able to get Wing Commander Gordon Turnbull, the psychiatrist who debriefed the hostages held in the Lebanon, to analyse sensory deprivation in hostage situations.

Hallucinations due to dysfunction of an end-organ – tinnitus or musical hallucinations from the ear; sensations from a phantom limb – are triggered by the interaction of one or more factors, including the absence of normal stimuli from the periphery, distortion of information from spontaneous irritability due to the deranged or degenerate state of the end organ, alterations in the state of alertness, and coexistent disturbances of cerebral function. All levels of the nervous system, and even higher functions such as memory stores, mental imagery and psychodynamic factors, influence the content of organic hallucinations. A severed optic nerve commonly evokes flashes of light. Surgical enucleation. may usher forth visions of clouds, birds or angels. Phosphenes of sparks of light can be produced by pressure, sudden movements or traction on the globe. Concussion, retinal haemorrhage, cataracts or incipient blindness may excite dazzling photopsiae with visions of green forests, seas of colour, incessant golden rain or smoky panoramas of dramatic landscapes after the manner of John Martin. Klein (1917), Horowitz (1964) and others have abstracted into a series of simple elements hallucinations and illusions believed to arise from the eyes (entoptic visions) and argued that anatomical structures within the eye such as the retinal ganglionic network and luminous dust – normally filtered from conscious perception – can impinge on the deranged mind and are then misconstrued, often forming the basis of schizophrenic art. They quote as an example the mosaic cat paintings of Louis Wain.

If we are to explore the effects of altered vigilance or levels of consciousness, we need to look beneath the mantle of the cerebral cortex into the inner workings of the brain. For example in dementia, and indeed to a lesser extent in everyone, there is a progressive fall out of functioning cortical neurones. This cortical cellular abiotrophy is well compensated for socially.

Symptoms occur when lesions involve the association tracts and the coordination of behaviour with altered emotional responses and sleep patterns. The continuous process of filtering and selecting sensory information develops and matures from early infancy. The nightmares of childhood become less frightening, lapses of vigilance are rarer, and aberrations leading to dissociated functioning of sensory processing with dreams and hallucinations are fewer and of shorter duration. Normal individuals may experience falling or floating feelings and déjà vu, but such phenomena are characterized by their brevity.

Age and disease may disrupt and confuse the pathways which normally alert the brain and there may be disordered function of the reticulo-hypothalamic- thalamic- cortical powerhouse normally controlling our state of consciousness. With dementia, space-occupying lesions, strokes, infections, or chemical changes induced by faulty metabolism or drugs, confusional states with hallucinosis can occur. A blind hemianopic field may become colonized by imaginary strangers who remorselessly gesticulate. Persistent visual hallucinations of Lilliputian forms and brightly coloured kaleidoscopic patterns (Lhermitte's peduncular hallucinosis) may arise within the brain stem. Microdreams in the form of hypnagogic hallucinations as errors of cerebration during the intermediate stage between wakefulness and sleep may occur in normal individuals, with noises, calls, feelings, and visual impressions often in the form of geometric designs, brightly coloured lines or points of light, flitting nature scenes, faces and figures. They have been utilised in the art of Klee and others.

> Before falling asleep we recall a number of things, lines of the most varied kinds, spots, dabs, smooth planes, dotted planes, wavy lines, obstructed and articulated movement, counter-movements, plaitings, weavings, brick-like elements, scale-like elements, simple and polyphonic motifs, lines that fade and lines that gain strength (dynamism), the joyful harmony of the first stretch, followed by inhibitions, nervousness. (*Creative Credo*, 1920)

The hypnagogic hallucinations of children often reflect their fantasy world of monsters such as King Kong and Frankenstein and can be so frightening that they fear falling asleep, fight against sleep or wake in the middle of the night with night terrors. With mountain sickness, sleep at altitude is punctuated by frequent awakenings with hypnagogic dreams that have entered into the mythology of the mountains. Obstructive sleep apnoea and drunken sleep may produce phenomena which resemble the night terrors of childhood.

Pathological dream states include oneirism, hallucinatory twilight states, and various forms of depersonalization. Oneirism is a prolonged psychotic experience persisting for days or months; it is to confusion what a dream is to sleep. Although oneirism is often drug-induced, there may be a schizophrenic psychosis and a familial tendency in this respect. Consciousness is deeply disorganized. The dream is all the more vivid because the subject participates (sometimes with considerable motor activity) living through multiple scenic hallucinations, intense emotions, and disordered perceptions. He is held prisoner by his dream as if hypnotized and unable to free himself by waking. In twilight states (dammerzustände) the subject appears passive with marked psychomotor retardation, although experiencing the liveliest emotional involvement as he witnesses scenes frequently of an apocalyptic, literary, or historical nature enacted as florid visual apparitions entering the objective world which he continues to perceive. The episode may last 1-2 hours and terminate in a generalized convulsion. Our guide on a ghost tour of York had had such an experience in the early 1950, which I reproduce with his permission.

As an apprentice aged 17 he had been working in the cellars of the Treasurer's house installing piping for central heating. He was standing on a short ladder when he first heard the sound of a trumpet. He paid little attention to this, other than feeling the slight surprise that the sound of a brass band should have reached him where he was working, but the sound drew nearer and nearer, and suddenly the figure of a horse came through the wall. It was large and lumbering – its fetlocks heavy and shaggy.

He fell from his ladder to the earthen floor in a state of confusion and shock. More was to come. On the back of the horse was a man dressed in Roman costume, and behind him came a group of soldiers, not marching in formation, but shuffling in a dispirited way, with their heads down. He was surprised by their small stature and shabby appearance. He described in great detail the rough, home-made clothes they were wearing. The sandals, cross-gartered to the knees, were very badly made, and their kilted skirts, green in colour, gave the impression that they had been roughly dyed. They carried round shields (an unusual feature in the Roman army), long spears and short swords. The finest part of their equipment appeared to be the helmets, with fine plumes of undyed feathers.

Shocked and trembling, he rushed up the cellar steps to the ground floor. Here he stumbled against the curator who said, noticing his agitation, 'You've seen the Romans, haven't you?' This remark was of great comfort. At the suggestion of the curator, he wrote down what he had seen and was later astonished to find two other people had also left accounts giving identical details.

## Unusual Auditory Hallucinations
### A. Musical hallucinations

Auditory hallucinations may originate as release phenomena due to an abnormality within the ear (end-organ dysfunction); or as a result of focal irritability and dysfunction along the auditory pathways projecting on to the cortex. In their most elemental form they occur as simple ill-defined sounds such as single tones, bangs, ticks, clicks or whistles. With greater elaboration they assume a vocal quality and enter the realms of language. Elaboration of a different kind produces sounds with rhythmic or melodic properties achieving a greater or lesser degree of harmonic integration: from the ringing of bells, bands playing, fragments of well-known tunes, or, in a highly developed form, taking on the gigantic proportions of a symphonic or operatic work. Emotional and multi-modality assimilations within the music may build up synaesthetic and experiential relationships.

Rather than supposing a spectrum of increasing complexity, it is perhaps more accurate to depict the wide range of auditory hallucinatory experiences as a Venn diagram involving four overlapping circles: sounds, vocalizations, music and mixed hallucinations. The aetiology of musical hallucinations is no different from that of other auditory hallucinations, being associated with end-organ dysfunction, epilepsy, vascular, space-taking and degenerative organic disorders, alcohol withdrawal states and psychoses. We also know that sounds termed 'oto-acoustic emissions' are released naturally from the ear spontaneously or as a result of specific stimuli. They are rarely audible to other people; but, using sophisticated apparatus, they can be utilized to confirm that a newborn child is not deaf.

My colleague, Professor Douglas Mitchell, defines music as a definite, reproducible auditory experience, universal to all human societies, which has the potential to induce a feeling of pleasure and satisfaction in those who hear it. It also possesses a unique capacity to evoke feelings associated with a wide range of human experiences by evoking natural sounds, by mimicry, by tone-painting and sound pictures.

Elaborate musical hallucinations are not that rare in people going deaf, but are far, far less common than the sibilant sounds and whistles of tinnitus. Most neurologists can quote a similar example to a patient of ours aged 56 who woke in the early hours of the morning to the sounds of revelry, apparently from an adjoining house. The noise consisted predominantly of country and western music, with a hubbub of conversation in the background, and prevented her getting back to sleep. Over an hour, the music changed to traditional Scottish pipe music and then to hymn singing. She knew that her neighbours were not in the least religious and could not understand the development. She woke her husband and daughter, who heard no noise. Only at that stage did she realize she was hallucinating. During this time her consciousness was clear and her judgment and affect unimpaired. There was no vertigo, deafness or any other vestibular symptom and no headache. There had been no change in her normal behaviour apart from anxiety engendered by this occurrence. Auditory and neurological investigations were all normal.

Another lady, aged 78, who had been deaf for years without tinnitus, developed musical hallucinations when she moved into a flat near where the Gas Board were using a pneumatic drill. She started to get headaches and a severe pain over the right eye. The hallucinations were of three tunes: 'Happy Birthday', 'Holding the Shoe' and something else. They were troublesome to her. If she were mildly depressed, the hallucinations would be particularly annoying, monotonous and repetitive. Her hallucinations were resistant to treatment with anticonvulsants, sedatives and antidepressants. She often played her radio loudly in an attempt to banish them but this was rarely helpful.

I have already quoted the lady who, after a left-sided stroke, developed a lesion on the other side of the brain, with tunes from the Latin Mass which she tried to suppress. Auditory illusions and hallucinations can occur in a setting of alcoholic withdrawal or relative abstinence following chronic drinking. Dante Gabriel Rossetti, addicted to chloral, alcohol and opiates, complained of the 'chiming of cobwebs', though his mind was otherwise clear at the time. In many patients similar brief rhythmic sounds may be interspersed with accusatory and paranoid vocalizations that bear a close resemblance to some schizophrenic states. Rod Duncan contributed one such example to our paper on *Hallucinations and Music*:-

> Three days into a voyage in the North Sea, a 33 year-old fisherman noticed an irritating background noise which he could not characterize and did not immediately identify as an hallucination. This became more and more obtrusive, developing first into a buzz of conversation, then into a succession of pop tunes with chat from a disc jockey between them. He was able to recall some of the tunes, recognizing them as being currently in the charts, and identified the disc jockey as Tony Blackburn, a radio personality he particularly detested. Following this he developed the persistent and fixed idea that his wife was being unfaithful to him and became violent, demanding to be put ashore.
>
> On admission to the local hospital, the patient was alert, oriented and physically well. It transpired that he was a moderately heavy drinker and had been on a binge since his last trip, having necessarily abstained from alcohol after leaving port. He did not go on to develop frank delirium tremens and his auditory hallucinations and paranoia regarding his wife's fidelity resolved completely over several days.

Musical hallucinations have featured in the lives of several composers: Bedrich Smetana, who is believed to have had syphilis; Hector Berlioz, who took opium; and Robert Schumann during his developing madness.

## B. Hallucinations in Prelingually Deaf Schizophrenic Patients

Schizophrenia, as opposed to schizophrenic states arising from physical illness, is regarded as *the* psychiatric illness: the illness of the mind. And yet there is an interminal search for a physical basis for the condition. Definition of the condition remains difficult, for the fundamental fault lies in the processing of thoughts and information. This in turn results in impaired or delusional perceptions and fragmentation of the ego-boundaries. The combination of a thought disorder and fragmentation of the ego-boundaries may be inhibitory or dysinhibitory. If dysinhibitory, there can be an extraordinary release or press of thoughts, often incongruous, patterned or stereotyped, sometimes spoken, often written, may be drawn, and characteristically in the form of a heavy annotation of texts. Delusions, illusions and pseudohallucinations merge and intermingle. Sensory experiences emanating from the body, skin, viscera and genitalia may undergo delusional blending, and, with loss of the boundaries that normally demarcate the inner personality from the outer world, the patient may feel himself possessed. Concentration is affected: thus he may discuss around and around a topic unable to reach a conclusion. At times the apparently enriched content of his thoughts may appear totally unrelated to his previous intelligence. Thus ruminations frequently involve higher flights of conceptual thought, leading to a prevailing concern for the world and life in general or to religion, psychology, philosophy, art or literature. Thoughts may be attached to other people, often leading to an accusation of a paranoid type. Many will shy away from other people, aware that their thought processes impair communication. Others find a loosening of associations resulting in a 'word salad', in klang rhymes, grotesque puns, and knight's-move connections or jumps of thought.

Positive symptoms are always easier to recognize than inhibited symptomatology. It is particularly difficult to detect a thought disorder where the means of communication are rudimentary. Thus, in the presence of muteness the diagnostic decision must be deferred and even in patients with normal communication, such symptoms are particularly intangible and difficult to define.

Although hallucinations occur initially in only 75% of newly diagnosed schizophrenic patients, they form the most tangible evidence of schizophrenia. It is the nature and quality of hallucinations and delusions that is

particularly characteristic of the disorder. The hallucinations of schizophrenia are distorted by delusional systematization. Auditory hallucinatory manifestations are most common, with, in descending order of frequency, olfactory, visual, somatic and tactile perceptions. Thus hallucinations of a visual type are present in only 3-4% of schizophrenics. Schneider utilized the specific forms of auditory hallucination in defining his first rank symptoms of schizophrenia:-
1. Voices, anticipating the patient's thoughts or repeating his thoughts out loud (thought-echo),
2. Voices, discussing the patient or arguing about him, referring to him in the third person,
3. Voices, discussing the patient's thoughts or behaviour, often as a running commentary.

Rarer forms of hallucinations described in schizophrenia include functional hallucinations, which only occur in the presence of another stimulus, and extracampine hallucinations, which occur outside the patient's sensory field. Thus a patient may hear or see something happening in another town.

The Whittingham Hospital just north of Preston was at one time one of the largest psychiatric institutions in the country. I have already referred to its rail link. The long nightingale wards have gradually closed down. I used to visit the main hospital, the Langdale unit (a forensic psychiatric unit for violent patients), and the Psychiatric Unit for the Deaf to provide a neurological opinion on selected patients. At one time the Unit for the Deaf was unique – the only one in the country. It has since closed and moved to Pendlebury in Manchester. The Pendlebury unit and that in Birmingham, among many now in existence in various parts of the country, have taken on the name of the Unit's superintendent and consultant, Dr John Denmark. I formed a special collaboration with Dr Denmark and with his successor, Dr Brendan Monteiro, which enabled me to study patients of special interest within the unit. These included those admitted as deaf, whereas in reality, when examined in depth, they had central language disorders, such that they might regard their native language as though it were foreign, with the same understanding as though it were Chinese. However, my attention was particularly engaged in studying the hallucinatory phenomena of prelingually deaf schizophrenics – i.e. those with lack of hearing for speech from birth or whose loss of hearing occurred in the first year of life. I was able to fulfil this interest with the help of various members of the unit.

   Profound deafness from birth or early age presents an enormous barrier to the development of both speech and language and the majority of prelingually profoundly deaf people are linguistically retarded with unintelligible speech. Finger spelling consists of spelling out each word, letter by letter, using different configurations of the fingers of one or both hands to represent the letters of the alphabet. Manual sign languages of deaf people involve the use of the hands and arms to convey the meaning of words and concepts. Sign languages differ to some extent from country to country and are different in syntax and grammatical construction from the native spoken language. Some deaf people who use manual communication methods have a good command of verbal language, while others are seriously retarded linguistically. The former will usually employ a combination of finger spelling and sign language, while those with poor verbal language will use sign language with additional gesturing and mime. The little speech they have will have developed at school and skills in finger spelling and sign language will have developed within their own community. But in adolescence and adult life they may be cut off from their peers and their speech skills may atrophy if they fail to find a sympathetic audience. Psychiatric breakdown at this stage is not uncommon.

It is claimed that schizophrenia among the profoundly deaf is no more common than in the community at large. Given the numbers who fail in the wider world, I would have expected far more deaf schizophrenics, but it is a supposition that I have been unable to test out. Given the communication problems of prelingually profoundly deaf patients, and especially their limited language, psychiatric diagnosis is extremely difficult. Dr Denmark and his social work assistants not only need to master sign language and finger spellings, but have to recognize the dissolution of such skills where these have occurred and if necessary build up the signing ability of their patients before they can reassess and make a diagnosis. These skills, which they most certainly did possess, are remarkably rarely found.

I was able to take patients who had complained of hallucinations and interview them with the help of the deaf social worker – Frank Warren or Kathleen Wilson. Several interviews were required and after discussion it was often necessary to reinterview or to ask Dr Denmark to reinterview to try to establish exactly what was happening. As expected, the frequency of the different types of hallucinatory experiences differed subtly from those of their hearing contemporaries. The frequency of haptic hallucinations, passivity phenomena and delusions often of a paranoid type was similar. Visual hallucinations, which are rare among hearing schizophrenics, occurred in 10 out of 12 patients: some of the experiences were classical scenic hallucinations but others were more accurately described as visuo-verbal hallucinations, as though the visual picture had been substituted for a verbal commentary. Non-auditory modes of communication familiar to profoundly deaf people, such as writing on the wall and sign language, were described among the hallucinatory experiences of 3 people, but invariably in association with 'auditory' experiences which were described by 10 out of 12 patients. Voiced experiences, whether presenting as a running commentary on the subject's thoughts or behaviour, as voices in discussion or as specific instruction addressed to the patient, differed widely in their clarity.

If we examine some of the case-histories, there is no doubt as to the schizophrenic nature of the experiences; the hearing component is less certain:-

1. A married female complained by sign language that she was frequently wakened at night with 'talk . . . talk'. She explained that there were men and women in her chest. She could not see them but could feel them talking and her chest was heavy when they talked. Someone in her chest wanted to marry her. She could not recall what they were talking about. When asked how she knew the voices were male and female, she replied, using sign language, 'Because they were having intercourse'. She could feel the 'wet and bumping'.

2. A younger woman with poor speech but with good manual communication skills complained that her husband was trying to kill her and that the police had hushed up an attempt to poison her. Subsequently she developed delusions of a religious and grandiose nature. She believed that God had spoken to her and told her that someone wanted to kill her. She stated that she had tubes in her ears and her vagina; that she had defecated a black-backed, yellow-fronted flea, and could not eat quickly because her stomach was full of fleas.

When questioned about her encounter with God, she said she was shocked as she had not seen him before. She said that there was a globe-like world and that God was behind the world. She saw his head and shoulders. She could see his lips moving and heard 'like voices' for 5 minutes. When pressed, she insisted that she heard (finger spelling the word 'heard') not lip-read. God spoke like a bell, very fast, but she was able to understand what he said. God said 'rich . . . quick . . . blood . . . steal . . . take blood of rich people'. God told her someone would die. It was the only time she 'heard' speech.

3. A 55 year-old entertained various paranoid ideas involving his brother, whom he accused of stealing things. He had the locks of his house changed to prevent his brother entering and had turned the clocks and mirrors to the wall because he thought he was being spied upon. He denied that he was mentally ill but complained of stomach trouble and was constantly bothered by voices. He complained that for 8 years voices had constantly

talked to him. He believed the voices were female but was unable to elucidate further.

4. A 34 year old, who had neglected his personal hygiene and become aggressive, entertained a number of strange ideas and believed he had seen Christ. He was frequently observed signing and smiling to himself and when questioned, explained that he could hear a voice communicating with him from London. When asked how, being deaf, he could talk to someone in London, he explained that he could see the person.

5. A 65 year-old female whose speech was unintelligible, but she was able to give a fair account of herself by sign language and finger spelling, claimed she could hear voices and a man talking to her, telling her to do this and that, talking bad (dirty) about man and woman. She heard noises of people talking in different parts of the house but she did not know what they said. She would remove her dentures and make mouthing movements in front of the mirror. After her first admission, she was afraid to return home as there were faces on the wall, floor and furniture which could look at her and laugh. In some way which she was unable to elucidate, they would talk to her and influence her to talk to herself in the mirror. She had involuntary mouth movements (oral dyskinesias) which she interpreted as talking to herself from her throat and mouth. She was adamant that it was talking and that she did not lip-read her mouth in the mirror.

6. Perhaps the most telling example is a lady to whom God spoke but St Theresa signed, suggesting a primacy of oral communication.

Before the possible significance of auditory hallucinations among deaf schizophrenics can be discussed further, certain caveats must be considered in detail. Firstly, hallucinations in schizophrenia differ intrinsically from classical hallucinations, being neither mental images nor true perceptions but liable to distortion by delusional systematization. Thus a relationship may be made without adequate proof in a bizarre delusional context. The information may be correctly schematized but the schema shift their inter-relationships, forcing the subject to develop a complex and interlocking argument. In hearing schizophrenics, the auditory hallucinations are frequently accompanied by activation of the muscles of phonation, reflected in most cases by electromyographic activity of the vocal cords and in some instances by actual subvocal speech, i.e. the voices emanate from their own speech apparatus. Hearing schizophrenics describe their hallucinations as anything from vague mumblings to distinct speech, usually addressed to the patient in the third person.

Secondly, the major problem in accepting the possible auditory nature of the hallucinations of deaf schizophrenics is not psychiatric but linguistic. The language ability of the majority of profoundly, prelingually deaf people is limited. The process of education, even with augmentation by a hearing aid, demands ideal conditions, much reinforcement and constant repetition. Simple concepts such as 'in, on up, under' are grasped with difficulty, vocabulary acquisition is tedious and when lip-reading, it is still necessary to guess nine out of ten words. Such communication skills as a deaf adult is able to retain may atrophy through lack of encouragement and, especially if he has a psychiatric problem, he is recognized as an isolate with whom it is difficult to establish a mutual method of communication.

Offset against these considerations, which demand circumspection, are a number of factors that support acceptance of the reality of their experiences. Man has had the capacity for hearing and vocalization for thousands of years. Damage to the peripheral hearing organ does not inevitably mean disruption of the central pathways and nearly all profoundly deaf people retain some residual hearing. Thus pure tone audiography may show that a person who inaccurately or incompletely hears occasional speech syllables is probably not entirely devoid of auditory experience. The speech audiogram occupies only a part of the wider range of appreciation of musical and other sounds. Thus a person incapable of hearing human speech may have experienced the sound of a horse trotting, a clap of thunder, a bell chiming, or even a dog barking.

Whilst one cannot accept the auditory descriptions at their face value without further questioning, and even then add the consideration of delusional systematization, one has to explain the insistence of the deaf patients themselves that the communicated experiences did not involve speech reading or sign language. When pressed for an explanation, only one admitted that she did not know how she could hear voices, another said that it was 'queer talk – not signs' and others were adamant that they had heard and not lip-read the experience, finger spelling the word 'heard' with great emphasis.

Using the analogy of epileptic auditory hallucinations, it may be said that the specific hallucinations of schizophrenia, in both hearing and deaf schizophrenics, are chemically excited in the region of the dominant temporal lobe. Throughout man's evolution, language has been forged on a vocal-auditory system intimately connected with thought processes, and the deaf person is not exempted from this development. A deaf child learning to communicate through gesture shows no clear cerebral dominance. If sign language is learnt, even though the means of communication are visual, the left hemisphere, in right-handers and in the majority of left-handers, becomes dominant.

## The Role of the Neurologist

Small neurological hospitals were founded at the end of the 19th century to treat conditions such as epilepsy, stroke and paraplegia neglected elsewhere, but most neurological work was performed by general physicians in the 'fever units' and larger hospitals. Individual neurologists established their speciality by their expertise with the lumbar puncture needle to examine the cerebro-spinal fluid and, with the ophthalmoscope, to diagnose papilloedema (swollen fluids behind the eye indicating similar swelling within the brain). In London they might travel from hospital to hospital for this purpose. In other parts of the country, as in Liverpool, they also declared themselves by their expertise with electro-encephalography. European neurologists typically combined the practice of neurology with that of psychiatry. Although some neurologists were able at one stage to obtain psychiatric degrees relatively easily, the combination never took off in Britain.

Many neurologists confined themselves to their specialized hospital, performing essentially a referral service elsewhere. A few were attached to neuro-surgical units, especially during the Second World War. However, even after the War most appointments throughout the country were for general physicians with an interest in neurology. They had a large number of beds and were on emergency take for all general medical conditions. The development of neuro-radiology, and to a lesser extent of electro-encephalography and electro-physiology, meant that neurologists needed to work alongside neuro-surgeons. Patients who have undergone myelography, angiography or air-encephalography cannot safely be transferred from one hospital to another and neurologists were faced with the choice either of leaving such tests to the neurosurgeons, realising that some patients would have negative findings and their journey would be wasted, or to work alongside the neurosurgeons, cooperating with them in planning procedures so that a rapid transfer could be made if an operation were required. As the tests became more sophisticated, this meant separation from general medicine into combined neurological and neurosurgical units. It also meant that the neurologists would have fewer beds. To some extent, the number of beds they had was related to the flow of patients through neuro-x-ray, allowing for the fact that neurosurgical emergencies commonly took precedence over routine neurological tests.

The change from physicians with an interest in neurology to pure neurology has never been fully accepted by the Royal College of Physicians. With increasing specialization within general medicine, so that in many centres gastro-enterologists, for example, are not on emergency take, the College is concerned that there are too few consultants sharing emergency work, and it is calculated that 20% of emergency admissions to general medical wards have a neurological content. Neurologists, not on take, do not see admissions with encephalitis, meningitis, subarachnoid haemorrhage, status epilepticus or strokes. They may see them as referrals at a later stage. The problem is twofold. If neurology is to advance, then the neurologists must keep up with the increasing sophistication of their diagnostic techniques. Secondly, having combined with neurosurgery into 'neuroscience units', they no longer have the required number of beds nor the supporting staff to take the influx of emergencies that come into general medicine. Strenuous efforts are made to try to deal with 'the take problem' but the total number of neurologists throughout the country until very recently has been pitifully small compared to other countries in Europe and North America.

The other change that has taken place is in the frequency with which cerebro-spinal fluid examinations by lumbar puncture are performed. At one time, to come into a neurological ward and not receive a lumbar puncture was exceptional. Nowadays, because it is preferable and advisable to perform a CT or other scan first, relatively few lumbar punctures are needed. Procedures have changed. Thus if meningitis is suspected, more often than not a CT scan is followed by the use of a broad spectrum antibiotic; and lumbar puncture is delayed to reduce the risk of displacement of the brain (coning) from brain swelling (cerebral oedema).

Most neurology is in fact performed in the out-patient departments or in seeing patients referred on the wards of other specialities. Many urgencies, possibly needing rapid admission to hospital, were seen as domiciliary visits at home. Home visits provided a rapid means of assessing the social conditions of the patient, and other family members who might not accompany the patient to the out-patient department could also be questioned. There was a further advantage in that one knew the area and circumstances of the people who were one's potential patients. The modern consultant, who works purely from hospital, lacks this essential understanding of his 'client population.' Domiciliary visits have to be fitted in between sessions or in one's spare time. A surgical colleague, doing a rare home visit after a night and day operating, fell asleep in the patient's home whilst waiting for the patient to come down stairs. On one occasion, asked to see a parkinsonian patient in a complex of interwoven houses in a village, I was led into a room by one of the neighbours and examined a patient who appeared more arterio-sclerotic than parkinsonian – this mistake is often made. I was later telephoned by an irate relative to say I had examined the wrong patient. I made sure when revisiting the place that the G.P. was in attendance. Ideally they should be and when I first started, more usually than not they were present; but over the years fewer attend along with the specialist. In fact, when I first started, it was rather like the membership examination, watched over, then questioned immediately on one's findings. One learns that there is 'none so queer as folk'. Visiting one farm on the Pennines (it had been snowing there but nowhere else) I was shown into the drawing room, festooned with photographs – not of the family, but of their prize sheep!

I have already referred to the fact that for many years I did out-patient work in 5 different hospitals and visited over 60 hospitals within my area. As scanning procedures have developed, it has become less necessary to admit patients for in-patient investigation, and the number of neurologists has at last started to expand, so that each district general hospital is meant to have its named neurologist, preferably dividing his time between the DGH and his neurological centre. Many tests such as CT and MR scanning can now be done at outlying hospitals but the technical standards, discussion before they are performed, reporting by general radiologists rather than by specialized neuro-radiologists, and above all, the opportunity for discussion at an x-ray conference between neuro-radiologist, neurologist and neuro-surgeon, cannot be as good as at the main centre. Despite administrative pressure not to see patients as domiciliary visits, and the expansion of the consultant grade, neurology still remains a peripatetic speciality with few neurologists working from just one hospital.

Neurologists in future are likely to come up against central government to an increasing extent. On the one hand through the management of trauma victims through all the stages of litigation, early treatment, rehabilitation and the provision of care and special provisions within their homes, they will dictate the money spent on one group of the disabled and thus influence national provision and concern for other people with disabilities. This is the route which will cause government to look and not turn away from their responsibilities. The other aspect for the future of neurology will be even more confrontational. New and expensive treatments are being developed for hitherto incurable diseases: AIDS, multiple sclerosis, motor neurone disease, Huntington's chorea; there will be a stage when the justification for using new drugs will be ethically questioned, a stage when two or three drugs in combination, as in tuberculosis or leukaemia, will be advanced, and finally, we hope, radical cures which may involve a life-time of prophylactic treatment. Spasticity and cerebral palsy will be managed with new techniques which, as with botulinum toxin, may be very expensive. Decisions for prioritizing treatments may not necessarily rest with governments. Thus they may be leant upon by the European Union authorizing new treatments, thereby increasing the pressure for their use from patients and their carers.

### Cerebro-vascular Disease

Most strokes are admitted to general medical wards and as the patient improves, many are transferred to stroke units providing rehabilitation and return to the community. For the majority of stroke victims there is little additional help which the neurologist can provide. Functional assessments are done by physiotherapists and occupational therapists based on aids to daily living. Aphasic speech disorders and swallowing difficulties are assessed by speech therapists, but after their initial assessment and advice to relatives, aphasia is best helped by neighbours and friends, who will encourage the stroke patient to try to speak in an atmosphere where they are not inhibited by their mistakes. The role of the neurologist is three-fold: to see that no treatable form of stroke is overlooked, to advise on the general running of stroke units, and to see that every potential development in diagnosis, early rehabilitation and in alleviating symptoms such as overcoming spasticity is properly tried and evaluated.

The major cause of strokes is hardening of atheroma (arterio-sclerosis), rendering the blood vessels hard, thickened, irregular, with ulceration of their inner layers; and there is a 600-fold increase in the incidence of stroke with advancing age from 10 per 100,000 below 35 years of age to 6,000 per 100,000 over 75 years. Risk factors are well known. The general population are well advised in this regard. Control of raised blood pressure is the most serious factor, heavy smoking comes next, followed by alcoholism, obesity, heart disease, previous ischaemic attacks (e.g. transient ischaemic attacks which do not amount to a completed stroke), diabetes, high oestrogen contraceptive pills, disease of other blood vessels, thrombotic tendencies as from polycythaemia, and hereditary factors with a positive family history of strokes. Arteriosclerotic strokes swamp all other forms of stroke. But other forms of stroke exist and many of the risk factors can be specifically reduced.

Strokes can occur in early life. By the use of ultrasonography, they may be detected in the foetus. Hemiplegia in early childhood may be produced by infection, usually in the presence of dehydration and malnutrition. Thrombosis can involve the veins over the brain or there may be septic thrombi lodged in the carotid artery. Especially in the tropics, sickle cell disease and parasitaemia (including cerebral malaria) are recognized causes of strokes. Cyanotic heart disease (blue babies) with blood flow across the heart from right to left allows septic or thrombotic emboli to enter the systemic circulation Associated sludging and thickening of the blood from polycythaemia can produce both venous and arterial thromboses. Blood dyscrasias, leukaemia, thrombotic and bleeding disorders can upset the delicate balance to cause haemorrhage or blood clotting, often as their presenting feature. Intra-cranial vascular malformations may cause spontaneous bleeding and weakness of the walls of arteries cause them to dissect, as in Marfan's syndrome or homocystinuria. The early circulation to the brain consists of many tiny blood vessels, later replaced by a few larger arteries. But in Moya-moya disease (the term literally means a puff of smoke) the primitive and inadequate pattern of blood vessels persists with areas of the brain under-perfused.

Traumatic hemiplegia can occur at all ages: from baby battering, from penetrating injury to the tonsils thrombosing the carotid artery, as when a child falls with a pencil in its mouth, or due to gymnastic exertion with over-stretching of the neck, rotation of the head and stretching of the vertebral arteries. Hemiplegia due to trauma to the neck vessels may be delayed until a thrombotic or embolic event occurs 24 hours after the initial insult.

It might be presumed that the risk of stroke between the ages of 15 to 45 is higher in women due to the thromboembolic risks associated with pregnancy, the contraceptive pill, deep vein thrombosis and the complications of childbirth, together with the higher risk from migraine in females and the use of drugs for dieting. However, certain counter-balancing influences explain the approximately equal sex incidence for strokes among young adults. Alcohol consumption is positively associated with cerebro-vascular disease and the incidence of strokes in men aged 35-64 is directly related to the number of fluid ounces of alcohol imbibed per month, increasing fibrinolytic activity, shortening the bleeding time and increasing the components of factor VIII. Heroin addiction is just one form of hard drug usage which carries a high risk of cerebral infarction and thromboembolism from endocarditis or injected impurities.

Young males, more so than others, take risks and a major source of cerebro-vascular accidents in that age group arises from physical factors and a sense of adventure – exposure to trauma, adverse environmental conditions. A young marathon runner developed a stroke, presumably from dehydration with body heat loss and excessive tissue breakdown. Near-drowning accidents may give brainstem strokes. Strokes and death at altitude occur in the Himalayas from mountain sickness. I had three such cases in close succession. A 22 year-old gamekeeper who developed dizziness, neck pains and an unexplained left hemiparesis on the grouse moors, a 38 year-old windsurfer with post-concussive aphasia, and a 33 year-old Catholic priest home from Jamaica, where he had been scuba diving. After diving at 35 feet for approximately 35 minutes, he surfaced rapidly, sustaining a painful perforation of his right ear drum. He went down again and resurfaced more slowly but 2 days later developed a left hemiparesis. After treatment in a decompression chamber to a depth of 165 feet with no change in his symptoms, he was transferred to a hospital in Florida. Scans showed two areas of infarction which had occurred after dissection of the right carotid artery with embolism into the brain. A recent article in the *British Medical Journal* highlights the risk of multiple brain lesions in scuba divers from emboli entering the arterial circulation via a patent foramen ovale in the heart.

Even in the elderly, many kinds of stroke are eminently treatable. Cranial arteritis (inflammation of medium sized blood vessels) involves the major vessels in the neck and their branches, such as the ophthalmic and central artery to the retina. This condition constitutes a neurological emergency, because loss of vision or thrombosis of the basilar artery can develop rapidly, yet be treated and prevented by the use of steroids. Long-term treatment for eighteen months or longer with prednisolone and immunosuppressive drugs is required to dampen down the inflammatory process and prevent its progression. Meningovascular syphilis can be treated, as may emboli from infection of heart valves (bacterial endocarditis). And it is in the elderly that hyperviscosity syndromes – leukaemia, macroglobulinaemia, myelomatosis, primary polycythaemia and polycythaemia secondary to lung disease, with a slow, sluggish, and slugging circulation, are most commonly seen.

The range and diversity of traumatic injury causing rupture, dissection or thrombosis of the blood vessels of the neck and skull-base need to be restated. The trauma may be direct or indirect, as from penetrating injuries, such as javelin injuries to the carotid, strangulation, atlanto-axial dislocation, cervical manipulation, yoga, whiplash injuries, head banging, skiing injuries and motor cycle accidents. Symptoms are particularly liable to develop in the presence of congenital abnormalities. Indeed, loops, kinks and coils, and arterial dysplasia, as from pseudoxanthoma elasticum, fibromuscular dysplasia or the Ehlers-Danlos syndrome, may predispose to thromboembolism in the absence of trauma or atheroma. Any source of infection – bacterial, viral, fungal, – especially with altered states of immunity, can cause thrombotic lesions. The arteries can be inflamed from such conditions as Takayushu's disease, which narrows the origins of the carotid and vertebral arteries, Behcet's disease with hyaline degeneration of small vessels, or collagen diseases such as polyarteritis nodosa or systemic lupus erythematosis (SLE). Cardiac arrest, blood loss, fat embolism, atrial myxoma are just some of the less usual causes of infarction. Blood clots under the skull such as subdural haematoma, bleeding around the brain (subarachnoid haemorrhage), are common stroke disorders, invariably referred to the neurosurgeons. An example, by no means unique, involved my sister, who was on anticoagulants because of thrombo-embolic disease. She slipped at the sea-front, landing on her bottom and over the next few days developed a subdural haematoma with increasing headache and almost lapsing into coma. Surgical treatment had to be delayed until the INR (anticoagulant ratio) had returned to normal.

Neurologists are often called in to diagnose lacunar strokes About one in five strokes results from injury to small perforating arteries and arterioles along with the development of microaneurysms in the deeper, non-cortical parts of the brain and brainstem. These small lesions may occur from bleeding, clotting or softening of tissue or a combination of these. In the past the usual cause was raised blood pressure but increasingly other causes are recognized. It may be necessary to do more than one CT scan to show the lesions. Their interest lies in the fact that they produce small discrete lesions or symptom complexes – a pure motor or sensory stroke, articulation defects affecting speech combined with clumsiness of a hand, movement disorders with continual gross throwing or flinging of an arm, or palsies of the ocular muscles.

Alvarez coined the phrase 'small strokes' for episodes which may pass unnoticed clinically, but result in a slow deterioration of mental or physical functions. These may occur with high blood pressure in the Binswanger syndrome, where there is multiple infarction subcortically. The end result is one of considerable morbidity, including a progressive subcortical dementia. Until recently the condition was more commonly diagnosed at post mortem than in life. Transient ischaemic attacks, defined as lasting less than 24 hours but usually lasting minutes, have been the subject of much investigation. The most common cause is platelet emboli arising from the surface of roughened arteriosclerotic plaques on the carotid arteries passing to the brain, where they break up before permanent damage is done or the ophthalmic artery giving amaurosis fugax (transient blindness). Occasionally pieces of the dispersing embolus can be seen with an ophthalmoscope in the blood vessels of the retina. It is now accepted that if there is gross narrowing of the carotid artery (over 75% stenosis), surgery is the advised treatment but aspirin reduces the risk by speeding up the breakup of platelet emboli in other patients. Emboli can arise from other sites, such as the heart valves, and as fat emboli from fractures. The first air-raid victim in London during the Second World War was a landlord of a pub in Camberwell, who, hearing the air-raid siren, rushed downstairs, falling, fracturing his femur and dying of a fat embolism.

Vascular insufficiency may mimic transient ischaemic attacks or result in strokes. The blood flow may be insufficient to maintain function and this can be a problem, especially with the basilar circulation to the back of the brain and brainstem. A classic example of this is the subclavian steal syndrome, a term suggested by Miller Fisher, where narrowing of the subclavian artery lessens flow up the vertebral artery, so that when an arm is energetically used the person becomes light-headed and weak. The existence of this syndrome was first proved by James Toole, who injected a radio-opaque dye directly into the heart.

A diagnostic rarity is the locked-in syndrome affecting the ventral part of the brainstem. There are several causes. If the result of a stroke, most patients die within a few days or weeks. Following migraine, recovery is known. I have had one patient with multiple sclerosis who has had the locked-in syndrome for 10 years. He is taken to football matches and great care is taken to keep his interests up. Alexandre Dumas in *The Count of Monte Cristo* (1844-5), describes the case of M. Noirtier de Villefort, who sustained a brainstem injury from a duel. There is a scene where he calls a notary for a will to disinherit his granddaughter if she marries into the d'Epinay family.

> M. Noirtier was sitting in an armchair, which moved upon castors, in which he was wheeled into the room in the morning, and in the same way drawn out again at night, thus enabling him to see all who entered the room, and everything which was going on around him, which would otherwise have been impossible. M. Noirtier, although almost immovable and helpless as a corpse, looked at the newcomers with a quick and intelligent expression, perceiving at once, by their ceremonial courtesy, that they were come on business of an unexpected and official character. He was placed before a large glass which reflected the whole apartment and permitted him to see, without any attempt to move. Sight and hearing were the only senses remaining, and they appeared left, like two solitary sparks, to animate the miserable body which seemed fit for nothing but the grave; it was only, however, by means of one of these senses that he could reveal the thoughts and feelings which still worked in his mind.

The expression and movement of the eyes, upward or down, was used as a sign language to indicate yes, no, etc.

> Three persons only could understand this language of the poor paralytic.

Except for the rarity of a traumatic cause, this is a faithful description of the life of a person with a locked-in syndrome.

> Well sir, the rupture of a blood vessel destroyed all this – not in a day, not in an hour – but in a second.

Emile Zola in his early novel, *Therese Raquin* (1868), a grim tale in a nightmarish Parisian setting, provides a possibly more authentic case:-

Madame Raquin suffers a stroke.

> She stopped in the middle of the sentence, open-mouthed, gaping, feeling as if she were being strangled. She tried to shout for help but could utter only raucous sounds. Her tongue turned to stone. Her hands and feet stiffened. She was struck dumb and motionless. For a few days Madame Raquin kept the use of her hands and could write on a slate and ask for what she wanted; but her hands went dead too, and it became impossible for her to raise them or hold a pencil. From then onwards, she had only the language of her eyes, and her niece had to guess what she wanted.

Therese was the only one who knew how to grasp the old lady's wants.

> She could communicate quite easily with that imprisoned mind buried alive in a dead body.

At first Madame Raquin was happy.

> She had learnt to use her eyes like a hand or mouth, to ask and give thanks, and in a strange way made up for the organs she had lost.

However, her happiness changed to hatred when she learned how her beloved son had died. Often when the couple were tending to her,

> she made frantic efforts to utter some cry of protest and put all her hatred into her eyes.

Finally, the murderers commit suicide by poison in the living room

> The bodies lay all night twisted and sprawling on the dining room floor in the yellowish light cast down on them by the shaded lamp. And for twelve hours, until about noon next day, Madame Raquin, stiff and silent, contemplated them at her feet, unable to feast her eyes enough, eyes that crushed them with brooding hate.

**Parietal Lobes, Rehabilitation and Disability**

The hallmark of Macdonald Critchley's career, more so than his writings on aphasia or dyslexia, has been his book on the parietal lobes, which, he claimed (and has been proved right) was 'the first and probably the last book' confined to that subject. The parietal lobes are concerned with body image, often shown clinically as neglect of the left side of the body or visual field. I remember as a child a painting done by a patient during an attack of migraine in which the right side of the picture was complete but the left side sketchy and incomplete. I have since seen many other similar pictures done by patients with parietal lobe tumours and, most appropriately, my last health service patient had a fully developed parietal lobe syndrome.

Disorders of body image usually give rise to negative features – neglect, inattention, or even denial – or more rarely reduplication of a part. An arteriosclerotic and hypertensive patient of mine whom I followed for many years developed pins and needles and cramps down the left arm and leg. For periods of 30 minutes or so, he felt as though he had two left arms, one outstretched, the other bent at the elbow. These episodes were present for at least 6 years.

In testing for negative features, firstly one establishes that the patient can see an object to his left or feel sensation down the left side when one stimulus is applied. If, then, bilateral stimuli are applied, he will see and recognize that on the right but ignore and not comment on that to the left. Thus, it may be possible to touch the right hand and left cheek simultaneously and the patient recognizes only the touching of the right hand. Neglect may take several forms. The patient, in dressing, may not get into his left trouser leg. He may bump into objects to his left. He may not eat from the left side of his plate and the nurse will turn it through 180 degrees. He may suddenly shout out, failing to recognize his left hand as his when it comes into view. He may feel that the left half of himself is another person lying in bed with him.

Defects arising from the dominant hemisphere are less easily demonstrated as they are likely to be obscured by associated speech impairment or other related phenomena. But there is a syndrome (Gerstmann's) from the dominant angular gyrus with abnormalities in writing, calculation, right left disorientation and inability to name and select individual fingers (e.g. if one touches the ring and index finger, he would not be able to say that the middle finger lay between them).

The present lack of concern among neurologists for higher cognitive disorders extends to the parietal lobe. In the past I have heard neurologists such as Eric Jewesberry and Raymond Hierons lecture on the parietal lobe purely from their own experience. When I wished to include a chapter on awareness of body image in my book on the *Neurological Boundaries of Reality*, I had the greatest difficulty in finding someone to do so, not just from the U.K. I eventually found a person who had written on the parietal lobes but I virtually rewrote the chapter myself when editing it. However, at the World Congress of Neurology in Vancouver, there was an exciting talk by K.M. Heilman describing various forms of neglect and how it was possible to show neglect other than across the midline.

Discussion of parietal inattention, neglect or denial is germane to the previous examination of strokes. Paralysis alone seldom accounts for a patient's incapacity and may contribute little to it. The overriding defect may be a change in intellect or some potentially reversible neurophysiological disturbance. These mental barriers to recovery have a disparate effect on the two hemispheres: patients with lesions of the left hemisphere make better recoveries than those with right-sided lesions, and each hemisphere provides a different challenge. Non-dominant parietal dysfunction, concerned with man's perception of his environment, may cause neglect of the affected limb, denial of the motor deficit, and bizarre conceptual defects. Such defects may be overlooked and – tragically – active treatment stopped because the patient is thought to be confused, uncooperative, or lacking motivation. By contrast, left-hemisphere damage may be obvious and interpreted, incorrectly, as giving a poor prognosis. Disturbances of language are readily apparent. Far from denial of illness, the patient may be depressed, and there is a danger that a comprehension defect, depression and clumsiness may be labelled as dementia.

The word apraxia is used when a person is not clumsy as such, but unable to perform specific tasks. Apraxic defects most commonly arise from left-hemisphere damage, occasionally from the non-dominant hemisphere, and often involve both sides of the brain. They can occur developmentally in children or are acquired as from a stroke. There is an inability to perform purposive or complex movements, despite intact mobility, sensation, and coordination. Its basis is uncertain. Perhaps it is due to loss of the capacity to permit the previously organized automatic performance of tasks. The complex movements may be language-dependent in so far as they are a response to commands. Or there may be impairment of kinaesthetic memory or feedback or a failure to process information at a normal rate.

If neurologists have neglected previous interest in higher brain functions, they can rightly claim to have taken over rehabilitation – an aspect of neurology sadly lacking in the past. Neurologists are now being appointed specifically with an interest in rehabilitation. I feel that such work can be soul-destroying unless it can be linked to a unit performing active research. For ten years I looked after a Young Disabled Unit. This was originally planned as a residential unit for the disabled but it was soon evident that it could be of greatest use if its primary purpose was assessment and rehabilitation. It could provide holiday relief for carers, at the same time upgrading activities such as transferring from bed to chair or improving mobility. What it could not do was to help those on the waiting list for admission. The mix of patients on such a unit is very important. It could not be used for brain-damaged patients with behavioural disturbances and aggression, for whom special units are required. Nor could it be used for Huntington's Chorea. We have, on occasion, had to take patients with both these disorders but fortunately there are now units with the necessary expertise to look after them. However, there are still too few specialized units and there is usually a waiting list for admission.

Equally important is the need to expand centres for the disabled providing advice, appliances, some rehabilitation, legal and social service help. These were advocated by the Royal College of Physicians; and the Department of Health suggested they should be set up in every health district, but no money was forthcoming. Although they are costly, the development by the U.K. of appliances – from hosiery to mobile chairs and home improvements – could have considerable export potential. With the help of business people, people with social service and physiotherapy expertise, and doctors working voluntarily, and indeed the Trust Board of the local hospital, I set up such a unit but it had to close after two years through lack of grants.

How can patients, such as those with stroke, be rehabilitated? A lot is being done but there is much scope for research. Rehabilitation should start from the time of admission of the patient to hospital, even when they are in coma. Experience has shown that patients supposedly in coma do hear something of what is said at the bedside, and what they hear is important. When examining or nursing such a patient, it is worth saying aloud words of encouragement, suggesting a reasonable prognosis. The family sitting by the bedside should be encouraged to do likewise. The use of tapes, for example, recordings of the sounds and songs of their origins. As they recover, there should be adequate space around the bed. Pictures, mobiles, sound-tracks, radio or television can help. And the number of staff with blurred roles, keeping the patient clean, passively moving affected limbs, making sure the patient can see around him/her, is vital. They should be sat out of bed when the time comes, moved for a change of view, go down to the gym, have hydrotherapy. Developments are occurring in the use of botulinum toxin in lessening spasticity. With improvement, mental stimulation is important, in short bursts initially but with encouragement to do crosswords, to read or discuss what they see on TV, etc., while realizing that they will tire quickly until their concentration can be built up. Doctors are not necessarily the best motivators for rehabilitation but all the ward staff, from the cleaners and odd-job people to others with more authority, should feel that they can help and have a positive role.

Unfortunately governments are never likely to provide enough money to help all trauma and stroke victims to return to the community or to an active and independent existence. The pressure for effective change comes from litigation, where, for example, the victim of a road traffic accident advised by an expert in charge of his case can obtain sufficient money for the best rehabilitation, home improvements and retraining, supervizing its suitability at every stage.

## Migraine

> I'm afraid. A red hot poker bores through my left eyebrow.
> Stained glass colours dance and shimmer before my eyes, blurring my sight.
> My face, my lips, my head grow stiff and numb, then prickle and stab,
> with pins and needles. Cold terror clutches me, and reeling nausea.
> Oh. Allah! Mohammed! Oh, Mary! Mother of God!
> Undo this strap that tightens round my head.'
>
> Anon.

A neurologist, especially if he has to deal with every aspect of his subject, comes under pressure to run special clinics for parkinsonism, for epilepsy, for migraine, and for many other conditions. These are worthwhile if they are backed by special funding, and if there is a specific project which can be carried out – for example studying tremor and the early response to laevodopa – and if it can be useful in the training of junior staff. But one has to balance this against the fact that one may be giving priority to certain patients whose needs do not require such priority. Migraine clinics have been condemned by some people on the assumption that migraine is a middle- or upper-class disease. There is a decidedly romanticized view of the so-called migrainous personality. Thus Dr Alvarez, an American physician wrote:-

> The prime characteristics of migrainous women are a small trim body with firm breasts. Usually these women dress well and move quickly. Ninety-five percent have a quick eager mind and much social attractiveness . . . many have luxuriant hair . . . these women age well.

The story is told of how a neurologist, hearing from the boy's mother that he had severe migraine, entered the examination room with his screed in full flow . . . 'that an attack is a reminder of human frailty, involving the brightest, hardest working and most obsessional, in short the achievers in society . . .' only to be confronted with a child with Down's syndrome (mongolism). The work-a-day neurologist knows that migraineurs are an exceedingly heterogenous group . . . some have allergies, some have not; some are hyperactive, some are obsessional, some are sloppy; some are brilliant and some are simpletons. In fact, there is a high incidence of migraine with Down's syndrome, possibly related to anomalies in the vasculature and ligamentous laxity at the back of the head.

There is a migrainous constitution whereby migraine can be a life-long disease with different manifestations at different ages. Children may present with biliousness and indigestion (abdominal migraine), cyclic vomiting or headaches associated with nosebleeds; adolescents with paroxysmal headaches, menstrual headaches or basilar migraine. The young adult usually has some respite from head pains but muzzy heads may replace a full blown migraine, which can take the form of a hemicrania such as Kipling had in his early years*, focal attacks with facial weakness, visual loss, numbness or weakness down one side of the body more prominent than the headache may predominate in adult life, and in the elderly vertiginous episodes may have a migrainous basis.

Migraine may also take other forms known euphemistically as 'migrainous equivalents' but may often be more aptly described as 'migrainous metastases' as for example with a patient of mine who illustrates that migraine need not be a straightforward disease.

> Twelve years ago, she had attacks of migraine with muddling of words and difficulty thinking of names. Five years ago she began to have attacks of paroxysmal tachycardia. These attacks have become more frequent and are accompanied by tingling sensations in the left arm and leg and temperature loss in the left foot. She is also mildly dysphasic, especially when reading phrases out to a class.
>
> The attacks begin when she is relaxing or they wake her at night. She is short of breath, then the heart starts beating violently and she has an urge to drink a lot. Her face flushes and she feels she wants to defecate. After a while her heart may slow and this is often accompanied by shivering. With the nocturnal attacks she may wake to find her arms and legs dead (either side or both together) and she has nausea. The attacks occur capriciously, though they come rather more often just before periods.

Migraine is usually thought of as occurring suddenly, triggered by emotion, changes in routine, exertion, or, in about a third of those affected, by foods, tyramine in pickled herrings, yeasts and cheese, betaphenyl-ethylamine in chocolate, histamine in cheeses and drinks, octopamine in citrus fruits, and hydroxytryptamine in tomatoes, pineapples, and bananas. Pre-menstrual migraine is well recognized and people may feel especially lively the night before an attack. Less recognized is the hypothalamic build up which may precede an attack, starting even days before the onset of headache. Increased thirst and water retention, yawning, mood changes and increased appetite with a desire for certain food may occur. An example of

---

*Do you know what hemicrania means? A half headache. I've been having it for a few days and it is a lovely thing. One half of my head in a mathematical line from the top of my skull to the cleft of my jaw, throbs and hammers and sizzles and bangs and swears while the other half – calm and collected – takes note of the agonies next door. My disgusting doctor says its overwork again and I'm equally certain that it rose from my suddenly and violently discarding tobacco for three days. Anyhow it hurts awfully – feels like petrifaction in sections and makes one write abject drivel.

hormonal changes is provided by Pamela Hansford Johnson in *The Humbler Creation*:

> It was true that, for her, the end of an attack was marked by involuntary weeping. These were tears she was quite powerless, with all her iron will, to check; tears scarcely of pain or of exhaustion, but of disappointment that this thing, which had tormented her for years, was never going to leave her alone, or to shorten its course by half an hour.
>
> 'Then you had it yesterday,' said Maurice, sitting down on the edge of the bed.
>
> 'Under control yesterday, even through that awful drive back. But I couldn't handle it this morning'.
>
> Kate had suffered from migraine headaches as a young woman, had virtually lost them during the whole of her happy marriage, had found them again a year after her husband's death. Unlike her sister, she had never been a Christian; once she had tried to be, as a resort against pain, but had found it no good. She felt some resentment towards the God in whom she did not believe because He could not, or would not, check these agonies.
>
> She had spoken to Maurice about them often, as if clinical discussion helped. The day before an attack occurred, she often felt unnaturally well; she had come almost to dread that sense of wellbeing. The moment she began to see in the air tiny dot-and-tail phantoms like germs or tadpoles, constantly dropping down out of the range of her vision, and soaring up into it again, she knew that nothing could help her, that she must go through with it; but she could never keep from hoping that, just this once, she would escape.
>
> She had confessed to Maurice, in a final weakening moment, that, for her, migraine was sometimes associated with violent sexual excitement; that was the worst thing of all. Once or twice she had attempted to ease it, only to find the attack prolonged and herself sickened by self-disgust. Indeed, there was something totally disgusting underlying this misery, something obscene in the remorseless clenching of the blood vessels, the hot blood tumescent in the vein, the triumphant conquest of will by agony.

This account is not far fetched. I have encountered at least six patients who have related similar experiences of sexual excitement and frustration with migrainous attacks; but such experiences are rarely sought and infrequently volunteered.

In an examination of the hypothalamic origins of migraine, associated with hormonal cycles, let-down headaches at weekends, smells, low blood sugar, emotions and altered mood, I felt that an underrated mechanism was the thermo-regulatory system controlling brain temperature during physical exertion. The blood flow to the brain remains stable with exercise and after an initial rise in temperature, there are various mechanisms such as sweating and panting to control the temperature, in animals and man. However, headaches can result from exertion, particularly in unfit people or with short distance races – 200 to 400 metres – whilst long distance runners get headaches if they miss a training session. My view was supported by Otto Appenzeller, who confirmed that endurance 'cures' migraine, but the same athletes who normally run 7 to 9 miles per day at a 7 to 9 minutes pace per mile will, if they miss a day, get a return of the aura but usually enough warning to send them out again for their daily jaunts. He also tested them out at altitude, examining the endorphin system. Others have found, as with mammals and other endotherms, that vigorous forms of activity have the effect of stabilizing cerebral thermo-regulation. Arthur Ransome, for example, used to go on a 30-mile walk to recover from a severe migraine. In his autobiography he writes:

> I was troubled at that time with violent headaches, for which I found walking the best though a painful cure. I used to set out from my studio half-blind with pain and, stumbling resolutely on, would find the pain lessening and at last gone altogether. One day with one of these headaches I set out from the Rue Campagne Premiere and walked out by the Lion de Belfort to the fortifications, when, though I found my headache slackening, the fine spring evening made me unwilling to turn back.

The warning or aura phase of migraine is most easily explained using the vascular hypothesis whereby vasospasm affecting large blood vessels of the external or internal carotid circulation or the basilar artery causes vascular impairment to the eye or part of the brain. This is followed by vasodilation with stretching of the structures around the brain and tension of the scalp and other muscles resulting in headpain. In some patients the two phases can occur simultaneously with swelling of the walls of the blood vessels, narrowing their lumen and allowing kinins and pair-provoking substances to seep out into the surrounding tissues. Migraine is defined as an episodic headache with total freedom between attacks. The symptoms last two to thirty hours, though they may be prolonged by anxiety, depression or tension, and they must be accompanied by either gastro-intestinal (nausea, anorexia or vomiting) or visual disturbances or both.

The initial symptoms may therefore take several forms. A prime, though rare example, is the tête-bêche effect, a term borrowed from philately, when one stamp in a row of stamps is printed upside down. The room is inverted so that people appear to be walking on the ceiling. Charcot, the great French Neurologist, described his own attacks:

> Mon Dieu! It is not surprising that one cannot describe the shock of the scintillating scotoma. Many times I have experienced it. The first occasion

when it happened I had, or thought I had, a firework display in front of me. Only later, from closer scrutiny, did I make out a sort of circle like one of Marshal Vaubain's fortifications with its salients and recesses.

In the USA a truck driver on a five-lane highway developed total blindness during a migraine attack and was guided to safety by a passing car using citizen's band C.B. radio*. An English neurologist described his partial loss of vision when an attack occurred as he was driving in central London. Another sufferer whom I saw described a hemiplegic attack waking him in the night with stiffness and numbness of his right arm and hand and numbness of the right leg lasting 90 minutes. The following year he had an attack with features of transient global amnesia. Following a two-day headache, he experienced a severe shooting pain in his head and his face went blotchy. He went to a shop, cannot remember parking his car and cannot remember the purchase. He came to himself 2 hours later $1^{1}/_{2}$ gallons of petrol short, some miles away, feeling very cold with his vision bad. When he looked at objects, they moved out of focus and floated. He may have had a small stroke, as can happen with migraine, for there was a residual speech impediment and fronto-occipital headache.

In childhood especially, a limb may appear longer or shorter than usual – the Alice in Wonderland or Alice and the Mushroom effect. (Lewis Carroll describes many phenomena which have been judged to relate to migraine, but it is equally possible that his experience came either from 'magic mushrooms' or from photography. He himself had migraine but there are no descriptions from his diaries which suggest that elaborate phenomena were part of his migraine attacks). An example from my practice concerns a 20 year-old lady who was sitting having tea. She stretched out her hand and found that it seemed to have grown. She then found that she could not see to her right and was unable to see her children sitting on the settee. Then the arm, from the elbow to the finger tips, appeared numb and her speech became garbled. The right side of her mouth went dead and gradually the symptoms improved, the thumb being the last to get right. The whole episode lasted 20 to 30 minutes. She then had a headache over the right temple which lasted until the next day.

Linnaeus (1707-1778) had doppelganger sensations with his attacks. The precipitants of his migraine were common enough: the result of drinking a glass of sloe gin, alcohol – sour wine in particular – cold weather, or strong winds, or even a sharp disappointment. He recorded how, through a

---

*C.B. radio can be extremely helpful to handicapped or disabled people unable to leave their homes as a means of contact with others.

gardener's stupidity, some long desired cochineal insects brought back for him from Surinam were destroyed before he could get sight of them. But it was the prodromes of his attacks which were especially noteworthy. He would see a very vivid image of himself, situated in natural circumstances and behaving in a natural fashion. He would enter his study to find his spectre seated in a chair writing or reading. Once he entered the lecture theatre prepared to take his class, but saw someone standing at the lectern and turned away, only to realize he had been looking at an hallucination of himself. Or as he wandered through his garden studying a plant or picking a blossom, he might see some little distance away his alter ego performing the same actions.

There are a few dicta indicative of migraine: a unilateral headache with symptoms down the same side of the body, an attack which wakes the sufferer from sleep, poorly localized pain in the teeth involving half the upper or lower jaw, aphasia combined with dysarthria and numbness of the mouth or lips, a cyclic tendency with attacks either under stress or as let-down headaches associated with holidays or weekends, and a particularly devastating headache after a long interval of freedom.

I have referred to hemiplegic migraine or hemianaesthetic migraine with weakness or sensory loss down one side of the body, the progression of symptoms taking minutes rather than seconds as in an epileptic attack. There would appear to be two types of hemiplegic migraine. One with a family history of simple migraine and the weakness occurring as part of the aura: the other with a family history of hemiplegic migraine and the weakness persisting for hours or days with and after the head pain. An increase in attacks after taking selective serotonin re-uptake inhibitors such as prozac enabled a clear diagnosis to be made of hemiplegic migraine in a Lancashire family in Lancashire, in whom it had previously been unclear whether the attacks were epileptic or migrainous. Before the advent of CT scanning, there was always a problem whether to investigate a person with hemiplegic migraine with angiography and the possible risk of infarction (stroke) as the result of the diagnostic procedure.

Lesser forms can occur such as facio-plegic migraine, when migraine can be associated with a recurrent facial palsy. A common form of migraine seen in adolescent girls and with a strong menstrual tendency was described by Edwin Bickerstaff, a neurologist in Birmingham. Visual phenomena may be negatively described as dimming or loss of vision, or positively as flashes or blobs of light or dark, devoid of colour and so intense as to blot out vision. This stage is rapidly followed by vertigo, a taste at the back of the tongue, clumsiness and unsteadiness, tinnitus, by a speech defect which is undoubtedly dysarthric, and by tingling in the hands and feet, and sometimes around the mouth. These symptoms last 10 to 30 minutes and are followed by a severe headache. At the height of the attack, consciousness may be lost. This is the most common cause of loss of consciousness with migraine but migraine also has the doubtful reputation of causing the most prolonged forms of loss of consciousness, particularly in childhood and in certain families. If I may quote just one example:-

A 21 year-old law student collapsed on five occasions and was semiconscious for hours. The episodes would start with a nodding of the head and rolling of the eyes, which she would try to keep open but would feel generally weak. She felt the jaw receding and as though the jaw and ears were dropping off. Her head felt four metres from her stomach and her arms went as long as possible. When she was semi-conscious after slumping to the ground, she smiled, cried, had mixed emotions but could not speak at all. Beforehand others noted that she went pale and her head went down on to her chest, her hands went cold and she was like jelly. The first episode of loss of consciousness lasted from 10.30 to 3.30, but usually they lasted for about an hour. Coming round, she had a very bad headache and neck pain for several days up to a week. This head pain involved all the head except for the right parietal quadrant, though since going on Prozac she has had an attack in which she has had a sharp pain with a burning sensation shooting across the right parietal region. Her eyes have felt very hot and have fluttered.

She was right-handed, had allergies to cheese, was on the contraceptive pill and complained of indigestion, but was basically well before the attacks and there was no relevant family history. She was tall, quite heavy round the hips, rather pale, tender round the head with a normal blood pressure and negative examination.

The other main theory of the causation of migraine is Sicuteri's central biochemical dysnociception – a disturbance of the endorphin system in the brainstem and elsewhere. This theory, grudgingly accepted as a possible hypothesis, explains attacks with fasting, at altitude, with exercise and with sleep, and the tendency to vomit with attacks. It is presumed that there is a hypersensitivity in certain circumstances to various stimuli.

I do not intend to give a comprehensive account of migraine. Confusional episodes, visual field defects, unequal pupils can all occur during migraine attacks. In the past a condition known as status hemicranicus, where one attack follows another, was described. It is probable that the likely diagnosis was benign intracranial hypertension, a very different syndrome. Rebound headaches, with severe prostrating attacks, loss of weight, sleeplessness, anorexia and depression, are most commonly the outcome of excessive medication, leading to migrainous disability. Severe headaches akin to migraine can occur in footballers due to heading the ball, during sexual intercourse, or following whiplash injury. Headaches with vomiting and migrainous features after a whiplash injury are often more persistent than more mundane post-traumatic head pains. Ice-cream headaches are due to intense cooling of the nasal passages. Ice-pick headaches, sudden sharp pains which are too short-lasting to be accessible to treatment, occur more frequently in migraine sufferers than others, and sudden explosive headaches without other features, though frightening, are usually harmless.

Migrainous neuralgia has many features distinct from migraine. There is a male preponderance. It is strictly unilateral, around, in and behind an eye. It is of agonizing severity, lasting up to 2 hours at a time, but recurring with at least one paroxysm every 24 hours. The timing of paroxysms may be such as to earn the epithet, 'clockwork headache'. Bouts last approximately 6 weeks and may be followed by intervals of freedom for 6 months. Alcohol or smoking may possibly trigger attacks. The eye waters, may become bloodshot and the nose or one nostril blocked. Treatment can be difficult but inhaling oxygen and subcutaneous injections of ergotamines can help.

The treatment of migraine itself can be by avoiding trigger situations. During an attack, pressure at certain sites can help and prophylaxis include yoga, biofeedback and acupuncture. Often an anti-emetic, if necessarily given separatedly, may settle the stomach and permit ingestion of analgesics which are not normally ingested during an actual attack. Herbal preparations such as feverfew, devil's claw and dandelion are effective in many people, but, as with drugs, are not devoid of side-effects.

### Sleep singing, watches and bioelectrical phenomena

Over several years I contributed leaders, signed and unsigned, to the *British Medical Journal* and *Lancet*. I refused to let myself be typecast, stating that I was prepared to take on any stimulating neurological topic. As a result I was also asked to contribute to the B.M.J.'s question and answer column, replying on: the risks of lumbar puncture if a CT scan could not be done, environmental and occupational related factors in Parkinsonism and the Steele-Richardson-Olszewski syndrome, how long to use steroids in temporal arteritis, increased hunger after stroke and loss of appetite after cerebral haemorrhage, household pets, viruses and multiple sclerosis, amphetamines for fatigue in multiple sclerosis, the cause of relapses, atonic bladders and whether multiple sclerosis involving the bladder affects female orgasm.

I also contributed a topic of my own on sleep singing. My father for most of his adult life would sing in his sleep, usually a variety of songs from the musical halls, trumpeting them loudly. There were similarities to Sacks and Kohl's patient with incontinent nostalgia who, given a tape recorder when high on laevodopa, recorded many songs from the musical halls, which she was unable to do when the erethism wore off. A colleague had woken the house singing in his sleep German lieder just before an exam on the same subject and a psychiatrist had sung in his sleep until he married, when his wife managed to stop it. The replies I got back all related to people with various illnesses, whereas I had regarded it as a natural phenomenon akin to sleep talking, dreaming or perhaps sleep walking.

The most unusual question I was asked to answer ran as follows:

Despite increasing complexity in the manufacture of wrist watches, anecdotal accounts that certain people in illness, and sometimes in health, cannot wear a watch without affecting the function of that watch still occur. Is there any scientific basis for this phenomenon?

Lyall Watson in *The Nature of Things* (1990) quotes the replies I received and contributes the example of the reporter, John Gale,

> I am what they like to call a manic-depressive. When I am manic, my beard and fingernails grow faster. In depression, my hair lies down; when I am manic it stands up electrically, catching sensations like antennae. If I am manic, my watch gains five minutes a week; if I am depressed, it loses five minutes a week.

I replied that experts accept the phenomenon exists and that even quartz and pulsar watches are not entirely exempt.

Spring watches may be affected by changes in magnetic fields, temperature, atmospheric pressure, alterations in position, lubrication, and wear on moving parts. Faults may occur from irregular winding; if wound regularly to $1^3/_4$ turns, the balance is less likely to be influenced by the movements of the wearer. Dust or loss of lubrication will affect pivot friction, introducing gravity effects: the watch will go slower when hanging or on edge than when worn dial upwards. Vibration effects, as with thryotoxicosis, may cause inaccurate escapement. Rises in temperature are more likely to cause slowing, due to expansion of the hairspring and watches commonly go slightly faster in winter than in summer. Quartz watches with no moving parts may be influenced by aging or the crystal, thermal drift, and cleanliness.

These recognizable causes do not explain each individual circumstance; anecdotal accounts of altered behaviour of watches in pathological circumstances (during periods of sleep deprivation, hypokinesia, fatigue after arduous exertion, or prolonged emotional stress), temporary changes in the geophysical environment – solar activity, magnetic fields – or even with unusual work/rest programmes appear to share a common factor in alterations in the person's geomagnetic field. Changes may be measured by SQUID (a superconductivity quantum interference device) showing: (a) increased heterogeneity of skin potentials with areas of high electrical conductivity, (b) desynchronized or weakened amplitude of circadian fluctuations, and (c) short period oscillations in sympathetic/parasympathetic tone. The interaction of changes in personal geomagnetic fields and mechanical devices (watches, pacemakers) is poorly understood, with very little hard data available. (I would be happy to receive personal accounts of particular experiences with the wearing of watches in order to facilitate a more scientific inquiry at a later date.)

I am reminded that Salvador Dali's painting, the Persistence of Memory, is based upon a pun – La montre molle – which can mean 'put out your tongue' or 'the soft watch'. My attempt to explain the watch phenomenon resulted in 143 letters giving personal accounts of difficulties with both spring and electronic watches. Only two of the correspondents appeared to have read the original article in the *B.M.J.*: 85 had read the *Times* report, 5 the *Mirror on Sunday*, 1 the *Singapore Straits Times*, 13 the *New Zealand Woman's Weekly*, and 16 the teenage magazine, *Just 17*.

From the correspondence it was clear that the majority of people unable to wear watches without influencing the working of their watch were perfectly healthy. Occasionally several members of the family were similarly affected. Twenty-five healthy children and 77 healthy adults were unable to wear watches and 5 others reported aberration in time-keeping during pregnancy or immediately after childbirth, 2 were able to tell the time of ovulation by the behaviour of their watch, but this experience was not shared by their friends. Depression, anxiety, 'having an affair' and nightmares accounted for 13 reports and 30 were associated with various forms of physical illness, including raised blood pressure 2, changes in cardiac rhythm 4, cancer 5, abdominal surgery 3, and neurological illness 6 – 3 with fits, 1 with multiple sclerosis and 1 with Parkinsonism.

Particular attention was paid to the wearing of quartz watches. These were trouble free in 10 instances, but no better than other watches in 31. Travel clocks (3) and electrical appliances (5) could also be affected when the susceptible individual was in their vicinity but others found that they could carry a watch provided it was on a chain or as children wear a wrist watch, provided they wore some rubber between the watch and their wrist. When wearing electronic watches, two individuals experienced tenseness and one shoulder pain. Three people were unable to wear jewellery without it becoming discoloured and 15 readily experienced electric shocks: 7 stating that they could not wear nylon clothing and 2 that they had blurring of vision when near electrical appliances.

Geomagneticism has been known for a long time and various experiments performed to see whether placing, say a limb, in a magnetic field would speed the healing of fractures. I was also keen to see whether there was a practical way of measuring geomagnetic fields as an explanation of patients' complaints of pins and needles in their limbs in the absence of any alteration in sensory nerve conduction. Unfortunately the Squid apparatus and other lesser types cannot be adapted for this purpose.

**Drug-Induced Neurological Disease**
Napoleon is reported to have said that 'I do not wish two diseases, one nature-made and one man-made', and Voltaire wrote that medicine is the art of putting drugs, of which we know nothing, into a patient of which we know even less. Any appreciation of one's subject should include a very clear knowledge and awareness of the potential adverse effects of the prescribed medications. It used to be said of neurology that there was very little treatment, and my Indian colleague, if he came across a slightly unusual drug which I had prescribed, would comment that it was a South Indian sex potion.

Side effects from drugs do not always relate to overdosage, though too enthusiastic a use of corticosteroids such as dexamethasone can reduce the water content of the brain, thereby permitting the expansion of any collection of blood over the surface of the brain. Inadequate treatment of meningitis with antibiotics can lead to aseptic meningitis and further diagnostic difficulties.

Drugs are potentially exogenous toxins and most clinicians acquire a wide practical knowledge of drug-induced disease. Drug trials and drug legislation cannot anticipate every interaction or unusual response from a particular patient, and it is essential that pharmaceutical research will continue to develop drugs which of their nature cannot be subjected to large trials, in order to combat rare diseases. Clinical potency may need to be offset against a recognizable hazard from undesirable secondary manifestations minimized by anticipation. Powerful modern drugs are inevitably prone to adverse reactions. With commonly prescribed drugs, equal consideration has to be given to therapeutic potency and safety from adverse reactions, i.e. the drug selected should have the least risk of even mild side actions such as drowsiness or nausea. The risk of iatrogenic (doctor-induced) illness can be reduced by recording which drugs are prescribed, their dose and frequency and by documenting in the patient's record known drug allergies, sensitivity to drugs taken in normal dosage, coexistent renal, cardiac, respiratory or liver disease, psychological aspects and any genetic disorder. Even so, awareness of common drug interactions may not be enough to protect a patient with porphyria from a peripheral neuropathy precipitated by barbiturate administration. Similarly, any list of drug-induced effects cannot be totally comprehensive, but may serve to alert the physician to potential hazards with allied drugs or in comparable situations.

Both young and old vary in their tolerance of drugs. For a minority of children the earliest challenge may arise from drugs which cross the placenta from the maternal to the foetal circulation. The result can be respiratory depression, floppiness, or convulsions after birth. Convulsions can also occur in breast-fed babies whose mothers are taking indomethacin. For the majority of children the earliest risk is from vaccination, unmasking any constitutional weakness and given at a time of considerable susceptibility to intercurrent infection met for the first time. It may be very difficult, even if there is a chronological relationship, to prove that an encephalopathy has been caused by a vaccine.

Recognition of particular drug reactions may be helped by noting distinctive patterns of involvement, perhaps causing gastro-intestinal or haematological symptoms along with a galaxy of neurological effects. To establish the toxicity of a drug, a definite association between therapy and the development of toxicity must be shown. The diagnosis is relatively easy when toxicity develops soon after treatment is started, occurs in several patients and its severity is in proportion to the dosage administered. It may be reversible on stopping the drug, but appear again if the drug is inadvertently given on a second occasion. With allergic reactions the toxicity may occur as part of a more generalized hypersensitivity reaction. Finally, the disorder may be produced experimentally, even if overlooked in the original drug trials. Difficulties arise where a drug has been used intermittently with safety for several years before being prescribed on a more regular basis for a different condition. The long term effects of steroids, for example, may be to enhance the risk of osteomalacia, fractures and vertebral collapse. Advances in therapy, e.g. renal dialysis, may require the use of drugs in a new situation and uncertainty arises whether pathological changes are produced by drug usage or by an unusual clinical situation.

One of the worst examples of drug misuse I came across was in a post office worker who, along with other members of the family, developed a viral meningitis. He was admitted to a local hospital where the junior doctor, given the latest antibiotic, chose to give the dose, normally given into a vein, into the intrathecal space around the spinal cord. The patient had a series of convulsions and I was phoned to advise whether it was worthwhile trying to wash out the drug from the spinal fluid. The patient went to Manchester and some months later he was demonstrated by my neurological colleague there, Laurie Liversedge, who showed him a £5 note and placed it under a saucer. A few minutes later he was told he could have what was under the saucer if he could say what had been put there. He was unable to do so. He failed to recover and I saw him at regular intervals. He used a pocket device to remind him of even the simplest task.

Several times a year I would see patients on anticonvulsants who became toxic due to overdosage. Faults might have occurred with prescribing. Thus a patient on Phenytoin 300 mg daily might also be prescribed Epanutin (or Dilantin) 300 mg daily, the practitioner failing to recognize that one is the generic name and the other the pharmaceutical name for the same product. Alternatively, serum levels of a drug may be enhanced by a reduction in weight or fluid loss from a diuretic, altered by other drugs which induce enzymic action, speeding its breakdown or compete, blocking its attachment to blood proteins or to renal clearance. What may also happen is that a patient who takes his drugs irregularly comes into hospital with an unrelated condition and is given the drugs in full dosage. A patient taking an anticonvulsant usually has a fine nystagmus — often a clinical guide to the fact that the drug is being taken — but when toxic, there is coarse jerking of the eyes, unsteadiness (ataxia), and perhaps slurred speech, drowsiness, weakness, and confusion. These symptoms can readily be reversed by stopping the drug for a few days and restarting at a lower dose. It is usually wise to support one's clinical judgment by obtaining a blood level, but over-reliance on drug levels can, of itself, be dangerous. Comparisons between units testing the same samples showed vast variations (up to 40%); thus clinical judgment can be more reliable. However, a drug level can check a patient's compliance. Regular drug levels, taken under the same conditions, can check interactions of drugs as in clinical trials; and as the level approaches the toxic level, the number of fits can actually rise. All too often junior doctors take low blood levels as an indication to add further drugs, whereas the aim of treatment is not to treat a blood level but to reduce and prevent the occurrence of fits. Traumatic events may break thorough any number of drugs and cause an attack.

A less common and less readily diagnosed syndrome produced by toxic levels of the same drugs is choreo-athetosis. This condition is seen most often in those who have had brainstem damage from kernicterus (jaundice of the newborn). They also respond to drug reduction. Blood levels are not an indication of the possibility of long-term effects from the drugs, e.g. loss of cells from the cerebellum.

Although I had written on drug-induced neurological disease, real involvement in this topic arose when we were referred three patients with a rare peripheral neuropathy from the cardiac department of a neighbouring hospital. The patients were all between 55 and 65 years of age and were being treated successfully for angina with perhexilene maleate. They had wasting of the proximal limb muscles and a glove-and-stocking sensory loss. The spinal fluid protein was grossly raised. The condition appeared progressive and despite stopping the medication, one of the patients died.

Perhexilene, which has since been withdrawn, was an important cardiovascular drug whose unique properties represented a major pharmacological advance. In addition to reducing the frequency and severity of anginal attacks, it lessens the likelihood of dysrhythmias and possesses the ability to reduce exercise-induced speeding of the heart rate. It has other useful but less important properties. Unfortunately some patients are slow metabolizers of the drug and after 2-3 months, accumulation leads to generalized weakness with a tendency to stagger. The symptoms disappeared on lowering the dose but reappeared when the dose was increased However, 'these patients preferred to continue perhexilene in spite of this side reaction as they wanted to remain angina free'.

As a result of submitting this report to Bryan Matthews, Professor of Neurology in Oxford, for publication in the *Journal of Neurological Sciences*, I was asked by him to make a major contribution on neuropathies due to drugs in the *Handbook of Neurology*. The *Handbook*, to date, consists of 70 volumes, each of which can, with difficulty, just about be grasped by one hand. I will select some of the more interesting aspects.

Isoniazid, a drug used in the treatment of tuberculosis, is metabolized in the liver, and, like perhexilene, slow acetylation can occur, inherited as a recessive gene. The trait is widely distributed among Europeans and Africans, but almost unknown among Eskimos and Japanese. High blood levels increase the liability to develop polyneuritis and other signs of neurotoxicity. Fortunately we know that the neuropathy of isoniazid is the result of deficiency of a vitamin B6. Similar neuropathies can occur with hydralazine and penicillamine. Vitamin B6 exists in nature in three forms which are interchangeable – pyridoxine, pyridoxal and pyridoxamine. Complexes are formed between pyridoxal and the drugs, resulting in vitamin deficiency if supplements are not given. But pyridoxine overdose or abuse, when health-conscious people, such as the novelist Barbara Cartland, take hundreds of vitamin pills on a regular basis, can also lead to a neuropathy – indeed, one somewhat similar to perhexilene neuropathy, with a high spinal fluid protein, proximal myopathy and peripheral sensory impairment. Another novelist, Agatha Christie, wrote a detective story, *A Pocketful of Rye*:-

> I'd be prepared to bet on what the poison was.
> Indeed?
> Taxine, my boy, Taxine.
> Taxine? Never heard of it.
> I know. Most unusual. Really delightfully unusual. I don't say I'd spotted it myself if I hadn't had a case only three or four weeks ago. Couple of kids playing doll's tea-parties – pulled berries off a yew tree and used them for tea.

Her writings did not stop the development of a plant alkaloid, taxol, derived from the bark of the pacific yew tree for use in the treatment of cancer of the ovary or breast when other treatments have failed but at the risk of a reversible peripheral neuropathy with pins and needles in the majority of patients.

Army service in the Far East meant that I was not involved in the prescription of thalidomide, used as a mild hypnotic for 5 years before its catastrophic embryopathic action caused its withdrawal from the market. Pamela Le Quesne (Paddy Fullerton, to her contemporaries) was the first to report that it could also cause an irreversible peripheral neuropathy. It is probably not widely appreciated that thalidomide continues to be used in dermatological practice for prurigo nodularis, discoid lupus, the vasculitic complications of lepromatous leprosy, pyoderma gangrenosa and colitis. Whereas the intermittent use of thalidomide as an hypnotic caused neuropathy in 0.5% of cases, its continued regular use has increased the incidence to nearly 50%. Its present use is on a named patient basis and carefully weighed against the patient's overall prognosis.

I referred, much earlier, to Pink disease, a marasmic and irritating disease of infants, assumed to be due to a virus or to nutritional deficiencies but eventually shown to be related to the use of mercuric teething powders. In the 1950s an epidemic disease called SMON (subacute myelo-optico-neuropathy) started to occur in Japan, increasing in frequency until 1970, with more than 10,000 cases, after which cases were reported over the Far East and even in the U.K. Like Pink disease, it was initially thought to be due to a virus.

SMON is characterised by diarrhoea and abdominal pain followed by painful numbness of the toes. Sensory loss may then develop, spreading over the lower half of the body and producing an ataxic gait. Half the patients also develop motor weakness in the lower limbs and a quarter some visual impairment. Other disturbances include raised blood pressure, blood cell changes, sugar in the urine and a green tongue. The disease follows a chronic relapsing course in 19%, with persisting painful dysaesthesiae in 93%. The full syndrome is rarely seen outside Japan but may cause an acute confusional state with toxic brain damage, isolated visual loss or a neuropathy.

An association was made with 'travellers' diarrhoea' and possibly the treatment used. In 1970 a ban on the sale of all halogenated hydroquinoles in Japan led to a rapid reduction in the number of reported cases and it was subsequently confirmed that SMON patients ingested clioquinol more often and in much larger amounts than did non-SMON patients. Apparently the Japanese are extremely bowel conscious and given to taking large quantities of medications to settle their digestive tracts. Clioquinol is absorbed from the small intestine and its neurotoxicity depends on decomposition of the conjugated form and chelation with iron and other metals. The chelated form is then taken up by neural tissue, where it produces destructive peroxides. There are many other gastro-facient drugs taken regularly containing aluminium, calcium, magnesium, copper and bismuth and these interact with clioquinol with a tendency to reduce the clinical severity and the risk of motor disturbances. Aluminium-containing drugs modify the risk of visual disturbances but can lead to an unfavourable clinical course in other respects.

After this paper came out, a new syndrome was reported with an old drug. Colchicine has been used for more than 200 years in the treatment of gout with a wider application to several rarer diseases. The well known side effects of colchicine are gastro-intestinal irritability, diarrhoea, loss of hair, bone marrow suppression, and transient mental confusion. It may also contribute to renal failure in gout. For years there has been experimental evidence that colchicine can cause neurological damage but this had never been reported in humans until Kuncl and colleagues in 1987 reported colchicine myopathy and neuropathy. This occurred in a setting of renal failure and with regular standard doses of colchicine taken for six months or more. They argued, convincingly, that in this situation, symptoms are not infrequent but tend to pass unrecognized or are misdiagnosed. There is an intermittent or progressive weakness of the muscles of the upper part of the legs and arms with suppression of deep tendon reflexes. Patients were unable to rise from a chair or lift objects above shoulder height and, on direct questioning, they also described slight numbness in their hands and toes. The diagnosis could be confirmed by chemical tests of muscle enzymes, electromyography and muscle biopsy.

Kuncl identified two reasons for diagnostic error. Patients were assumed to have a uraemic neuropathy due to the renal failure or an inflammation of muscle known as polymyositis. However, not only did the tests confirm their diagnosis, but stopping the colchicine could lead to a reversal of symptoms.

## Motor Neurone Disease and Disorders of the Spinal Cord

I was grateful once again to Professor Bryan Matthews. On this occasion for inviting me to be co-editor with him of the neurological section of the roll-on post-graduate magazine *Medicine International*. He also suggested that I wrote the section on the spinal cord and this was to lead to my editing not one but two textbooks on the subject. I had previously written the section on Motor Neurone Disease for the same magazine. I was pleased to boast that I had written on Motor Neurone Disease when a new colleague, (now Professor) Douglas Mitchell, joined the department. His M.D. thesis was on motor neurone disease, concentrating on rare element involvement, toxicology and epidemiology of the condition. At interviews some of the lay members looked aghast at his C.V., which stated he belonged to the Free Radical Society and another with a Russian name – both related to the investigation of the toxicology of disease. In Preston, his work on the condition was supported by Professor Ian Shaw at the University of Central Lancashire, who is primarily a toxicologist, and they shared Ph.D. students.

Motor neurone disease is a most horrific and lethal condition and I was happy to pass my patients over to him for drug studies, phone-in and other follow-up advice. The diagnosis is for the most part a relatively easy one but, to be absolutely sure and to begin the process of counselling, the patient and his/her family, admission and investigations including muscle biopsy are essential. With Douglas Mitchell I wrote on one of my hobby-horses, 'The explanation and management of neurological conditions'. He needed research funds, not only from the Motor Neurone Disease Association, where he was chairman of the medical advisory panel, but from local charities started by relatives of sufferers. As chairman of the Trustees, I found myself at a village fete introducing on the same platform the host of the Television programme Mr and Mrs and the drag artist, Danny La Rue! I also went to small hotels in Blackpool where the Independent Hoteliers raised vast sums of money for charity and amid the floral hats and elaborate cakes, each recipient had to rise to their feet to explain what their charity did and achieved.

When later I made a definite decision to edit a book on the spinal cord, confirmation of my role as a practical physician, I collected a group of possible contributors and approached the Oxford University Press. They were initially helpful but suddenly baulked at the delay in completing the list and dropped the project. I therefore approached Springer Verlag and their series editor, Michael Swash. He was keen that I had some North American contributors. I agreed but felt that the only way to do it satisfactorily was to have a co-editor. I approached Michael Aminoff, whom I had known when he was a student at University College Hospital. He agreed to provide a chapter but not to edit. Donald Calne, with whom I had seen patients in preparation for membership and was now in Vancouver, also felt preoccupied but suggested Andy Eisen, who proved an excellent choice. He had qualified in Leeds but after a rather inauspicious start in medicine and feeling he was getting nowhere, decided to go to Magill, where he joined the neurophysiological department. After three months his chief said that he was leaving and asked Andy to take over. Professor Eisen is nowadays one of the leading neurophysiologists in North America.

The Spinal Cord had been very much the Cinderella of the nervous system until the advent of non-invasive scanning techniques. There was always the danger of a missed diagnosis and the 'strike rate' of correct diagnoses from the history and again after examination has always been lower than for other parts of the nervous system. Until the advent of MR and CT imaging, the key investigation was the myelogram. The injection of contrast medium into the spinal arachnoid space can theoretically be done in any radiological department but, if the patient has then to be transported a distance for surgery, with the alteration of pressure due to the injection, 'coning' can occur with downward pressure of the brain endangering life. I became particularly aware of this whilst at Maida Vale, where a Senior Registrar had returned from New Orleans, where he had been a consultant, and had got a consultant post at various small hospitals south of London. He had the problem of when to transfer his patients for investigation, losing them in so doing. If he transferred and the investigations were negative, he would lose face; if too late he would be equally to blame. Wisely he obtained another post at the Midland Centre for Neurology and Neurosurgery near Birmingham. We had a similar situation in Lancashire. Patients were seen in regional clinics in outlying hospitals. However, within our unit we had an agreed policy that myelograms would not be done except at the centre and the neurologists would inform the neurosurgeons, allowing them to give their own opinion on the case, before proceeding. They in their turn would try and operate as necessary as soon as possible. Other neurologists elsewhere are far less fussy in this respect and many neurosurgeons are prepared to wait months after myelography before operating.

Trauma to the neck can take many forms. Spearing injuries from head-on tackling in American football can lead to transient quadriplegia. The danger of neck trauma in such diverse sports as trampolining, steeplechasing and rugby union have meant that the governing bodies of these activities have been prepared to alter their rules. Central cord lesions can occur. A farmer was hit on the head in a gale by a chimney pot and sustained an injury to his neck with weakness of both hands and arms, some respiratory distress but very little weakness of his legs. Rheumatoid necks can disintegrate with pannus formation, dislocating the odontoid peg, which can intermittently or permanently impair the circulation of the basilar artery and 'pith', the brainstem and spinal cord. Paraplegia can result from neck or lumbar injuries in the home, with sports, but particularly from road trauma. The recognition and dangers of spinal compression were ably expounded by one of the neuro-surgeons at Preston, Nihal Gurusinghe. Finally the management depends on rehabilitation and functional aids for walking, diaphragmatic stimulation and artificial respiration.

Surgeons tend to be reluctant to operate for radiculopathies of the cervical spinal cord unless a very definite improvement can be foreseen. One such example was that of a deaf blind man of 62 who had progressive numbness of his left hand over 8 years and of his right for three years. As the symptoms progressed, he had further stiffness and limitation of neck movement, so that he was unable to appreciate the presence of other people in the room by vibration of the floor boards. There had been some hesitancy of micturition and a tendency to fall backwards and to the right. His main problem was that of reading braille, which was now too fine for him to appreciate. He tried Moon's type, but even that was difficult. His normal method of communication was using sign language to the left hand. He had to transfer to the right hand, and finally found he could hardly communicate at all. Otherwise his memory and intelligence were good.

He had had an accident at the age of 19, becoming deaf and temporarily blind. There was an initial recovery of eyesight followed by progressive blindness. He had had no other illnesses. On examination, he had no sense of smell, had an artificial right eye and a gross cataract of the left without any pupil reactivity, but a normal corneal response. There was bilateral nerve deafness. He had lost bulk in the right deltoid and infraspinatus muscles. He was unsteady on his feet with brisk reflexes in upper and lower limbs. Sensation was lost to pinprick and touch from the right shoulder to the hand and from the left elbow, with loss of two-point discrimination in both hands. His blood pressure was raised.

There was calcification within various arteries in the neck and the myelogram showed a narrow vertebral canal with numerous disc indentations. He was operated upon with a cervical laminectomy. Objectively there was little improvement in the sensory changes in his hands, but the patient himself was aware of some improvement and was once more able to read.

The spinal cord rarely makes headlines. The severely disabled may be written off as paraplegic or tetraplegic. Little attention is paid to the patient as an individual, his/her personality, drive, abilities. I was able to look at a group of patients handicapped with the most severe disabilities, who nonetheless contribute actively and brilliantly to society and set an example for us all.

## The Motivation of Mouth- and Foot-Painting Artists

My patient is tetraplegic, not even able to bend one finger. Furthermore she has a painful, stiff, virtually immobile neck. She moves from room to room in an electric wheel-chair activated by her chin. Yet she is one of this country's leading mouth-painting artists, whom I have known for 20 years. When I first met her she was walking awkwardly with elbow crutches and accepted the diagnosis of multiple sclerosis with understandable reluctance. She had been a maths teacher and for 4 years tried to continue as a home tutor. An exacerbation of her illness rendered her tetraplegic, wheel-chair bound, with little back or neck movement and no movement of her hands or arms. Recourse to all manner of labour-saving devices did little to hide the practical problems this entailed for her husband and her family.

Unable to leave the house while her husband was working, she became bored. She had been brought up to believe that if you are bored it is your own fault, you must get on with something useful. She had a POSSUM device and taught herself to type using her mouth, making 'loads of mistakes'. She enrolled in evening classes in order to meet people, taking a course on writing for pleasure. Her stories were published. Further stories were asked for but she was not physically capable of the effort required. She started drawing and found this easier.

At this time there was a perceptible change when she visited the out-patient department. Questions concerning treatment and developments in multiple sclerosis became fewer. She was more positive, the liveliness had returned to her face, and she would explain her latest ventures. Later I was to see small, but painstaking and artistic, samples of her work. She made a typically wry comment when sending me an example of her work: 'I thought you would be interested in a new skill I've found. The fastest jaw in the West!' At this stage she sat in an easy chair and had a drawing board attached to a towel rail. She prepared headed stationery, which was shown at a trade fair and came to the notice of the Mouth and Foot Painting Artists (MFPA). She was given a scholarship to attend classes. The classes were a help socially and overcame her reluctance to use colour, but she disliked others bustling about on her behalf, preferring to work unaided as much as possible.

The back room became a studio, uncarpeted so that she could manoeuvre the electric wheel-chair, controlled by movement of her chin on a suitably shaped bar. Her husband designed a mobile easel with an electric motor which she could activate with her brush. At first she used a tiny brush or pen, holding it between her teeth in a cork, but the cork made her teeth go brown and a beechwood holder has proved more suitable.

She had to overcome other obstacles. The neck pain and limitation of movement meant that despite the mobile frame, her paintings were necessarily small. Subject matter was also difficult. Flowers were always a stand-by though they provided a limited choice. Whenever they travelled, her husband would photograph trees, houses, a horse and landau, etc., which she could copy, until her confidence built up, freeing her perspective. She broadened her scope, doing sketches of London buildings for a conference programme. Her husband obtained a turntable from a shop display unit so that she could paint on ceramics. She would meticulously apply gold leaf or blow a pattern with a mixture of milk and paints. Once they met her standards, they were fired on a small kiln.

By now she was meeting and becoming inspired by other disabled artists, feeling that if she tried harder she might just manage to emulate them. Within 5 years her work had developed and she was accepted as a member (partner) of the MFPA. She was able to tell me that she was receiving a regular salary, could set aside any reliance on welfare, and that her husband had taken early retirement to look after her. Besides presenting her own work, she has organized exhibitions of mouth- and foot-painting artists in various parts of the country.

The MFPA has often been criticized as being too commercial in its approach. Its main funding comes from sales of Christmas cards and calenders. Most of the art is conventional, stylised, with a limited appeal to the middle aged and elderly. Artists working under handicap do try for exactness rather than for abstract conceptual designs, though several have also produced more modernistic works. I have been grateful to the Association for allowing me to interview a dozen of its members up and down the country. Most of the members interviewed are well-known, as are their disabilities, and I have their permission to report on their medical aspects. Nonetheless I prefer to record them with alphabetic symbols. For most the MFPA has proved to be a helpful partnership:

> It is a perfect form of patronage. As a student you are helped by a scholarship. As a member you contribute as and when you can to their Christmas and

other outlets. In addition you may exhibit and sell your paintings and you are free to develop your own artistic direction. No matter where you live, you get an equal monthly salary, which makes you independent of welfare.

The stated aims of the MFPA include making contact with all people who are either artists who have lost the use of their hands through accident or illness, and who paint with the brush held in the mouth or the toes; or people who, having been born or become disabled, wish to learn to paint and support themselves through the sale of their work, thus helping disabled artists attain self-respect, creative fulfilment and financial security.

The worldwide Association of Mouth and Foot Painting Artists was founded in Liechtenstein in 1956 by Arnulf Erich Stegmann (1912-84). He developed poliomyelitis when aged 3, losing the use of his arms and hands, attended art school from the age of 15, studied under Erwin von Kormandy, and earned his living as a professional painter from the age of 23. He began as a street artist, sketching portraits of passers-by, pen in mouth, at amazing speed. However he resented coins thrown at his feet and dressed elegantly so that his true worth was realized. He set up his own publishing firm to sell artist's cards and graphic works but was arrested as an enemy of the state when the Nazis came to power in 1934 and spent 10 years in gaol. In 1944 he was forced into hiding. After the War he restarted his publishing company. Combining with other MFP artists whom he sought out, he formed a cooperative with full professional backing to provide commercial outlets for their products, enabling MFP artists worldwide to receive a regular monthly salary.

There can be no greater contrast with my patient than 'A', who runs the MFPA art gallery at Selborne, Hampshire. Selborne was the home of the 18th century naturalist Gilbert White who published the *Natural History of Selborne*. A is very extrovert. A victim of thalidomide, he has full mobility but no hands. At the age of 10 he went to Treloar College at Alton in Hampshire, studied normal subjects for 7 years and decided he could only do art. He then went to the Hastings College of Art to do a year's foundation course, then to Brighton to do expressive art.

He goes skiing and drives a specially adapted car. He took a sabbatical year to work for CRYPT (Creative Young People Together), helping disabled youngsters with artistic talents. After which he taught art at Treloar College. He worked with business in the community and became a student in 1986 with the MFPA. He also did voluntary work with maladjusted children and is buying a property next to the gallery on his own initiative as a disabled workshop.

He is married to an art student and chose Iceland for their honeymoon, attracted by the fact that in Reykjavik there is a National Union of Disabled People with a specially designed building, complete with a bank of carers, compartments for rent, a gym, swimming pool and craft room. He has to meet people and dislikes working on his own. His flexibility and quick movements are very striking and he will demonstrate how he can take a cigarette and light a match using his toes. He takes photographs with a shoulder attachment he designed so that he can work it with chin and teeth. As a painter with a penchant for bright colours, he is equally adept with mouth and feet, but prefers to use his mouth as more exact, using his feet for charcoal drawings as the charcoal does not taste nice.

B was a talented gymnast. He joined the army and served as a physical training instructor before going into show business as part of one of the top balancing acts in the country. Part of his act consisted of balancing by means of his left arm on a table whilst he juggled hoops with his feet and played a harmonica with his free hand. This part of the performance ended with a somersault from the table. Whilst rehearsing in Manchester in 1961, he somersaulted as usual but his foot caught in the ropes of a wrestling ring which had been erected on the stage and he fell, fracturing his neck at C5-6. He had no use of his hands and found his arms atrophied, so that he was unable to drive even with a specially designed steering wheel. However for 6 months he worked at revitalizing his muscles by means of exercises with weights attached to his arms, enabling him eventually to drive as well as an able-bodied person.

At this stage he became a theatrical agent with his brother but he then developed post-traumatic syringomyelia with ascending cavitation of the centre of the spinal cord, making his arms and hands again useless. Around this time someone asked him, 'Did he paint'. He gave up the theatrical agency. With a very positive attitude and the discipline from work as a an acrobat, he taught himself to paint from a book, modelling himself on Constable. He has always liked outdoor scenery, never copies, does several sketches and takes occasional photographs. He takes ideas of trees, etc. from books but never exactly copies. He holds the brush in his mouth and is able to move his neck and mix paints. His canvasses can be large, with 6 or more paintings on the go at any one time. He trained a dog to pick up and fetch for him.

When I saw him 5 years ago he was recovering from a bedsore and he has since died from an extension of his syringomyelia.

C represents a very severely handicapped patient with respiratory difficulties and a story very similar to the well publicized Elizabeth Twistington Higgins of *The Dance Goes On*. At 18 she had an audition for Sadlers Wells but was too tall and took up nursing instead. Two years later she married. However at the age of 23, she developed poliomyelitis, her husband left her, her 2 year-old was adopted by her sister in law, she lost her house and lost her babe stillborn. For 10 years she was in hospital, learning to type whilst in an iron lung. She was later to remarry only to be widowed.

She remained constantly in an iron lung for 2 years and then learned frog breathing, which enabled her to sit in a wheel chair using a Thompson Pneumabeld portable respirator during the day and the iron lung at night. She learnt to use a mouth stick to operate an electric typewriter. As an artist, she was self-taught from school with an interest in ballet paintings and painting animals and birds in oils. She can only hold a brush for a limited time as she cannot breathe while painting. In 1964 she won 1st prize at an International Art Exhibition at the Kennedy Institute in America. She used to take 3 weeks to do a picture, painting in bits as she cannot always reach all of the canvas. But full membership of the MFPA came after 18 years because of continued ill-health. Eventually she was able to write to the authorities to say that she no longer required assistance as she had become financially independent and had even bought her own house. She has two caring assistants and travels by means of an ambulance which takes her chair and respirator.

About the time I saw her, her health had deteriorated; she had fallen out of a respirator after a recent chest infection and hurt her hip. A rotatory iron lung was being used to enable her to receive physiotherapy to her back. Because she was spending more time in the iron lung, she was concentrating on a story about the supposed adventures of her dog, which was stolen and eventually recovered. The apotheosis of her indomitable spirit was shown in 1990 when she had a garden party with a pig roast and buffet for 130 people to celebrate her 33rd year of breathless happiness.

D wears a rugby jersey when painting. He was a carpenter until he broke his neck at C4 playing rugby. The lesion was a partial one, allowing movement of his upper arms. He typed and wrote before taking up painting. In fact for many years he would spend his time idling in the pub until he went for short-term care to a Young Disabled Unit where he was encouraged to start painting. He was never tutored but did attend an Adult Education course for beginners in art. Relatives of a foot painter nearby saw his work and sent to the MFPA and he acquired full membership within $2^{1}/_{2}$ years. He is married to an osteopath and owns his own house, using a workbench made by a friend.

When painting, he uses a gumshield on his lower teeth to hold the stick, putting pins through the paint brushes to hold them firmly and turn them. He tried painting in oils but found the brushes were difficult to clean and the smell of oil and turpentine gave him headaches. Nowadays he uses acrylics and water colours, with a particular liking for snow scenes and trees. Acrylic paints can be mixed with water and have a dramatically shorter drying time. He is mildly red-green colour blind and eschews red where possible. He will take up to 4 months on a work, painting in amazing detail.

E, older than the others, had congenital deformities and despite many operations, had very limited use of hands, arms and legs. His story illustrates the very poor conditions under which people of his era with handicap were treated. When I saw him in his 70s he had bilateral cataracts, was virtually blind in his right eye and virtually immobile. He has since died. He was institutionalised from the age of 3 and remained mainly in orthopaedic hospitals until 14. After many operations, he was fitted with leg irons and taught himself to walk with a waddle. At 17 he entered a poor law institution and at 19 a home for incurables and cripples run by monks in Yorkshire. He taught himself to paint postcards, which he would try to sell for a shilling each, but his mates made fun of him, regarded his pictures as a joke, and would pour water over them. Despite being able to walk a mile, he ended up in a Cheshire home in Hampshire. Here, at the age of 30, he was taught by a reputable artist (an A.R.A.), had to unlearn what he had done up to then, learnt perspective and developed a good colour sense. He became a full member in 4 years.

Despite this background, and even as a child, he always thought 'how am I going to earn money?' He tried to learn French so that he might become an interpreter. Whenever possible, he preferred to paint out of doors and was always pleased to be surrounded by children. He liked raising and giving money to schools and arranged a balloon race to this end. He was particularly pleased (chuffed) when a newspaper recognised his charity, providing £4,000 for a school extension given by a local artist, and making no mention of his disability.

F is a little annoyed at his slow recognition by the MFPA after being a student for 12 years. He regards himself as only 10% disabled but was born with arthrogryposis and after many operations was enabled to walk with a waddling gait but has no use in his arms. He uses his mouth to light cigarettes, pick up a glass, look after the children, change their diapers, and cook for the family. Part of his education was in a normal school. Because his grandfather was an artist, he enjoyed art lessons though he had no ambition to become a professional painter. He had hoped to join other members of his family working in a factory making ejector seats.

He and his wife are upset because the neighbours think they had the house, car and internal decoration from welfare, whereas they paid for it all themselves. He is perhaps the most innovative of the MFP artists. He does anything but portraits, and likes drawing animals and birds in action, e.g. shooting with spaniels. He likes to go night fishing and has an abiding interest in lizards, dogs, parrots, gerbils and chinchillas. He is intrigued by fantasy and futuristic painting, as with Salvador Dali, and will wake at 1-2 am to paint and work for several hours by himself in water colours or oils. He prefers water colours as easier to clean than oils. He has had many pictures exhibited and a rabbit character of his has taken off in Japan. Another of his fascinations is with cars and he is in great demand to customize VW Beetles, decorating them with his designs.

G was advised when at school to go to Art College but went instead into his family's butchering business before becoming an explosives expert in the Army. His accident was caused diving into a swimming pool in Spain. He was the only one I saw who went straight to painting rather than doing writing or typing first. I found him religious, born again, mildly schizoid and depressed. He was, in fairness, recovering from a chest infection. The tetraplegia has rendered him unsteady, for which he wears a support. He feels he has an increased sense of smell, taste and vision, but although he mixes his own paints, the smell affects him. He admits to considerable frustration, which he sometimes works out in paint.

I was mildly surprised to be asked to see H, rather than a better known artist who lived near him. H was a farm labourer and dyslexic, though not unintelligent. He had a motor cycle accident aged 20 with an incomplete lesion at C4 allowing slight movement of his right biceps and triceps. He can even wheel his chair with his right hand and can move his neck well. He was in Oswestry for 14 months and for many years had been unable to sit because of pressure sores and toxicity. There had been a recent fracture to his leg. His balance, like that of G, is poor and his clothes have been carefully cut by his wife so that the support bands do not show.

He disliked reading and would make a fool of himself typing, but now uses possum devices and the computer mouse to provide a word check. He was in a rehabilitation centre for 2 years, where he met and married his wife, a physiotherapist. He spent years watching T.V., very bored and depressed. Eventually, to break the monotony, he would stay in a Cheshire Home for 2 weeks out of every 6. Here he met John, a mouth artist, whom he used to watch for hours, noting his enthusiasm. But he could never paint at school and never thought he could paint. He now has a restricted area, self-designed, with an easel he can raise and lower. Most of his paintings are based on photographs. He has designed a camera platform with elastic bands to hold the camera and uses mouthpieces and washers to take the films. He uses a palate to mix the colours and can clean the brushes himself.

'I' was the one genuine foot-painting artist I met. He did not share the facility of the Danish foot artist able to use a blow lamp with her feet. He was a spastic athetoid with difficult speech, no use in his hands, knock-kneed with an awkward gait and appeared intelligent. From 9 years of age he was anxious to earn an independent living and tried initially working on his father's car, but saw no future as a mechanic. He won prizes for drawings in local competitions and came to the notice of Peter Spencer of the MFPA. He was essentially self-taught but got a further education scholarship to attend art school. He still receives a student's stipend drawing portraits and landscapes. His wife, also spastic, takes photographs.

J did not enjoy school, where he played truant, but was good at painting, woodwork and reading. He worked as an engineer and then in the building trade. But a car accident on ice resulted in a C5-6 injury to the neck such that he can move his arms and hold a cup in his left hand He was in hospital for 9 months, four of which were on traction, and then attended Stoke Mandeville. Before attempting to paint, he tried mending watches and clocks using a spanner in his mouth. He used a mouth-stick to turn pages of a book and later to use a sewing machine in order to make clothes for his children.

He was initially self-taught, copying from books and painting by numbers. He borrowed books on painting from a nurse and took drawing lessons. He painted the tail on a donkey and did a canvas for a village play. Like Edward Burra, he applies water colours and oils thickly on the canvas, tending to paint very much on his own, undisturbed, concentrating on boats and animals. At one stage he poisoned himself with bamboo mouth pieces which were impregnated, but now uses cigarette holders for his pens. He can now afford a battery operated chair and spends much of his time visiting schools on behalf of the handicapped.

**The Spectrum of Mouth- and Foot-Painters**
From the limited group just described, publications of the MFPA and the seminal work, *Canvases of Courage*, it is evident that mouth- and foot-painters necessarily come from diverse backgrounds with differing innate abilities, educational achievements and initial prospects. The varied aetiologies of their handicap fall into three distinct groups: congenital malformation and deformity; acquired and potentially progressive illness, and traumatic injury. Mouth artist 16 congenital; 20 acquired; 27 traumatic. Foot artists 9 congenital, 4 acquired; 2 traumatic.

Despite the obvious diversities, my interviews led me to acknowledge that in most respects they had developed similar aims and motivations, borne for the most part from a shared experience, and often encouraged by their rehabilitation specialists. Those born with deformities were at risk of frank rejection, as illustrated by Christy Brown's biography, *My Left Foot*. All four with congenital deformities asked themselves at an early age: 'how am I going to earn money?' as a means of obtaining self-esteem. For others the initial trauma of their condition led to a reactive depression and required long periods of treatment in a succession of hospitals for secondary infection, remedial operations and gradual rehabilitation to a wheel-chair existence. Despite the activities of occupational and other therapists, all were frustrated by the inevitable boredom of their situation. They concentrated on the use of possum equipment, often by blowing and sucking and only later by means of a mouth-held probe. Few thought they possessed artistic ability.

Many attempted alternative means of employment. The move to art was often accidental, following on the skills learnt wielding a pen held in the mouth. Some took up painting tentatively to while away the time and were self-taught from books. Others were able to obtain expert tuition. Very often they were encouraged to enter local competitions with the result that their achievements came to the notice of the MFPA. Such recognition would lead to financial assistance in the form of scholarships, enabling them to attend art lessons. The prospect of financial stability and commercial support has meant that in most cases those with the necessary ability have preferred to drop other forms of employment and concentrate on developing their talents as painters.

It may be assumed that a necessary prerequisite for the development of their art is that their health should have reached a stable plateau. This would appear not to be the case. Four of the 10 described were in a state of recent convalescence, recovering from pressure sores, a fractured leg, pneumonia, and chest infections and a fifth was awaiting cataract surgery. Often early experiences with oil paints and turpentine near the mouth made them ill and determined their preferences for acrylics and water colours. All but the most agile obtain greater control over their brushes by means of holders.

Painting even a short vertical line with a mouth-held brush is necessarily a slow business. Those with congenital malformations or amputations may have full neck movement and achieve a fluidity which the others find difficult. Others had truncal ataxia and had to be stabilized in a wheel-chair, and one could only hold a brush for a limited time as she cannot breathe freely when painting. A picture may take 3 weeks or even 3 months to complete and may often be done in bits, permitting a section to dry before continuing. The initial aim must be for precision. Those who can paint the biggest canvases have the advantage that a subsequent reduction in scale can minimize inaccuracies, whilst a small picture, if amplified, will increase any inaccuracies.

The traditional outlet for mouth- and foot-painting artists has been the Christmas card and calendar, and most of the artists aid the association with this work. Several not only keep a photographic record of their work, but use photography to provide copy for their art. One can readily identify particular skills, such as the use of perspective through which a particular artist's work stands out. All except Erich Stegmann, who founded the MFPA internationally, avoid portraits. How many sitters would have the patience to model for a mouth artist?

The two most striking impressions from the interviews is their motivation and the mutual help their organization provides. To listen to them talking, singly or as a group, is to eavesdrop upon enthusiasts. Some are by nature extroverts; others must work alone, but none of them show an introverted involvement in their condition as exhibited by Edvard Munch, Frida Kahlo or even Richard Pope (Norwegian, Mexican and Canadian artists). There is little jealousy; rather a mutual respect. They may feel depressed at times and are certainly prepared to reject anything which fails to come up to expectation, but this is not reflected in their art. They accept that recognition depends on high standards, compatible with those of any other artist. They are agreed that their motivation in no way arises from their illness but was probably inherent and developed from their early discipline and training. The development of increasing self-esteem, which is the other aspect of motivation, is a gradual process.

It is, of course, relatively easy for the more mobile to be expansive but others are outgoing in different ways. A positive attitude to their art is seen among those who are students as well as among full members. They also have a degree of financial stability and are able to do much without recourse to welfare. There are probably some students who will never be able to qualify as members. Early success in competitions or in having a rabbit character accepted for sale in Japan does not guarantee rapid advancement. One of the finest artists had to wait 18 years. Clearly there will always be controversy as to what constitutes an adequate standard, but it does not appear to impair the essential motivation of the artists.

## Sarah Biffin

I became intrigued by the medical story of Sarah Biffin, the first known British mouth-painting artist, born in 1784 with only residual proximal portions of her arms and legs. We normally associated phocomelia with the embryonic effects of the drug thalidomide but phocomelia can arise as a genetic defect or secondary to other drugs, toxins or infections about which little is known. My curiosity was aroused by such questions as her survival at that time, her means of locomotion and manner of painting and eventually the cause of her death.

I was not alone in my research. Far ahead of me was a retired teacher, Winifred Laybourne, who was a member of the Dickens Society. Sarah was mentioned three times in his novels:-

*Nicholas Nickleby*, chapter 37. (1839)

Mrs Nickleby makes her classic reference to the 'gentleman in the next house'. There can be no doubt that he is a gentleman and has the manners of a gentleman, although he does not wear smalls and grey worsted stockings. That may be eccentricity, or he may be proud of his legs. I don't see why he should not be. The Prince Regent was proud of his legs and so was Daniel Lambert; he was proud of his legs. So was Miss Biffin. She was — no, added Miss Nickleby, correcting herself, 'I think she had only toes, but the principle's the same'.

*Martin Chuzzlewit*, chapter 28. (1844)

Mr Pip repeats what 'the Viscount' had said to him. 'There's a lot of feet in Shakespeare's verse, but there aint any legs worth mentioning in Shakespeare's plays, are there Pip? Juliet, Desdemona, Lady Macbeth, and all the rest of 'em, whatever their names are, might as well have no legs at all, for anything the audience know about it, Pip. Why, in that respect they are all Miss Biffins to the audience, Pip.'

*Little Dorrit* chapter 18 (1857)

Mr Merdle came creeping in with not much more appearance of arms in his sleeves than if he had been the twin brother of Miss Biffin.

I also found a quotation in *Household Words* volume V, p. 119 concerning pottery.

How when a figure shrinks unequally, it is spoiled — emerging from the furnace a mis-shapen birth: a big head and a little body, or a little head and a big body, or a Quasimodo with long arms and short legs, or a Miss Biffin with neither legs nor arms worth mentioning.

It is possible that Dickens had met Miss Biffin. There are several possible venues: London, Liverpool, but perhaps Brighton is the most likely. He had a vast circle of artistic friends and went out of his way to meet oddities such as the dwarf, 'General' Tom Thumb and three deaf and dumb children: Laura Bridgman, Oliver Caswell and Sophy. At one stage he must have lived close to Miss Biffin in London, and could have visited her later in Brighton or Liverpool.

Sarah was born in East Quantoxhead in Somerset. In the course of my researches I wrote to the Rt. Hon. John Biffen*, who kindly put me in touch with his old tutor, John Lawrence and his wife, Berta Lawrence, a Somerset author with scholarly works on Coleridge and Wordsworth. The word 'biffin' is the name of an old and excellent variety of kitchen apple, often sold in a dry and flattened state with a red colour; from beefin – ox for strength, referring to the apple's colour. Partridge also gives other meanings from about 1840: an intimate friend or old fruit; cf. ribstone (a cockney form of affectionate address) and piffin.

The village of East Quantoxhead is one of the most picturesque and best preserved villages of the North Somerset coast, associated with the Luttrell family from the Norman Conquest. Berta Lawrence in *Quantock Country* places Sarah's birth in idyllic surroundings in one of those thatched cottages that have a tiny footbridge spanning the stream outside their gate. In fact, her birth took place above the village near the highway from Bridgwater to Minehead, where there were two small cottages with mud floors and thatch, and a common entrance passage between them. Today, they form one house, Townsend House, and a sign on its walls indicates that before the Second World War, it had provided board and lodging for members of a cycling club. Further up the hill, adjacent to the highway on the opposite side, was the farm belonging to the Luttrell estate where Henry Biffin, Sarah's father, worked as a labourer.

We learn that Sarah was baptized within a week of birth, was of a lively happy disposition. She was intelligent, with surprising independence and ability not only to draw and paint, but to perform tricks with needle and thread. She could even tie knots in thread with her tongue, sewed with extreme neatness, and cut out and made her own clothes.

In her early teens she received her first lessons in art from a Mr Emmanuel Dukes, and in return gave him a written agreement to remain with him for 16 years and to travel around and exhibit her talent and herself – she was only 37 inches in height – at country fairs and circus side-shows. At the age of 15 she appeared at Bartholomew Fair in London. Her act consisted of signing her name, making small landscape drawings, and, for an extra three guineas, painting a miniature portrait of the customer. She had a long-handled pen and brush which she scooped off the table with her tongue, and putting the end under a pin on the top of her right shoulder she then used the pen or brush by moving it with her lips. When not in use, her pens and brushes were slipped into loops on the shoulder of her dress. Her

---

*Another Sarah Biffen, wife of John, was at one time secretary to my cousin, Sir Julian Critchley M.P.

performances were all the more exhausting because they were given in front of a crowd of spectators to prove that it really was all her own work. It seems that she was treated with the utmost kindness by Mr and Mrs Dukes, but a good deal of indignation was aroused when it came to light that she received only £5 a year in salary in addition to her keep.

The next stage in her story is that nine years later, once again at Bartholomew's Fair, the Earl of Morton, Chamberlain of the Queen's Household, stopped to watch her and was so impressed that he ordered a portrait of himself. He thought it possible that there was some trickery about the whole business, so after each sitting, he took the miniature away with him. Finally convinced of Sarah's talent and delighted with his miniature, he showed it to King George III. The King was very philanthropic where the arts were concerned and touched by the exploitation of Sarah. He commanded William Marshall Craig, one of the best miniature painters of the day, to instruct her. Although she remained with the Dukes for the agreed 16 years, she was awarded a medal by the Society of Arts in 1821 for her delicate, beautifully coloured miniatures and was patronized in turn by George III, George IV, William IV, Queen Victoria and the Dutch royal family. She later moved to Liverpool, where she had many patrons. It is probable that she had planned a journey to America from there, but she died in 1850. In later life she appeared as an educated person, thus William Holland, in his *Diary of a Somerset Parson* (1817), states that she spoke very well and sensibly.

I wish to paraphrase the main aspects of her medical history. For a child with a serious deformity, born in the 18th C, to have survived much beyond her birth must have been something of a marvel. Many a midwife of that period would have ensured that she did not do so. Everywhere, with the possible exception of Wales, even the birth of twins was regarded as an abnormal event. It was assumed that one twin had been fathered unnaturally. Deformities and monsters were regarded as auguries or portents of potential evil. The likelihood is that the birth occurred unattended: quick, easy and very probably unanticipated. Mrs Sarah Biffin was already 37 years of age and although she had two further children (5 in all), an early menopause was not uncommon and presumably was thought to be the cause of her amenorrhoea.

A possible clue to her survival is that she took the same name as her mother. Had the mother entered a phase of puerperal depression and the worried husband insisted that nothing be done to avoid upsetting the precarious health of the mother? Alternatively, it is possible that a young child saw the babe and took to it as a doll, making it even harder for those who felt otherwise to ensure that it reached God's care without too much fuss and bother. The mother could have had strong, perhaps unusual, religious beliefs, or the vicar might have pronounced on the birth ensuring that no harm came to the child. Almost certainly the child was recognized in its early years as a burden which the parents, and possibly the wider community, could ill afford to maintain. They were probably glad when the Dukes took over her future care.

We do not know precisely about her limbs except from portraits and observations, many of which were possibly inaccurate. One writer who referred to an article in *The Lancet* in 1891 of a similar person comments that:-

> probably she had some vestige of the lower limbs, but did not use them to any great degree. Still, to judge by the experience of others since her time., if she had feet of any kind she would have used them to bounce herself into a sitting position. She must have continually surprised her family by demonstrating some new accomplishment they would never have dreamt of teaching her; rolling along the floor . . . possibly bouncing herself along.

My own views, again dependent on others with similar problems, are somewhat different. She was born with short stubs of arms and legs. Her tiny spine would have possessed serpentine mobility and probably remained subtle until the last years of her life, when she became chubby with increased intra-abdominal fat. As a child she may have been able to wriggle along the floor, sit upright unaided, or bend double to lift an object off the ground with her tongue. We do not know the shape of her vestigial legs. Did they span out with her buttocks to provide a stable four-cornered rest, or were they slightly below her buttocks, necessitating a compensatory adjustment of her spine to achieve a balance? Such factors come into consideration when we discuss how she handled a brush or pen. The varied accounts are by no means straightforward.

> She must at first have held pencil or brush in her lips, but a self-portrait in her middle years shows Sarah with a brush slung or hooked to her shoulder, and a circular advertizing her as a skilled painter of miniatures stated that 'she executes her drawings by her shoulder with the assistance of her mouth.'

She may well have changed her method in later life, perhaps persuaded by William Craig. The use of the shoulder would obviate the risk of poisoning herself with the oils and turpentines needed for miniature painting. Movements of the shoulder independent of her trunk or neck could have been more stable than movements of her tongue or mouth if her balance was in any way precarious. What is difficult to understand is the suggestion that the end of the brush was firmly held by the pin on her shoulder and the movement of the brush on the surface to be painted then executed by control of the middle of the brush by her lips. Such a posture would necessitate holding her head at angle to the portrait. Her tongue would certainly be free from contamination by the paints, and there would be no means of counteracting any inadequacy of balance. I venture to suggest that all her life the more delicate brush strokes were performed by her mouth and lips alone but that some of the lesser strokes could be achieved by shoulder movement directing the brush.

Lastly, her mode of death: in her sixties, 'age overtook her, exertions of extraordinary kind grew painful and she fell into poverty.' Late self-portraits suggest that she was putting on weight with subsequent loss of mobility. almost certainly breathing became difficult and after a longish illness she died in the autumn of 1850 aged 66 years. Her death certificate gave the cause of death as Disordered Stomach, Breaking up of the Constitution. From what is known of the associated defects coexisting with phocomelia, and the little evidence we have concerning her medical condition, with laboured breathing in the latter stages, a reasonable supposition is that she had a congenital weakness of her diaphragm with resultant herniation of the abdominal contents upwards into the thorax, presumably pressing on the left lung.

I sent a copy of my article on the mouth- and foot-painting artists to various people thanking them for the help I had received. In return I received a letter from Col. Walter Luttrell, who said he was particularly interested in my reference to Arnulf Erich Stegmann.

> Before the war my mother returned from Germany with a remarkably accurate drawing (pen and sepia ink) of our coat of arms which had been done 'by a German artist with no arms the pen being held in his mouth'. More than that she did not know, having just spotted it – to her great surprise – in the window of a picture shop. I wonder whether by any chance it had been done by Stegmann, and if so why he (or any other German artist) had decided to draw the quite intricate coat of arms of an English family! I left the picture at Dunster Castle when I gave the place to the National Trust.

PART III

# WIDER HORIZONS

### Examining for Membership

NEUROLOGISTS SEE PEOPLE at two levels: a medical discipline dealing with both homo and sapiens. People are seen mechanistically with respect to their physical state, how intact or otherwise are their nerves, blood vessels, sense organs and vital functions. They are also examined with respect to their capabilities, their higher functions, intellect, behaviour, thoughts (abstract and concrete), sensibilities, volition, expressive abilities – facial expression, warmth to others, executive skills in speech, writing, manipulating machinery, or self-expression through the arts. Notice is taken of their self-esteem, stability, ethics, aesthetic sense, drive, empathy and mood. Neither level of observation can be neglected but the balance may vary. I have always been attracted to the cerebral, but the more mundane form the basis of most of my everyday practice and I have been happy to write, perhaps increasingly so with time, on topics such as coma, spinal cord compression, subdurals, carpal tunnel syndromes, trigeminal neuralgia, function of the autonomous nervous system and the liver.

We are also required to run our departments, plan for the future, make sure that the investigations are appropriate and helpful; and cooperate with our colleagues and with the administrators trying to make sense out of directives from above. Thus, a consultant is increasingly involved with administration and in committees. I have spent years on administrative committees, research committees, post-graduate committees, ethics committees locally, and with regional and national committees mainly concerned with neurology. I was also elected to the Council of the Royal College of Physicians to serve for three years. On the revered council, still run on masonic lines, one is very much the small fry. The elected members sit at the far end of one table, away from the top table of President, Registrar, and Treasurer. There are other officials – Censors, Vice-Presidents, College Officers, Heads of Faculties more highly placed, and three years allows one to have a listening brief, rarely to be in a position to say something worthwhile. The grass-roots opinion is better presented, better stated, more vigorously said, by the committee of regional advisers. What I was able to observe was the excellent response, particularly by Dame Margaret Turner-Warwick working singly and through the joint colleges, to the political pressures placed upon the medical profession. No white paper was allowed to ignore medical training and the essential freedom of clinical opinion.

I was surprised at the end of my time on the College Council, perhaps because I had not thought seriously of the possibility, to be asked to be a membership examiner. This meant examining in general medicine as well as in neurology. There is, in every speciality, considerable overlap with other aspects of medicine; but there are also domains unexplored since one's early training, even sometimes since one's pre-qualification training. I found that my general medical colleagues examined on the neurology they learnt as an undergraduate, omitting such topics as cervical spondylosis*, neuropathies, therapy or imaging techniques which have developed since. I can only assume that I behave similarly with respect to general medicine. Certainly aspects of immunology, renal disease and endocrine gastro-enterology have developed enormously yet have had little direct bearing on neurology.

> Now Eli was ninety and eight years old and his eyes were dim and he could not see, And the messenger said Israel has fled. And it came to pass when he made mention of the ark of God that he fell from off the seat backward by the side of the gate and his neck brake, and he died; for he was an old man and heavy.

But the U.K. colleges were keen to have neurologists aboard, especially those working in District General rather than specialized hospitals, who could examine both general medicine and neurology. I noticed that those chosen had mostly written textbooks in their subject. Perhaps they were chosen because writing a textbook on neurology also entails revision of those aspects of neurology which overlap with general medicine. Some examiners believe that one should never examine on one's subject, but for the reasons I have stated, I believe that one should mix one's questions, aiming at the same level of knowledge by the candidates across the board.

There are six examiners for the clinical at each hospital. On my first occasion the local examiner was an old friend with whom I had looked at membership cases in the past. As a novice, I was paired with the senior examiner. There is also an examiner from the Scottish colleges. Candidates firstly take a 'long case' i.e. a patient with a full history whom they also examine in detail and are given plenty of time for this purpose. Such cases are rarely discriminatory. They enable the candidate to settle. However quite a depth of specialized knowledge may be required of candidate and examiner. The short cases, covering several body systems: cardiology, chests,

---

*Except for certain people in the medical profession, cervical trauma has been about a long time. 1 Samuel 4 v. 15 and 18.

abdomens, rheumatoid diseases, neurology, and skins, have changed little over the years and the techniques required are those I learnt when I took membership. Endocrine diseases, though often shown, are usually too clear-cut to be of value at this level. Eyes – looking at fundi (the back of the eye with an ophthalmoscope) – can be difficult; though if the patient has had laser treatment, it is almost certain that the underlying disease is diabetes. However, a diabetic fundus can be useful as an examination test if the question asked is 'Here is a patient with diabetes who has come up to the clinic for routine reassessment of his eyes. What can you see and what needs to be done?' Candidates may also be asked to treat a collapse or cardiac arrhythmia on a dummy, commonly known as Resuscitation Annie! Properly used, this can be a most revealing part of the exam. The short cases are still the major discriminators – pass or fail. Lastly there is a viva, done after the clinical cases in England but separately and even before the clinicals in the Scottish colleges. One used to start by checking how a candidate is likely to deal with an emergency and then to test their wider knowledge. Lately this part has been revamped so that one must spend time checking on statistics, ethics, communication skills or social issues. The result is that the viva score has less and less impact on the final decision whether to pass or fail.

I am not giving away any secrets in stating that both examiners mark each part of the exam independently before comparing scores and reaching a common mark. We are told whether we are doves or hawks after the exam and how close to the mean our marking has been. I have always been very slightly dovish; which is quite gratifying when one returns to an exam after many years. But I have argued against the marking system which favours the higher-marking examiner. My reason is that those who are the more generous are often those with the least knowledge of the topic asked, and assume that the candidate is giving a correct answer, which may be far from the truth.

The exam system is not ideal. All examiners are anxious to get away from the old system whereby approximately 40% of candidates fail part one, and 40% of those taking the second part also fail. Bad fails on a second occasion are often counselled and a further attempt delayed. To my mind, especially realizing the expense of the exam, no candidate should ever attempt it without going on a course first. Many with knowledge fail themselves. When this is purely through nerves it is a great pity. It may be that nerves have caused them to make up signs which do not exist or over-interpret other signs. This is perhaps a failing which they need to eliminate to be safe clinicians. There is the occasional candidate, who may be extremely knowledgeable, who is failed because the patient is handled roughly.

For the examiner the exam is a learning occasion, not just seeing how another hospital handles patients. Examiners, to my mind rightly, obtain CME points for examining (CME = continuing medical education). The process can be tiring, examining twelve candidates each day for three and a half days; though in the past the exam apparently lasted a full week at just a few centres in London. We arrive before the candidates. We learn the layout of the patients in the ward. We meet, introduce ourselves and examine the long cases first thing in the morning and again in the early afternoon. We then see and examine the short cases and meet to discuss the merits of the physical signs. The best patients are often those admitted acutely to the ward but if their condition is unstable, so that they may need urgent treatment or are not fit enough to be examined by several candidates, they are returned to their ward and alternative patients are found. One patient, I remember, had a hypoglycaemic attack and started to undress and walk out. Other patients, usually from outside, may have lost their physical signs by the time of the exam. Patients will have given up their time to come and do so voluntarily to further medical training, so that one cannot just reject an individual because the physical signs are not good enough. Therefore it becomes the duty of the host examiner to find something to examine every patient on so that he/she is not ignored. Occasionally, however, this can prove disconcerting for the candidate. Patients may also arrive with totally different signs to those described in the examiners' crib and discussion between examiners is vital. Many examiners will examine a short-case patient before checking with the case summary to make sure that the presentation is a fair one for the candidates. On one occasion a difficult neurological patient arrived late. I had to demonstrate the physical signs in front of the other examiners and it was then my duty to examine straightway on that patient or he would have been ignored. I doubt whether the majority of candidates know how well, or otherwise, they have done when they have completed the clinical examination. There are good reasons why candidates should not judge their success by the number of patients they see.

With a short case, the neurologist can be at an advantage. A patient does not need to have good physical signs to be a good examination case. To watch how a candidate examines the cranial nerves or does the reflexes, especially the ankle jerks, may be sufficient to tell his ability. Over enthusiasm in checking for 'clonus' could be grounds for failing a candidate. However it is rare for a candidate to be failed on just one system of the body.

Over the years I have been a host examiner more than once, a senior examiner, and on three occasions have been representative of the London College in Scotland. I was also asked to give an after-dinner speech at the conclusion of a membership course in Rochdale. A little wit was attempted, describing the candidate for the Irish membership, who wrote in asking to be passed on this occasion as he had written the best selling book on how to pass the membership! I was also asked by a female candidate how one should dress for the exam. Smart and conventional is the correct answer; but I was reminded of the Oxford finals when undergraduates wore black 'subfusc'. For the written part the girls wore dowdy clothing: for the vivas some wore low cut evening dresses!.

There is a sexist story about a candidate being asked, 'What are rheumy eyes?' 'Bed-roomy eyes?' she replied. One examiner of old had a glass eye which he would take out and clean or even drop on the floor if dissatisfied. He once asked a candidate which was his false eye. How could you tell? Because it had a hint of kindness! (Surely the story is apocryphal). Eye prostheses can be easy to tell or quite difficult. I will use patients with false eyes when teaching for membership but not in the actual exam. Apparently it is not on to use such a patient in ophthalmological exams. Another examiner who regarded himself as a friendly and mellow creature – and mostly he was just that – videoed his own performance in an exam, only to realise how aggressive he was in his questioning. The story is told of a candidate who had failed many times complaining that he always seemed to come up against the same examiner. On checking his complaint, his statement was verified, but the particular examiner had passed him on each occasion.

Being a host examiner has its own stresses. One works in conjunction with a senior registrar who helps find cases from one's colleagues. This is more difficult if one is a neurologist and works separately from the general medical wards. Unless patients have been used repeatedly for a course, they are usually very willing to oblige and take part. Not only is it necessary to have 90 or so patients ready, plus possible reserves; one has to decide whether the patient's signs etc. are testing at the correct level and how discriminatory they are. Certain diagnoses are so often found in the exams as to be of little value and are best avoided. A host examiner is probably asked to examine from his own base on alternate years. Finding suitable patients should theoretically be easy, using one's previous list, but it is quite surprising how many patients have moved elsewhere, died, or no longer have symptoms or signs of even a chronic condition.

The examination has been extended so that the MRCP (U.K.) can be taken in Hongkong, Singapore or Malaysia, with a regular interchange of examiners. Other countries such as India, now prefer to run their own examination (D.M. in a speciality) rather than a parallel exam to that in the

U.K. But more and more of the candidates are female and more and more from abroad. It is disappointing when an overseas candidate can answer brilliantly on a rare topic such as Creutzfeld-Jakob disease but gives a weak response when asked about the association of poverty and ill-health. My co-examiner was flabbergasted after four successive candidates appeared to have no social feel for their background.

The senior examiner has the task of seeing that all the candidates get their full allocation of time, that the marking system is understood and adhered to, and that he or she passes on the results to the college each day and attends the college to discuss the overall results and who needs counselling before future exams. With each part, unless the candidate has done particularly well, the examiners will have written comments on their performance.

Devising questions can be fascinating. I had one where a solicitor rings the consultant. A client is in his office wanting to sue a fellow rugby player who stamped on his face in a match. The solicitor is concerned because the client is grimacing continually and speech is becoming more and more difficult – possibly the onset of tetanus. Another examiner has a question about his fellow examiners going for a gourmet meal at a foreign restaurant. One collapses during the meal, another 4 hours later, another 24 hours later and a fourth 4 days later. What are the possible causes? I have asked the same question on more than one occasion to see what responses I could elicit: describe a medical emergency which in your opinion is poorly managed?

One 29-year old patient of mine was the source of several taxing questions. Her story began in March. When she was travelling around a bend in a car, the door opened and she nearly fell out. She developed weakness of her right side, which she ascribed to this accident. She then started to develop difficulty with speech and ataxia. She was admitted to another hospital. The MR scan suggested multiple sclerosis and she was given a three-day course of intravenous methylprednisolone with some initial improvement. However, within a week she relapsed with bilateral weakness and ataxia. The scan was, if anything, more positive but a further course of methylprednisolone did not help. She continued to deteriorate with swallowing difficulties and was admitted to us in June with a provisional diagnosis of atypical M.S.; tests for vasculitis were negative and our MR scan confirmed the diagnosis. Once again there was a poor response to steroids and she was given a course of cyclophosphamide. In July she deteriorated still further, despite steroids, cyclophosphamide sulphonamides, antibiotics and fungicides at various times. The pattern of lesions, both from the scan and clinically, appeared to involve the brainstem predominantly. She lost speech (aphonia) and respiration was irregular at times with apnoeic episodes. At this stage we felt under pressure how to continue medication, Her husband, a theatre technician with some medical knowledge, was extremely anxious and worried especially by our use of cyclophosphamide. We called in a professor from Glasgow as a second opinion. He agreed with our differential diagnosis but favoured a vasculitis, commenting that the plaques did not appear typical and were situated mainly in the brainstem. In view of her aphonia we decided to test the C4 count, which was zero, and it was clear that she was suffering from Aids. We confirmed with an HIV test and explained matters to her husband. Further scans suggested that her demylinating appearance was most probably due to progressive multifocal leukoencephalopathy caused by the JC virus (not Creutzfeld-Jakob) in immuno-compromised patients. We had effectively tried her on all the correct treatments but failed to stop the disease progression. She was transferred to a hospice at the husband's wish, where she died.

From the husband, who cooperated very fully, we learnt that she had had a candida infection of her throat in the previous October. She had been married in Spain – although she was to all intents and purposes English – she had two children there, aged 13 and 17. Her first husband had left her, his whereabouts unknown even to the Spanish grandmother. The questions were of an ethical nature. Were we correct in proceeding to HIV testing? Clearly yes. What risk was there to the second husband? Would it affect his work? The risk of transmission from wife to husband is low, approximately 20%. In fact he was negative on testing and agreed to a further retest six months later. What then about the children? What must they be told?. We felt that contact could be made via the second husband and grandmother; that they need not know full details but they should be tested as for visa requirements. The purist would probably not accept our approach but it is always useful to present candidates with a true-life situation.

The other part of the exam is written: straight MCQs for the first part and more complex short answers to case-histories or to picture quizzes in the second. The pictures used to be displayed on screens at certain centres but are now much more accurately reproduced as photographs. Groups of examiners meet in different rooms in the college to correct three or four of the questions from all the candidates. This is a fascinating procedure. The clarity of the question is discussed. How it might be improved in future. The accuracy of the answers given by the setting panel is checked and the marking possibly altered. A test group of – say – 50 papers are then marked and any queries discussed; after which the rest of the papers are marked, always checking an unusual answer with the other examiners. The thoroughness of this procedure is impressive.

Once retired, one's value as an examiner diminishes with time. But one is often given the perk of examining for the Irish MRCP, either in Dublin or Belfast. I did so in Belfast. This was my second time there and the atmosphere was so much easier although there had been bombs outside the Europa Hotel. I flew, as before, from Blackpool to the harbour airport, Belfast being one city where it is possible to land near its centre. The flight, however, was extremely bumpy. The one hospital still heavily guarded and protected was the Royal Victoria, but others seemed to require no protection. The examiners, as expected from both North and South, were delightful people as were the patients. Patients normally take an interest in the exam and often indicate to their friends how they feel each candidate has done, usually by means of thumbs up or thumbs down. One old man, a 90-year old with aortic stenosis, said as the candidate was about to leave: 'I haven't had a winner all afternoon' My fellow examiner was quick to point out to the concerned Indian candidate that the patient was watching the horseracing on his TV!

But a retired examiner, like an admiral, can still be called on to perform a further duty. I was initially asked to examine in Khartoum in 1998 as External Examiner for the M.D. Sudan. This journey however was cancelled by the Royal Colleges on advice as President Clinton had fired a missile at a factory just north of Khartoum. A later visit was cancelled because there was insufficient time to get visas, etc. This October, with adequate warning, I was ready to go but the weekend before I still had not received any tickets and frantic faxing was required. On the Tuesday I was told I would have to go to London to get my visa (I had already received a faxed copy). Fortunately there came a further fax stating I would collect my visa on arrival. Without this fax, I would never have been allowed on the aeroplane. The journey was uneventful although the plane from Frankfurt was apparently overbooked. And all was well when I was greeted on arrival. Within six hours I was examining.

The Royal Colleges are anxious for countries to establish exams which can be considered to be the equivalent of membership rather than cause them to come to Britain to take membership at the risk of being lost to an underdeveloped country. The MD Sudan is one such examination and for those wishing to take the membership also, it gives exemption from the first part. Despite the fact that there is a civil war going on in the far south of Sudan (Sudan is the largest country in Africa), the colleges felt that such cooperation is a force for peace, and there are signs that Muslim fundamentalism in Sudan is on the wane and that a more democratic regime is likely to develop naturally.

My co-examiners had all spent on average four years in the U.K. taking membership, often doing higher exams (an MD) or research. concentrating on units in Bristol and Newcastle. However, links with Britain had lapsed over the past 7 or so years. Women were well represented both among the examiners and the candidates and tended to wear a head-dress, but I found no one, medically or on the streets, using yashmacs. The difference from membership was that the MD was regarded as an exit exam, enabling the successful candidate to work as a consultant. There was, as expected, an emphasis on tropical conditions and there are well planned programmes in place for tackling these problems but finance is lacking.

I have a favourite question: what condition in your opinion is inadequately treated and why? My co-examiner answered 'malaria'. Khartoum is once again a malarious area because DDT is banned from use and the situation is compounded with drug resistant forms. TB is also rife, with HIV infected individuals and drug resistance. A condition causing concern and the subject of a seminar I attended was Rift Valley Fever, which from time to time spreads across Africa and has recently crossed to Yemen and Saudi Arabia. As one professor put it, viruses need no passports and mosquitoes no airline tickets.

A delightful aspect of the examination was a two-and-a-half-hour trip on the Nile with the successful candidates and their children, together with the examiners and those who had prepared the examination.

**Aspects of Art**
Medical aspects of art attract many doctors with numerous points of interest. Additionally, it provides the opportunity for doctors, brought up on rote learning, to acquire a feeling for culture. The anatomist can study depictions of the crucifixion. If the nails were hammered into the middle of the hand they would never take the weight of the body – merely tear the flesh. Hammered into the wrist, they would cause an ulnar nerve palsy with the fourth and fifth fingers bent. This correct position is most commonly seen in Spanish crucifixion scenes but not elsewhere. Likewise, in religious art, paintings of the Madonna and child, usually posed for by the artist's family, vary not only in the age of the child but how the child is held, almost invariably on the left side.

A seminal book on medical aspects of art is that of Patrick Trevor-Roper, *The World through Blunted Sight*. Red-green colour blind artists tend to depict objects shown in sunlight as red and in shade as green or brown (the sign of Liebreich). Artists with developing cataracts have an abundance of red vision (I have a picture by Tom Bradley, husband of the better-known Lancashire artist Helen Bradley, which shows just that); after cataract extraction, blue vision predominates. The myope will see reds in better definition than the blues; thus the Japanese have only recently adopted a specific word for blue. Oliver Sacks, in *The Island of the Colour Blind*, says that people devoid of cones in their retinae cannot respond to bright sunlight. They see better at dusk with their rods and peripheral vision. I am aware that my own colour discrimination in the red-green range is dependent on the quanta of light. Many artists are myopic. Would-be myopic artists, seeing light broken up prismatically into spectra by their glasses, develop a feeling for colour at an early age. An ophthalmologist in 1936 argued that without artists with poor central vision, Impressionism would not have been born. The Nazis, infatuated by the belief that all artists were degenerate, quoted a critic of the time who attributed the revolutionary technique of the Impressionists to their flickering eyeballs. Hypermetropes tend to under-use or under-value colour. Synaesthesia involves the natural or intellectual blending of colour and sound, or occasionally of other senses. Astigmatism has played a part in the art of Modigliani and El Greco. Correction of a more recent artist's distorted sight by means of appropriate glasses left him quite unable to paint in his established style. He complained that the unaccustomed clarity of detail and colour made him lose the effects of masses of colour and of the essential lines of contours and form which are marked in greater contrast when the vision is blurred. Hendrick Terbrugghen (1588-1629) heightens the pathos of his picture of De Ongelvige Thomas (the Incredulity of St Thomas) by giving the doubting saint a pair of rimless (NHS) spectacles. Cezanne, when losing sight due to diseased retinae from diabetes, required 115 sittings to paint Vollard's portrait, complaining that 'I hope to make some progress but the contour keeps slipping away from me'. Wyndham Lewis, with an enlarging pituitary tumour, had to hold his head very close to the canvas but was still able to produce a fine portrait of T.S. Eliot.

Hallucinations can be the basis of compelling pictures induced by drugs, in disease states and in schizophrenia; but they also occur naturally as do most examples of Di Chirico's metaphysical art. However, there is another aspect of art which appeals to the doctor. In the course of our work we are obliged to examine the boundaries of reality in terms of neuropathology or psychopathology, looking at man's highest mental functions – consciousness, emotion, memory, thought, perception and their expression through language – by studying the effects of trauma, drugs or disease, observing the results of enfeeblement, and using aberrations and malfunctioning to gain insight into the human mind. Art offers a very different facet of the human story: a chance to study the very best the mind and imagination can present, displayed in a form open to careful and leisurely analysis. Tolstoy's description of the generative process of all forms of art applies to artists from time immemorial.

> To evoke in oneself a feeling one has experienced, and having evoked it in oneself, then by means of movement, lines, colouring, sounds or forms expressed in words, so to transmit that feeling that others may experience the same feeling – that is the activity of art.

The plastic arts are the exteriorization of so many visual perceptions, provided not only by the quaint, the queer, the mystic over-much, the dismal and the dry, but often by those possessing the greatest talents and intellectual abilities. 'Art', so said Benedetto Croce, 'is ruled uniquely by the imagination. Images are its only wealth, it does not classify objects, it does not pronounce the real or imaginary, does not qualify them, does not define them, it feels and presents them – nothing more.'

One can admire the skill of optical illusions in art: the use of anamorphosis – often used by secret agents in the Elizabethan era – trompe-l'oeil, visual puns, impossible pictures and the paranoiac-critical works of Salvador Dali. Illusory movement, as in the art of Bridget Riley or Velasquez' spinning wheel, deceive the eye to heighten our enjoyment. Specific medical subjects: genetics*, sleep†, emotions, can be presented through the plastic arts.

An artist, to be successful, usually has to be an interesting personality. There is a tendency, when medical people write on art, to emphasize the pathological basis rather than the imaginative or intellectual aspect, which may, of course, have developed as an exceptional response to mild pathology. Violence exhibited by artists can be a fascinating aspect of the artist's personality. The Romanian, Victor Brauner, was preoccupied with mutilation of the eyes. He had painted a self-portrait in 1931 in which he showed himself with one eye crushed and his cheek covered with blood. He never knew what made him paint this way. On 27th August 1938, at a studio party, Brauner tried to separate two friends who were quarrelling, and was struck in the face by a bottle by Dominguez. His left eye was put out. Everyone was stupefied, and felt that Brauner had announced years ago that this accident was going to happen – the more so since in 1932, 'Mediterranean Landscape', and in 1935, in 'Magic of the Seashore', he had shown himself with his eye pierced by an instrument with the letter D, Dominguez' initial, on its handle. The picture also illustrates that in self-portraits, looking into a mirror, the artist invariably reverses left and right.

---
*c.f. AEH Emery Medicine, Genetics and Art, *Proc. Roy.Coll, Physicians* 1991 21: 33–42.
†*Sleep in Art*. ed. R. Potzsch, 1993, Editiones Roche, Basel.

I once gave a lecture, unpublished, on 'Art and Violence', one story from which illustrates many medical points:-

The biographer, Vasari, described the character of the various artists of his day: Raphael as urbane, Michelangelo as terribilita, and Benvenuto Cellini, best known for his salt-cellar made for King Francois I, as terribilissimo. When Cellini was languishing in prison, they planned to put some powdered diamond into his food. A diamond, though not poisonous in itself, is incredibly hard so that when pounded it still retains its sharp edges As a result, when it enters the stomach along with one's food, in the process of digestion the diamond becomes embedded in the lining of the stomach and in the bowels. Then, little by little, as fresh food comes in and presses it forward, the diamond pierces one's inside; and the result is death. If any other kind of stone or glass is mixed with one's food, it hasn't the power to adhere, and so it passes out with the food. Durante gave one of the guards a diamond of some small value. An enemy of Cellini's, Leone Leoni, was entrusted with the job of pounding it. However, he was very poor and the diamond was worth a few dozen crowns. He returned to the guard something which he pretended was the powered diamond and Cellini ate the powder with the food with no adverse effect.

Whilst Cellini was in prison, Leoni contrived to capture his post as engraver of papal coins but soon lost favour after an unfortunate incident in which he assaulted and permanently mutilated the Pope's jeweller. He was sentenced to lose his right hand, but was saved by powerful sponsors and his punishment commuted to serving as a galley-slave. He was later released by Charles V's greatest sea captain, the Genoese Andrea Doria, for whom the grateful Leoni engraved a medal.

Thus emancipated he continued to alternate criminal violence and exquisite workmanship. One of his victims was his own workman, whom he tried to murder. Later he attempted to murder Titan's much loved son, Orazio. After the Emperor Charles V's death, Philip II commissioned Leoni and his son Pompeo to produce bronze statues but Philip was excited by a new opportunity. One of his client princes, the Grand Duke of Tuscany, offered him a particularly choice marble statue. This was a life-size Crucifixion, which Benvenuto Cellini had lovingly made for his own tomb, but which the Grand Duke's predecessor had wheedled out of him. Philip accepted the offer with delight. Its arrival was celebrated like the coming of a great prince: no expense, no ceremony, was spared. and it was carried from Madrid to the Escorial with the utmost care by 50 porters; for the king could not entrust so precious a work to mere mules. But when it was unpacked and could be scrutinized, Philip's enthusiasm faded: the statue, he now discovered, had neither gravedad nor decoro – gravity and decorum – the two qualities, which to him were essential On the contrary, it was pagan, sensuous, even voluptuous. It was also naked. The pious king covered the sensitive area of the marble body with his handkerchief, which afterwards, we are told, was long preserved as a relic. Then he sent it to a dark chapel behind the choir and its intended place was left to be filled, in due course, by a more suitable Crucifixion, by the faithful family firm of Leoni and son. Thus Leone Leoni scored a last victory over his rival Benvenuto Cellini.

**Sleep Disorders**

My two index cases are: firstly an obese 18-stone prison warder who fell asleep with a bunch of keys on his lap and was told that he had to be cured within the month or he would lose his job; and secondly, an obese woman in her late 30s who had had ECT for depression in the past, was a restless sleeper, snoring and frightening her husband by breath-holding episodes in her sleep. She constantly awoke with a headache and was prone to making a lot of silly mistakes, such as putting milk in the oven or hot dinners in the fridge. She has an excessive appetite and is mildly hypothyroid. There are many other patients whose excessive daytime sleepiness has led to road traffic accidents or falling asleep on the hard shoulder of a motor-way. Sleep disorders have been a serious concern of the medical profession for over 20 years, yet when seeking a parliamentary question on the availability of resources for this problem, both the M.P. and the Under-Secretary who answered the written question assumed that this was a rather recherché, recondite matter.

One can agree that there are psychological causes, 'neurotic hyper-somnolence' in individuals who complain of life-long fatigue and excessive sleepiness, but there are also disease causes of hypersomnolence: Trypano-somiasis carried by the Tse-Tse fly, Encephalitis Lethargica after World War I, Hypersomnia (the Rip van Winkle syndrome), recurrent hypersomnia due to the Klein-Levin syndrome of periodic hypersomnia and excessive appetite in young adolescent males (as illustrated by the fat boy in Pickwick), occasionally in dystrophia myotonica, and in shift workers. Napoleon usually slept 4-5 hours a night, but after the battle of Aspern, his first defeat after 17 victories, he experienced invincible somnolence and slept for 36 hours without waking, so that his aides feared for his life.

Daytime drowsiness can be a serious condition without having a neurotic cause or a relationship to a clearcut illness. It may be responsible for subwakefulness with lapses of vigilance; falling asleep at the wheel of a vehicle, confused behaviour with silly mistakes and forgetfulness.

Narcolepsy, the best known sleep disorder, is defined as periodic irresistible day-time episodes of sleep, most frequently as the result of monotony, often at inappropriate times, and lasting 10 to 20 minutes. The person may fall asleep in an upright posture and remain standing; but Gelineau's original description adds to the overall picture.

> He said he felt no pain at the moment of being seized; only he felt a profound heaviness, a mental void, a sort of cloud circling his head, a heavy weight on his forehead and at the back of his eyes. His thoughts were muddled, then blotted out. His eyelids half closed and finally they closed; he slept; and all this very rapidly so that the preliminary stage of physiological sleep lasted hardly a few seconds... If standing, he tottered, staggered like a drunk; he heard people accuse him of drinking and laugh at him; he could not reply. He slumped down in a final effort, getting out of the way of horses and carriages.

Several writers in the past have considered that the narcoleptic syndrome is a psychological defence mechanism and have likened it to the primitive 'sham death' pattern utilized by other forms of life from caterpillars to possums. Physical examination and all investigations are almost invariably quite negative. Indeed, one is often struck by the person's splendid physical condition, with perhaps a tendency to obesity due to the inordinate amount of rest.

The full syndrome, Gelineau's syndrome, consists of a tetrad of narcolepsy, cataplexy – inhibition of postural muscle tone with instantaneous recovery; sleep paralysis – on waking or when falling asleep, lasting a few minutes, at most 30 minutes; and hypnagogic hallucinations – visual or auditory hallucinations, commonly mundane but occasionally frightening, immediately preceding or following sleep. Each of these manifestations can occur separately in normal people. Thus cataplexy can occur quite separately with loss of muscle tone in the absence of loss of consciousness. Loss of tone may be confined to a part of the body – the jaw or head – or generalized, so that the patient buckles at the knees or falls helplessly to the ground. The weakness comes suddenly, following emotional stimuli distinctive for that individual but inevitably associated with an element of surprise. Prof. Parkes has photographs of both the Queen and Prince Charles buckling at the knees from an apparent joke. Laughter is the most common trigger. For some it may be a hearty laugh of 'banana skin humour', for others a subtle joke that produces a fleeting smile; but anger, fear, excitement, suspense or frustration may be provocative stimuli for some patients.

A patient of mine in her 50s, with a 25-year history of mild narcolepsy, illustrates the problems which can arise from the associated features. She tends to fall asleep occasionally during the day and sleeps at night in a somewhat restless manner. However, if she is walking along a street and she is pleased to see somebody she has not seen for a while, she is going to smile and greet them, but has to turn away as she cannot speak. Similarly if she is told a joke, she has to turn away or she would shake all over. She has dropped objects from her hands and gone weak at the knees with such episodes. After dozing she cannot move straightway, though she can after a night's sleep and she wakes as though drugged. Sometimes when she is sleeping, she can dream that her husband has come back into bed with her and woken up to find that he has not returned.

Narcolepsy is now known to be a genetically determined disorder, associated with the DR2 HLA group, affecting 0.01-0.09% of the population. The onset is usually in early adult life, developing gradually over many years, but for some it may follow an antecedent infection, head injury, emotional shock or endocrine change. Very occasionally there may be a structural lesion. In a survey of 241 patients there was a 68% incidence of cataplexy, 24% of sleep paralysis and 30% of hypnagogic hallucinations. The condition is associated with REM sleep. There are invariably problems in treatment. Weight reduction can help as can avoiding heavy meals. Cataplexy can be helped by tricyclic antidepressants such as clomipramine. A mild hypnotic at night might improve nocturnal sleep and reduce daytime sleepiness. Stimulant drugs during the day to produce wakefulness are the mainstay of treatment but difficulties frequently arise in prescribing these necessary drugs because of anti-drug abuse laws. The prescription has to be written out in full for an individual case. Repeat prescriptions can be difficult. And additional problems may arise with general practitioners reluctant to prescribe and pharmacists to dispense.

A condition which is less well defined or recognized is sleep apnoea. An apnoea is a cessation of airflow at the level of the nostrils and mouth, lasting at least 10 seconds. The severity of the disorder is measured by an apnoeic index – the number of apnoeic episodes per hour of sleep. Although they can occur in normal sleep, recurrent episodes are most frequent at the extremes of age. Snoring, obesity, alcohol, and drug-induced sleep are significantly associated with an increase in the number of apnoeic episodes. Apnoea thus becomes a potential emergency with important theoretical overtones: responsible for a proportion of those dying with the sudden infant death syndrome, especially preterm or low-weight babies, underlying the association between alcohol and strokes in young adults, and an explanation as to why most people die in their sleep. The outcome of sleep apnoea can also be crippling cardio-respiratory illness.

Obstructive apnoea, which is a major cause of sleep apnoea, can take several forms. Obesity is a factor in at least 60% of patients. There may be upper airways obstruction due to polyps or enlarged tonsils, which can be treated surgically, genetic defects such as those giving bird-like facies, or weakness (hypotonia) of the muscles of the pharyngeal and laryngeal muscles, some forms of which may be treated medically. Tracheotomy may be required if the obstruction cannot be relieved by other means. Most episodes occur during non-REM sleep with lack of oxygen (hypoxia) being the trigger to the resumption of respiration. Primary sleep apnoea of central origin is an unusual condition that occurs as a result of an acute failure of automatic respiration, known eponymously as Ondine's curse, after the mythological water nymph whose human suitor was cursed to lose automatic functions whilst asleep. In a strictly scientific sense, Ondine's curse is primarily due to hypoventilation rather than to apnoea. Mixed syndromes of obstructive and central origin occur. Cardio-respiratory failure occurs due to persistent carbon dioxide retention with a decrease in total lung volume, and progresses to intermittent cyanosis, polycythemia, and cor pulmonale.

Milder forms of sleep apnoea can be reversed by avoidance of sedatives, avoidance of alcohol, weight reduction, correction of raised blood pressure, bleeding, if there is secondary polycythaemia, and propping up in bed at night. Intravenous respiratory stimulants may also be used in the short term. If the situation is life-threatening, CPAP (continuous positive airway pressure techniques) may be required. Air, or air and oxygen, is supplied via a humidifier. The pressure may be limited to the expiratory phase, which has the effect not only of abolishing the apnoea but of creating reflex stimulation of the muscles of the respiratory tract. Mechanical aids, inapplicable to obstructive sleep apnoea, may help considerably in the event of central sleep apnoea. These include diaphragmatic pacemakers, cuirass respirators, rocking beds and positive end respiratory pressure ventilators. Tracheotomy remains the safest procedure where diagnostic doubt exists and the patient is clearly at risk.

One of my concerns was sleep in relation to Parkinsonism. Dopa is one of the chemicals involved in the sleep-wake cycle. When laevodopa is initially given, patients sleep better. With bigger doses given throughout the day, daytime drowsiness increases and nocturnal sleep may be disturbed. Other factors are related to age and immobility. The tendency to restricted activity, relative boredom and dependence on others favours daytime sleepiness. The elderly may suffer from insomnia, lie in bed at night without attempting to sleep, try to sleep unsuccessfully at night or take to napping through the day.

The post-encephalitic forms of Parkinsonism were associated with prolonged sleep disturbances, characteristic slowness and episodic immobility.

**Medico-Legal Work**
I have a love-hate relationship with medico-legal work. The love is with the work itself, enabling me to see a variety of fascinating cases one would not otherwise see, and especially when I was the sole consultant neurologist. Medico-legal work and private practice kept me alert to questions which need to be answered. All too often in NHS work the patient would blindly accept what was said to them. The hate is with the legal system, archaic, inefficient and not really just. Ninety per cent of the work is settled, quite rightly, out of court. The court proceedings are acceptable for the most part, but the hanging around, the fixing and cancelling of appearances, requires urgent revision. A date has been fixed for a trial. The doctors on both sides are agreed on the evidence, but all must attend. The barristers may well decide before entering the court proper on the payment of damages and time lost off work by the plaintiff (all these are settled by a formula and may not be substantial in a particular case) But the proceedings nonetheless grind on with all the doctors being called in order to decide which side will be expected to meet the legal costs. From the medical point of view, it is like deciding how may angels can be balanced on the head of a pin.

Another aspect of legal boloney which causes annoyance is the misuse of medical opinions. Not only will lawyers search around, discarding reports which do not suit them, but they will lean on doctors to alter their reports once given. A doctor giving a report is a specialist evaluating the evidence without bias, in so far as that is possible. Doctors do tend to be supportive of one side rather than the other, but their report is their considered opinion, and not, as is the lawyers' role, one of primarily representing the defence or the prosecution.

The law's treatment of medical conditions can be very illogical. On a shop-lifting charge it only has to be stated that the defendant might have had an epileptic attack or might have been confused, for the charges to be dropped. I was amazed at the leniency with which a person was treated who had killed two others in a car accident when under the influence of drugs, speeding in a built-up area, driving without a licence in a non-roadworthy car (checked by his friend 'Acid'), with dangerously ill-matched tyre pressures.

Out of interest, at one time I analysed 650 patients I had seen for medico-legal purposes. The highest number (170) were head injuries due to road traffic accidents. I was surprised by the number of cyclists (20), motor cyclists

(17) and pedestrians (23) involved. The next most common, and very much anticipated, were whiplash injuries (120) in road traffic accidents. They have almost acquired the same social status as M.E. There were 6 train, one tram and one helicopter accident due to a mid-air collision. Injuries at work (106) form an important category needing assessment but there were also 9 accidents at home, accidents on fairgrounds, in shops, playing football and three people were electrocuted. Street accidents (26), tripping, falling into potholes, are regular subjects for claims, Some can be highly dubious. Falls occurred from ladders, scaffolding, roofs and on the dance floor. Forty patients (40) were seen as the result of assaults. Ten patients (10) involved drugs and toxic chemicals. Nearly a hundred (100) were seen for various medical conditions of which epilepsy (27) formed the largest single group, often in relation to driving. Multiple sclerosis was the next largest group (20) and conditions related to multiple sclerosis (8). Assessments were made with respect to employability, wartime, including P.O.W. experiences, and claims of medical negligence.

Unfortunately it can be rightly claimed that head injuries of all types are the most neglected group of hospital patients. They are usually admitted via casualty on to surgical wards. The way they are treated at the scene of an accident, the way they are transported, and await assessment in Accident and Emergency Departments add to their morbidity. Fortunately nowadays most hospitals have CT scanning and screening can eliminate subdural haematomas and other forms of bleeding; but, if found, patients are rarely treated in the admitting hospital but transferred to neurosurgical units, with further morbidity likely to occur in the process of transfer. If a patient is admitted to a surgical ward, bleeding from other sites, abdominal injury and fractures will not just receive priority, but may be judged the sole need for intervention and treatment and the possibility of a coexistent head injury totally neglected. Thus patients presenting for medico-legal reasons three months to two years later will not have had preliminary tests done, will not have been examined by a neurologist or neuro-surgeon, and most certainly will not have had a psychological assessment. Because the early management has been overlooked, rehabilitation will not have been started for speech or memory disturbances, emotional changes, coexistent depression, or retraining and readjustment for work or a normal life-style. We rely heavily on dispositions made in court, allowing money to be advanced for rehabilitation and American-style management of individual head-injured patients, to pressurize the health service into future improvements of the care of those with head injury.

A typical example is of a man walking down a country lane with his dog.

He heard a car and went up on to the verge but the car went out of control, up the verge and through a hedge. He vaguely remembers getting home. Next he remembers shouting at his wife and then waking up in hospital the next morning. Apparently five youths had stolen the car and after this accident had jumped out and run off. He was detained in hospital for five days with pain and swelling around his knees, below his left ear and an abrasion to his left hand. Though he had amnesia, there was said to have been no head injury. Over the next three months he had blackouts and headaches and was noticed to have hesitancy of speech. He returned to work after six months but made a lot of mistakes and forgot things which he had known for years. Medico-legal examination, nine months after the accident, revealed a flat affect, depression, a hesitant speech, poor arithmetical ability, lack of sense of smell (bilateral anosmia), and a reduction of his visual fields. Thus he needed readmission for basic tests which he should have had in the weeks immediately following the accident. The injury below the left ear certainly should have required investigation and if a proper history had been taken, they would have found that he had had a blackout 3 years before the accident.

I wish to quote the experience of a national hunt jockey who had a severe head injury at the age of 20, leaving him with a spastic quadriparesis, incoordination of his limbs, ataxia and a dysarthric speech on top of which he developed epilepsy. Contact sports, and particularly national hunt riding, are quoted by the boxing lobby as having comparable risks of brain damage to that of boxing. The governing bodies of such diverse sports as boxing, trampolining, steeplechasing, American football and rugby union have been prepared to alter their rules to reduce the risk of injury. In American football, 'spearing' or head-on tackling causing axial loading with a risk of fracture dislocation of the lower cervical spine has been banned, and in rugby union the number of flexion injuries to the neck in rucks and mauls has been reduced. But the risk can never be eliminated entirely. I reviewed transient traumatic tetraplegia in which a sports accident, usually with hyperextension of the neck, can cause 'neuropraxia' i.e. a transient loss of function from contusion of the spinal cord in the neck. There can be sensory changes with burning pain, numbness, tingling, and loss of sensation or motor changes with weakness or even complete paralysis, lasting 10 to 15 minutes though sometimes resolving over 48 hours. Usually there is an added factor, seen only after the accident, namely a narrow (stenotic) cervical vertebral spine. Each year a few rugby union players develop paraplegia and an American orthopaedic surgeon was able to contact 117 football players with paraplegia. I have been referred soccer players and my colleague rugby players (the reverse of our interests!) for assessment as to whether they should stop playing for several months or permanently because of less serious neurological problems. One such patient, in fact a rugby player, after numerous episodes of concussion, complained of blurred vision from a more serious accident and from that time onwards if he hit his head in tackle he would experience flashbacks of vision. Nowadays a soccer international who was injured in an aircraft crash during the War would never have been allowed to resume his international career afterwards.

Punch-drunkenness is a chronic traumatic encephalopathy which may occur as the result of repeated head injury. It leads to deterioration of the personality, impairment of memory, dysarthria, tremor, Parkinsonian features and ataxia; and imaging of the cranium may show loss of the septum pellucidum in the centre of the brain. It is essentially associated with boxing, though the incidence is high also among national hunt jockeys and to a lesser extent in other sports. The difference is that in no other sport is the aim to damage two of the most vital organs of the body, the brain and the eye.

Whiplash injuries are best discussed under the less emotive term, acute neck sprain. The majority are indeed associated with some form of road traffic accident, in 50% a jolt from another car running into the back of the vehicle in which the subject is seated, and therefore there is a compensation or litigation aspect. However, very few respond soon after any litigation is settled, making it probable that organic discomfort has occurred and that pre-existing psychological vulnerability is not a major factor. The major injury is to the soft tissues of the neck with resultant muscle contractions. Central core problems to the spinal cord are not a factor, Although the normal curvature of the neck may be lost and the onset of cervical spondylosis hastened, subluxations and disc protrusions are uncommon. Disc surgery is rarely required. Radiculopathies may occur due to irritation or compression of emergent nerve roots and vertigo, and even partial deafness can occur.

The injury is usually a hyperflexion injury but some rotation may have occurred. The major symptoms are usually neck pain and stiffness, coexistent neck and back pain, headache arising occipitally but often referred frontally, and pins and needles in the upper limbs. About half remit within 5 weeks but those lasting more than 9 months usually fail to remit. Pain may not occur immediately after the accident but develop over 24 to 72 hours afterwards.

The patients with the worse prognosis in my experience are older patients with cervical spondylosis which normally occurs in about 50% of people over the age of 50, those with preexisting neck problems and with headaches with clearly migrainous features. When examined, neck stiffness is noted, varying with the direction of rotation or flexion; pain when the neck is held in rotation for 30 seconds or more, and occasionally inverted or altered reflexes in the upper limbs. Early treatment is required with analgesics, a soft collar and physiotherapy, including short wave diathermy but not traction. Where there are persisting symptoms, an MR or CT scan is advisable.

The clinical problem is that many people lose their jobs because of the manifestations of a whiplash injury. Some return to light work and can later resume their normal occupation, and just a few develop more severe features relating to cervical spondylosis or even, in less than 10%, develop spasmodic torticollis. Rather than give the history of one such patient, who developed torticollis some years after two whiplash injuries, I will describe the fate of a lady with multiple subluxations (slippage of one vertebra on another) due to spasmodic torticollis. There was the continual danger than the cord could be compressed or even severed and she was referred for a Cloward operation, fixing the neck vertebrae from the front. Because of the constant movement, this was not a straightforward operation, and arrangements were made for treatment with drugs and a frame to quieten the constant rotation. Just as she was about to have the operation the surgeon died. We have found that high doses of botulinum toxin have controlled the further progression of the torticollis but she is now in a wheel chair, is under constant review, but is wary of future surgery.

There were weeks when dealing with assault cases appeared to be a very routine function. Assaults and mugging of elderly people at home and in the street rightly hit the headlines; but the vast majority of attacks are on people under the age of 21 and by 25 years nearly 50% may well have had such an experience, often associated with leaving pubs in the late evening or in the early hours of the morning. On Christmas Eve one person went into the pub toilet (gents) to find a lass in the middle of the room commenting on everyone and causing a fracas. He remonstrated with her, telling her she should not be there, and was immediately set upon by her boyfriend with a knife, slashing from the ear across the face. The boyfriend had been released on parole from prison on compassionate grounds because his grandmother was ill. There are plenty of horror stories, none more than that of a 60 year-old lady who suffered from another form of assault.

She was walking with her dogs along a public right of way near a caravan site where they were staying. In fact she was walking along a road where there was no fencing between the road and grazing land. A herd of cows crowded round her and the dogs and one literally raised its front legs and jumped on her, felling her to the ground; after which the whole herd attacked her and stampeded her. She was on the road at the time. She was knocked over several times and kicked many times but did not lose consciousness. As they kept coming at her, she eventually felt it safer to lie down, curl up and close her eyes. She was trampled over, sniffed and had to lie there until she saw a van coming in the distance. When it approached it was the farmer who owned the cows. He got out and with a stick tried to fight off the cows, but they attacked him and in fact he had the stick down one of the cows gullets and shouted to the lady to try and get herself into the van as they would only kill them both if he were to try to pick her up. She was able to drag herself to the van, got in, and he drove off straight away. He drove to the camp site and phoned an ambulance.

When seen in hospital, she was fully conscious and oriented. The major injury was a large laceration on her right calf with degloving of a crescent of skin based posteriorly and measuring 25 cm from end to end. In addition there were multiple soft tissue bruises on her limbs and trunk and two lacerations on the back of her head. She was also bleeding from her gums. After anti-tetanus and antibiotic cover, she was transfused with 2 units of blood and taken to the operating theatre. She was taken back to theatre for further treatment to the major wound two weeks later, prior to skin grafting. She was in hospital for five weeks and discharged on crutches.

I was asked to see her because of recurrent headaches and dizziness, word finding difficulties and poor memory and comprehension. Her personality had clearly altered with the accident and she was unwilling to go out of doors. She was fully investigated at the time but her neurological symptoms showed a gradual deterioration over time.

Sometimes it is not the most severe occurrences which cause the greatest problems but rather the need to decide to what extent an accident was responsible for the complaints. Thus a chef at a nursing home switched on some heated trolleys, one of which was faulty, and when attempting to disconnect it, his right hand touched the flex and he received an electric shock which threw him backwards. Apparently he was lying between two metal plates. He felt disoriented, with generalized pain and numbness involving his right index finger. About an hour after the accident he developed nausea and headache. Later that day he collapsed with vomiting.

Headaches persisted and 4-5 times a week would recur, associated with blurred vision, nausea and sharp pains above his eyes. Once or twice a week he would also blackout. He firstly gets a sensation of flashing lights and lines and feels the need to micturate, but when he gets to the toilet, he is unable to do so. He then feels slightly disoriented for 20 minutes and tries to lie down if possible. At the same time he may develop a pain in a fairly localized area over the left eye. As it becomes more intense, he feels faint and unsteady on his feet, or may vomit. The vomiting does not cause a blackout but the headache may do so. His wife says that he goes wobbly on his feet, his eyes go weird and roll, he goes stiff and his legs may jerk. He is unconscious for seconds or minutes.

There had been no previous history of migraine or epilepsy and the electroencephalogram was normal. Three neurologists were uncertain whether the blackouts were secondary to migraine or primarily epileptic and trials of anticonvulsant and antimigrainous drugs did not solve the problem. He appeared to be a stable person giving an authentic account. What exactly happens with an electric shock is rarely clear. It possibly spread only as high as the brainstem. Here blackouts can occur in association with migraine without affecting the EEG, which monitors changes over the cortex of the brain only.

When people have horrendous experiences in hospital the question of medical negligence not unnaturally arises. A whole series of questions have to be addressed. Were the doctors fully alert to the problem? Did they act quickly enough? Was the best treatment given – if not, why not? Was there any culpable action performed or was there something overlooked or neglected? I will cite as an example the experience of a lady 21 weeks pregnant, who developed abdominal pain. She became toxic and at operation was found to have a gangrenous perforated appendix. Despite the operation, she continued to have pain and vomiting. She was rehydrated and at a second operation was found to have subacute intestinal obstruction and adhesions. Two days later she developed cortical blindness and lost her babe. The cortical blindness was believed to be due to septicaemia producing intracranial venous thrombosis and was accompanied by fits. She was given various appropriate treatments but continued to have further fits. Nowadays, even if no charge for negligence had been made, there would have been an automatic audit, so that any lessons which could lead to the prevention of similar events could have been avoided.

## Lecture Tours

Jokes are made about professors. You can always tell a professor by his permanent suntan. What is the difference between a professor and God? God is everywhere: our professor is everywhere but never here! I cannot claim a permanent suntan and have done only a few lecture tours; but the experience is valuable. Like most people on lecture tours, I tend to stop very briefly at each place so as not to overstay my welcome. This makes for a hectic series of days, enjoyable but also hard work. I once did a few lectures in the States, ending in Albuquerque. Then headed for a conference in St John's, Newfoundland via Montreal. Between Albuquerque and Montreal I changed plane three times, losing my luggage, anxiously washing my effects, only to be woken by a fire-practice in the hotel which meant dressing hurriedly and going down the fire escape. The conference in St John's coincided with a visit from Prince Charles and Lady Di. The Royal Yacht was in the harbour with an iceberg behind it at the harbour entrance.

A visit to Russia coincided with the 2000 anniversary of the Christian Church and at the height of peristroika. In Moscow we visited a working church shaped like a cross, at the centre of which the priest was preaching on a small stand, giving the message of peace (Mir) and the resurrection. The people standing around him could certainly have touched his garment as in Biblical days. On one side of the nave was an open coffin. The onion domes of the churches were being gilded and restored. This was particularly so in Zagorsk – the religious centre of the Russian Orthodox Church. The churches were high, with a reredos filled with icons separating off the sanctuary. The congregation came forward to kiss an icon held by the priest whilst others sang unaccompanied by any instrument. Our conference was in Leningrad (now once again St Petersberg). On the first day there were a lot of Russian doctors. The top ones attended the dinner and we learnt that they flew everywhere to organize matters. Electrodes would be inserted over the surface of the brain in certain types of epilepsy and would remain there for weeks. Their talks consisted of lengthy explanations of why it was unnecessary to do sophisticated operations or procedures or use prophylactic drugs. After the first day, very few Russians attended. We asked to see the neurological wards but failed in our endeavour. If multiple sclerosis was recognized, it would probably be treated not in a hospital but at a polyclinic. Our attempts to visit such a place were blocked. We met a neurosurgeon who showed us one of three myelograms he had done that year and our request to see a hospital eventually took us to a cardiac rehabilitation centre, but nothing neurological.

The longest and most successful tour was of India, starting with a joint meeting of the Royal College of Physicians with the Indian Association of Physicians in Delhi. We then visited the golden triangle of Varanasi, Khajuraho, Agra, Sikandra, Amber and Jaipur with the College, before going our separate ways. My wife and I then went on our own lecture tour. We went firstly to Bombay where, besides formal lectures, I taught the students and was shown patients on the ward by the resident, who was later to come to Preston as our registrar. I also learnt how private practice works in India. The private hospitals are far superior to the public ones and have several grades of paying patient, but they are also obliged by law to take or investigate 15% of public patients. With more sophisticated equipment, this may mean that a patient can get a CT scan not otherwise available, and although patients may be selected for this test for their interest, it goes some way to rule out the inequalities in treatment.

Our next stop at Coimbatore was very demanding but probably of the greatest value. I attended the outpatients of the neurologist, Dr Pranesh, and saw patients with the Madras form of motor neurone disease – a slowly progressive form with accompanying deafness. We stayed in the Cotton Company's rest home and ate lovely vegetarian food off plantain leaves. What I did not tell my wife at the time was the experience of Dr Jack Foster and his wife when they stayed there. The kitchen had been overrun by rats, but being good Hindus, they did not kill them but caught them in traps and released them at the end of the garden, from which they duly returned, legging it back to the kitchen. One of my lectures to their Osler club was on Hallucinations and Art, which was given an upbeat commentary in the local press. My wife, who had not intended to lecture, was asked to lecture at short notice, and after a banquet a slide show of interesting cases was presented so that I might comment. Fortunately there were 20 or 30 such cases, so I was able to a degree to pick and choose on what I replied. We visited both the public hospital, where conditions were not good, and a splendid private hospital run by a manic surgeon, Dr Bakthavathsalam. He had gone to Europe to train but was urged back by his rich relatives, who bought the hospital for him. Although other consultants worked at the K.G. Hospital, he personally saw that every patient had the best treatment and investigation immediately on arrival. He also took us to three cinemas he owned, taking time to check the hygiene of the toilets. In his company we also visited silversmiths, a Hindu temple with the temple elephant, and a hospital practising Ayurvedic medicine. It is possible for doctors to receive instruction in Ayurvedic medicine as part of their formal training. To a greater extent than with alternative medicine in Britain, there are conditions which are well treated by this approach and they provide more rehabilitation than most Indian hospitals.

Before leaving Coimbatore we were taken on a tour of the Nilgris hill station by taxis. The taxis overtook on bends with gay abandon. Fortunately my wife did not see the tread on the taxi's wheels; but neither did I when I looked! Except for Dr Pranesh, who drove so carefully that you assumed he was avoiding every fly, driving in India is reckless with a high accident rate. Only sacred cows, who wander everywhere, are avoided. And on which side of the road do they drive? – answer, suicide. Other lectures followed at

Trivandrum, Pondicherry, and at both University Hospitals in Madras before we returned to Bombay via Goa.

A visit to Sri Lanka, with talks scheduled to coincide with the transfer of a CT scanner from Preston to Colombo, was severely hampered by the death of the brother of my host during the Sri Lankan elections. A return to Malaysia with the Royal College was far more successful. In Singapore the papers presented displayed the differences in disease patterns due to differences in employment, culture, foods and other factors between the various races. We then visited Malacca, which was much altered since my National Service days but still held for me the excitement of St Francis Xavier's mission to the Far East. There was a new road along the reclaimed sea-front and an excellent display of the houses of various parts of Malaysia. Malacca is the centre of the Babu Chinese, early Chinese settlers who are completely Malayanized. Malaysia now meant the opening up of the East coast, which was sparsely inhabited previously, and the addition of parts of Borneo made up the federation of states. Kuala Lumpur had grown without obvious change and before returning, we were able to spend some time on Penang Island. Here I had the opportunity for parascending along with some of the older College representatives in their eighties, and also the less pleasant experience of being stung by a jelly fish when swimming; but my leg soon recovered after resting.

My most recent trip was to South Africa. The college was careful to give degrees in South Africa to avoid the necessity of the recipients travelling to Europe and becoming lost to South Africa, which is suffering from an acute shortage of doctors. They were recruiting doctors from East Germany and Cuba whilst we were there. There were also inequalities of distribution. Far too many doctors had left the state service to go into private practice; and whereas the Cape Province was reasonably well off for doctors, there were serious shortages elsewhere. These social problems were highlighted in the joint meeting with the Medical Association of South Africa. In Cape Town itself we were impressed by the relative calm of the rainbow revolution and mixing of races, though they appeared wary of each other. It was hard to imagine the cathedral as the site of racial battles. The service, as always, was very much interracial though Archbishop Tutu was away involved in the Reconciliation Conference.

I gave a paper on Magnetic Resonance Imaging, many aspects of which surprised members of the College of Physicians, whose administrative duties had caused them to lose touch with clinical developments. For example, they could not understand that MR angiography did not need the use of a contrast medium. But for me the socially oriented papers of the South

African doctors, especially from Johannesburg and the remoter districts, were very poignant. I met up with a doctor who had been in Malaya doing National Service during my time at Sungei Patani, the Gurkha camp, from where many of our patients came to BMH Kamunting. He had then been a registrar at the Royal Free with me, and was now in Vancouver. Unfortunately he developed coronary pain and had to have a cardiac by-pass operation in South Africa before returning home.

For our visit along the Garden Route we had a Cape Coloured driver and an Afrikaans guide, both of whom ate and stayed with us in the same hotels and together provided a commentary on events. I cannot recollect the driver eating with us on other tours in different parts of the world. We visited all the usual places: vineries, tropical gardens, ostrich farms, caves, nature reserves, the Huguenot memorial and the attractive town of Stellenbosch, but also had a chance to see a little, admittedly, of the real South Africa. Shanty towns were well away from the places of work, but were being built up through contracts using local labour with heavy penalties attached if they failed to provide. We learnt however that elsewhere, namely, in Johannesburg and Kwazi-Zulu Natal, racial tensions were still very strong. But, as with Russia, it was fascinating to see a country in transition.

**Neurological Emergencies**
Most medical emergencies are defined in terms of a threat to life and indeed this is also the case with neurological emergencies. Deaths occur from cerebrovascular disease, including subarachnoid haemorrhage, intracranial haemorrhage, and infarction; from meningitis, encephalitis, trauma, neoplasia and states of altered immunity. But the brain may also be under threat in other ways. There can be a threatened impairment of a person's faculties, special senses or social acceptability. Patients may survive but remain in a persistent vegetative state, or with their physical abilities intact but with gross impairment of mental orientation or ability. Loss of consciousness is invariably a hazardous condition, and any threatened alteration to the level of consciousness a potential emergency. Vertigo, sleep apnoea, Jacksonian epilepsy or focal sensations arising from partial seizures are all conditions which carry the risk of impaired consciousness. An isolated syncopal attack may recur or can be prolonged with consequent cerebral anoxia. Yet again, emergencies may produce total or partial impairment of an aspect of physical control of the body. Employability or way of life may be dramatically changed. And lastly, emergency treatment may be required for unbearable pain.

The most precise treatment comes from finding the root causes of a complaint. Attention to detail cannot be jettisoned because of the exigencies of the case. History-taking and observation may have to be squeezed in between life-saving measures – clearing the airway, putting up a drip, etc. – but should never be squeezed out. With neurological problems, skilful history-taking provides the diagnosis eight times out of ten. If the patient is capable of giving an account himself, that account is probably the most exact, but relatives and eye-witnesses can often add substantially to the history and occasionally it may be necessary to range more widely into background factors.

The emphasis placed by many neurologists on the correct use of language is not misplaced. The terminology used when taking a history must be clear to both patient and doctor. The term 'blackout' first came into common use in World War II. It can as easily refer to loss of vision as to loss of consciousness. Sometimes local terms like 'half-faint' may be far more explicit and obviate the need for intense investigation. Dizziness does not automatically imply vertigo – an hallucination of movement. The patient needs to be questioned more closely as to whether he actually means that he feels faint, light-headed, woozy, 'mazey', floating, unsteady with 'sea-legs' or just ill. Some patients resent the term 'giddy' as implying lack of intelligence. Careful questioning may be required to determine whether loss of vision in one eye really means unilateral blindness or a loss of hemianopic vision to the right or left. If the patient is drowsy, confused or stuporose, most questions will need to be put simply so as to obtain a brief unequivocal answer. At the same time it is also helpful to encourage the patient to reply in short sentences, confirming that his speech is not aphasic. Where speech is not possible, an alternative means of communication, such as head nodding or lip movements, can be encouraged. Once the veracity of the answers has been checked, such methods should be used as fully as possible without tiring the patient. Even if the patient is not able to communicate and the conscious level is uncertain, it is advisable to make encouraging comments whilst performing the examination and every caution should be taken to avoid adverse statements pronounced near a supposedly unconscious patient.

A scientific approach to disturbances of consciousness has been dogged for many years by a profusion of terminology – clouding, confusion, obtundation, delirium, stupor and coma. The simplest and most understandable definition of coma is that of unrousable unresponsiveness. We now use the Glasgow coma scale to replace these terms, docketing the best motor and verbal responses and the ability of the patient to open his/her eyes, spontaneously, to command, or to pain. There is also a Glasgow outcome scale and refinements to the somewhat simple format of the coma scale have added greater awareness to our clinical approach. Management of the comatose patient is a combination of basic life-support procedures, achieving circulatory and respiratory homeostasis and cerebral resuscitation combined with a detective's approach to diagnosis. Thereafter specific treatments may be implemented. These may involve replacement of blood or fluid loss, correction of electrolyte imbalance, as in the dialysis dysequilibrium syndrome, removal of poisons, then giving a specific antidote, correcting vitamin deficiencies or coagulation defects, stabilizing the temperature thermostat, preventing liver failure, correcting endocrine disturbances, or treating raised or reduced blood glucose levels.

I have already explained that when examining, I like to question the candidates on what they consider to be poorly managed emergencies and why they are poorly managed in practice.

Hypoglycaemia in the insulin-dependent diabetic is usually well recognized and patients with diabetics are encouraged to experience a hypoglycaemic episode so that they can recognize the symptoms and the response to correction; but secondary causes of hypoglycaemia with drugs, underlying diseases, or other forms of endocrine failure, or coming on slowly with oral hypoglycaemic medications, may fail to be recognized and it may even be supposed that the patient has had a stroke caused by a cerebro-vascular accident.

The mortality from the common form of diabetic hyperglycaemic ketoacidotic coma (diabetic coma) is still around 10% for a variety of reasons. A common presenting symptom is abdominal pain, which may be treated as a surgical emergency. Vomiting may be misunderstood. Coma may be precipitated by coronary heart disease (myocardial infarction), cerebral infarction, Addison's disease or acute pancreatitis, each of which carries additional risks. There are concurrent physiological abnormalities which have to be corrected besides the high blood sugar level — acidosis, the presence of ketones, dehydration, potassium loss and concentration of electrolytes (hyperosmolarity). And finally, particularly in children, the brain may be swollen with cerebral oedema. Underlying causes must always be sought out as coma rarely occurs on its own.

The other form of diabetic coma (non-ketotic hyperglycaemic hyper-osmolarity) usually comes on slowly and is generally seen in the elderly with mild diabetes. It may be precipitated by infection, burns, or various forms of therapy. Dehydration is an important feature and thrombosis can occur, affecting brain, heart or limbs.

Raised pressure within the skull sufficient to impair the cerebral circulation ranks along with coma as a life-threatening emergency. The rapid relief of pressure, as by removing spinal fluid via a lumbar puncture, can lead to coning with downward displacement of the intracranial contents, blocking the foramen magnum between the cranial cavity and the vertebral column. The increased pressure may be mechanical, due to obstruction, from swelling of the cells themselves or due to a damming back of the circulation. The effects of raised intracranial pressure may be seen in 60% of cases as swelling at the back of the eye (Papilloedema). Causes include tumours, infections, trauma and haemorrhage. Structures may be displaced to give true or false localizing signs. Diagnosis without resort to investigative procedures may not be easy and pitfalls are all too common.

Occupational causes of coma include electric shock and Caisson's disease in divers or tunnellers. Survivors of electric shock may have bizarre gaits, which raise questions of hysteria, and differentiation may be difficult. The symptoms suffered by divers have been trivialized as niggles, staggers, chokes and bends but are in essence severe, with divers forced to give up their occupation on account of persistent problems ranging from personality changes and convulsions to numbness, paraplegia and bladder disturbances. With decompression, gas may form intravascularly within tissues such as the brain and spinal cord, or spread to distant parts as gas emboli. Treatment involves the use of hyperbaric oxygen raising the pressure to 2 atmospheres and gradually reducing it to a safer level in order that the autochthonous bubbles may be reabsorbed safely. This procedure may have to be repeated if initially unsuccessful.

Hyperbaric oxygen has also been used for patients with carbon monoxide poisoning, osteomyelitis, gangrene and after spinal cord injury, but in none of these has it gained general acceptance. In the early 1980s it was promoted by the self-help group called ARMS for the treatment of multiple sclerosis. Putnam in 1937 had suggested that microthrombi in the capillaries of the central nervous system might initiate the destructive process leading to primary demyelination. Philip James in Dundee resurrected this theory, suggesting that the lesions might represent areas of transient venous occlusion due to fat embolism. He speculated that this would cause focal hypoxia (lack of oxygen) damaging the myelin-sustaining cells and that hyperoxygenation was the logical treatment. But this theory is not supported by our knowledge of pathological changes following fat emboli. There is, however, just the possibility that treatment with hyperbaric oxygen may be beneficial through its effects on the function of the immune system. Not all criticism was scientific: he was castigated by a colleague in a neighbouring town as 'an enthusiastic ostrich'.

ARMS were responsible for setting up at least 30 decompression chambers throughout the country, installed outside hospitals and run by non-medical people, reportedly after one week's training. The local protagonist in my area, a patient of mine, was an Irish ex-diver with severe multiple sclerosis. When asked why, if decompression was so wonderful for multiple sclerosis, had he, who had been decompressed many times, developed the disease, he replied that he liked his pint of beer and had hurried the process of decompression for that reason!

The presumed beneficial effect of hyperbaric oxygen is limited to a relatively narrow range of pressures. Pressures higher than 2.5 atmospheres have been found to be toxic, especially to the central nervous system and the respiratory system and prolonged exposure at that level can cause swelling within the brain, destruction (central necrosis) within the spinal cord and acute pneumonia. Treatment can be given in monoplace chambers where the patient is removed from the direct attention of the supporting personnel. This can be dangerous due to the risk of epilepsy, the risk of which is higher in patients with multiple sclerosis than in the normal population. At a pressure of 2 atmospheres, ear pain and perforation of the ear drum can occur. In one study grommets were inserted prior to hyperbaric exposure. At lesser pressures the treatment is totally ineffective. The original claims were that 39% of symptoms improved, 54% remained the same and 7% deteriorated. The symptoms most likely to improve were bladder related. The assessment is necessarily subjective and no patient improved by more than two points on the Kurtze scale. This expensive and potentially dangerous treatment has lost its initial appeal.

## Multiple Sclerosis

I usually enjoy talking to patients' societies relevant to their diseases. I place such experiences along with domiciliary (home) visits as ways whereby one can learn more about the patient, their family and carers, than in the crowded outpatient department of a hospital. Whether it be to epilepsy, muscular dystrophy, motor neurone or M.S. groups, the learning process is in two directions. I am expected to talk for 10 to 20 minutes, outlining the disease, what can be done and its future. With multiple sclerosis, for example, one can give the experience on poliomyelitis – I remember just a few patients over the years and various friends and relatives afflicted – but it has virtually disappeared and the money and the research now aid a better understanding of other diseases such as multiple sclerosis. The same could happen to money raised in future for multiple sclerosis. After the formal talk, I answer questions for nearly twice that time and am then thanked. But that never ends the session. For the same amount of time again, I will find myself answering private informal questions as I meet the various groups around the room.

Questions can be difficult but the most difficult and embarrassing I had came from the back of the room from a patient of mine I recognized immediately. 'Does M.S. affect one's mind and the ability to do a job?' To most of the audience this may have seemed a very innocent query, but I had had to deprive this patient of his livelihood as a schoolmaster because, due to a rare frontal plaque, during school meals he would cause embarrassment by taking and eating food off a pupil's plate or transferring his food, unrequested, on to another's plate.

Patient's accounts of their disease can be most helpful. Jock Murray from Halifax Nova Scotia, an old friend who has also written on Dr Johnson's illness and is one of the Canadian authorities on multiple sclerosis, describes the illness of Barbellion, who wrote the *Journal of a Disappointed Man*; A doctor with M.S., Alexander Burnfield, has written on doctor-patients dilemmas in multiple sclerosis and in practical terms the personal paper by Sheila Milward written in 1984 has proved of great value when giving advice. The Multiple Sclerosis Society itself exemplifies how useful such a society can be in checking on all new research when or before it hits the headlines of the tabloids, and will investigate any suggestions. Reg Kelly, when he was head of the M.S.S. Advisory Council, said there were so many possible lines of research that they could almost equal the number of patients.

M.S. is the commonest neurological disease affecting young adults in temperate climates. Despite the tremendous variability of symptoms displayed, clinicians are naturally concerned to provide guidance on the prospects of continued employment and independence, the need for family and community support, and the eventual course of the disease. In 1980 I did a leading article based upon a French actuarial study published in the journal *Brain*. I wrote to the then editor of *Brain*, Charles Phillips, pointing out that some of the data published in that study were contradictory, but the general trend is clear. Seventy per cent of patients develop M.S. between 20-40 years of age. In their paper, onset with complete remissions occurs at 30 years, remissions leaving a residual disability at 34 years, and the progressive phase at 38 years, allowing a standard deviation of plus or minus 10 years. Eighteen percent are progressive from their onset. My impression since that time is that the prognosis has improved for most patients. One sees fewer bedsores or overwhelming infections in M.S. patients. I suspect that the improvement has not resulted from newer treatments but from better care, support for the skin, hygiene, etc. In the past also the diagnosis of M.S. was made using Charcot's triad of nystagmus, ataxia and cerebellar speech – all late cerebellar signs. We used McAlpine's diagnostic criteria dividing patients into definite, probable and possible M.S. Now with MR scanning, evoked potential tests and oligoclonal bands in the spinal fluid, we can diagnose most mild cases early on in their disease. In the past we relied on the Lange curve in syphilis and to a lesser extent for M.S. – with heights suggesting paretic (Paris), luetic (Lyon), and meningitic (Marseilles) neurosyphilis and a strongly paretic Lange, suggesting what was called Lupus sclerosis.

The causation is still unclear. The disease occurs in the Northern Hemisphere in temperate climates, higher in Orkney and Shetland than elsewhere in Britain, possibly related to genetic factors, possibly to diet, with a very real suggestion that the trigger factor is an auto-immune or allergic reaction to a virus – or to several viruses. It is possible that the type of virus, including the measles virus, may help determine the progression of the disease. I had to respond to the possibility that it could be caused by a virus transmitted by household pets, especially dogs. This is just one of the many factors which epidemiological surveys have looked into. Although there is some cross-reactivity between canine distemper virus and measles virus, the distemper virus has not been shown to be a factor.

Diet has been examined in detail. One can quote Falstaff on this subject:-

If sack and sugar be a fault, God help the wicked!
If to be old and merry be a sin, then many an old host that I know is damn'd;
If to be fat be to be hated, then Pharaoh's lean kine are to be loved.

In the 1960's Zilkha and Thompson at Guy's Hospital studied the breakdown products in the spinal fluid of patients with M.S. and concluded that unsaturated fatty acids might help. Sun flower seed oil was potentially effective in reducing exacerbations in a multi-centre trial but has the defect of being rather unpalatable. The story of Roger MacDougall is well known, A successful playwright, he contracted M.S. at the height of his achievement and was soon confined to a wheelchair. He went to a dietician named Hawthorn and was advised to follow a most stringent diet, cutting out all wheat germ or gluten. As can happen to about 6% of those severely incapacitated with M.S., he made a spectacular recovery. He subsequently went to California as Professor of Dramatic Art. The MacDougall-Hawthorn diet is essentially a composite one: avoiding wheat germ and all refined starches and sugars, with the addition of magnesium sulphate and vitamins, including oral vitamin B 12.

For several years about half the patients I saw were on that diet but more recently half take a high roughage diet with evening primrose oil – a more palatable unsaturated fatty acid than sunflower seed oil.

Certain symptoms – those relating to the eye, to the sensory system and hemiparesis – have a far better prognosis than paraparesis with ataxia. Many paroxysmal symptoms are poorly recognized. These include unilateral spasms of the limbs, sudden loss of power, unexpected falls, brief episodes of incoordination, double vision, hiccough, and showers of sparks on movement of the eyes. There may also be trigeminal neuralgia responsive to steroids along with tegretol. One patient of mine with familial M.S. had recurrent jerking of the legs, body and spine following a hip operation. The best known paroxysmal symptom is L'Hermitte's sign, the barber's chair sign. This occurs with bending the head forwards, when a shower of electric feelings pass down the spine or occasionally in other directions. It is a condition which can occur with other disorders which affect demyelinatin in the cervical spinal cord. – trauma to the spine as with whiplash, irradiation, vitamin B 12 deficiency, etc.

Another group of transient symptoms in M.S. are often referred to as Uhthoff's phenomena. Vision may improve when bathing in cold water. With exercise or hot water, symptoms may deteriorate. Morris Bender showed that a plantar response in doubtful M.S. may become extensor after a prolonged hot bath or shower. But Uhthoff's phenomenon is most often seen as symptoms deterioration after a heavy carbohydrate meal. Headache which can persist across the forehead, related to retrobulbar neuritis, may fail to be diagnosed because of the lack of accompanying features. Other forms of pain can be a feature of M.S. Many of these, as for example pain down the legs, respond very well to acupuncture.

New treatments are being tried in M.S. The patients selected for the trials of beta interferon are those with remitting relapsing disease – probably not the ones most in need of help. Relapses are treated as before with steroids, and the patients require daily subcutaneous or weekly intramuscular injections. The treatment is expensive, has side-effects and because of the insensitivity of the disability scales in M.S., reliance is placed on recognizing true relapses as opposed to decompensation of previous symptoms due to intercurrent infection. Although I have had quite a number on carefully monitored treatment, the early results have proved far from impressive.

Management of dysfunction of the bladder, which occurs in 50-80% of patients, has been one of the factors improving the quality of life of M.S. sufferers. In the past repeated infections spreading to the kidneys (pyelonephrosis) were the chief cause of death in M.S. They also lead to incontinence, excoriation of the skin, combining with friction burns to produce penetrating bedsores, and combining with infection of the feet to cause spasticity with scissoring of the legs, spasms (paraplegia in flexion) and contractures. It was in this situation that intrathecal phenol was used along with operations such as obturator neurectomy so that the patient could be properly nursed. There are now specialized neuro-urological clinics able to evaluate which treatment is most appropriate. In women an irritable bladder with detrusor hyperreflexia (i.e. an overresponsive sphincter) is the most frequent form of disability: in man an obstructive disability with detrusor sphincter dyssynergia is equally common. The bladder may also be a-contractile or show clonic sphincter contractions associated with spasms of spasticity. Voiding exercises to reduce any residual urine left in the bladder which may result in infection have proved simple yet effective for many patients. Infusions of capsaicin (derived from curry powder) is just one way by which bladder irritability can be reduced. Better control with drugs and treatments for dyssynergia and hyperreflexia of the bladder sphincters have made a considerable improvement but a Nobel prize is still awaited for the person who can correct female incontinence.

The great debate on multiple sclerosis was whether patients should receive the much vaunted interferon. The seminal study had been done in Canada and was presented at the World Federation of Neurology meeting in Vancouver. The wife of my co-editor on *Diseases of the Spinal Cord*, Kathy Eisen, was in charge of the monitoring procedure. Only a slight change was definable by clinical criteria but the MRI scan changes were impressive. In the North West, the Neurologists met to devise a common policy. We did not want just one person or one centre to be designated as expert in the condition when we had been looking after our own patients for years. As a jobbing neurologist, I for one can claim to have seen as many multiple sclerosis patients, parkinsonian patients, epileptic patients, etc. as the so-called specialist professors in any one of these conditions. We were therefore able to proceed with a monitored trial of a limited number of patients in all parts of the North West. Some patients reacted to the drug, others developed antibodies, and, as expected, despite public pressure, the results were far from impressive. I have often wondered whether Amantidine does not in fact produce as good a result with a lesser risk of side effects.

## Diagnostic puzzles
The health department would like all conditions to be quantifiable as 'consultant episodes' – to use their bizarre terminology. It is the patient whose story is not quite straightforward, who provides a diagnostic puzzle or the patient with hysterical symptoms; and one is obliged to exclude the

possibility of organic disease; or the patient involved in ligitation, where every conceivable test is required: these are the patients who monopolize the time, effort and funding of departments. Let us consider a characteristic diagnostic puzzle – symptoms which might be due to temporal lobe epilepsy, basilar migraine, hysteria or cataplexy.

The patient's episodes started 5 years ago at the age of 12. The episodes may recur up to six or seven times a day, but can clear for as long as two weeks between attacks. They start with a sickly feeling in the stomach and a sensation that she is doing the same thing again and again. This undue familiarity seems to be very much in evidence. She can also hear what is said but is unable to take it in. The attacks last for seconds or she may sit through a series of episodic attacks for about 5 to 10 minutes. Afterwards she feels light-headed, sometimes with a headache over both temples lasting for 30 minutes. She becomes forgetful. She can be dizzy and may fail to remember faces, places or names; or what happened last year. She also has a lot of nightmares with one or two recurring themes. She explained that she feels she is running down 'a side-less and ground-less' corridor. Someone is running faster behind her. She comes into a room with a settee and with pictures that terrify her. She always feels people are in the room with her, particularly at night time; and she walks in her sleep. She has been involved with seances and Jehovah's Witnesses.

In the past she has had cosmetic surgery to her ears. She is allergic to dust and prone to bronchitis. She is right-handed. She is a second child, weighed $6^{1}/_{2}$lb at birth, walked at 12 months, crawled normally and had normal milestones. On examination, she is a bit overweight. Her blood pressure was 130.80 and there are no abnormal neurological signs.

**Muscle Neurology**
Earlier on I referred somewhat rudely to muscle neurologists. One may wryly observe that muscle diseases, although they carry considerable intrinsic interest, sit uneasily in neurological textbooks. The justification is, of course, that the nerves work primarily through the voluntary musculature of the body, whereas their input comes from many and varied sources. John Walton, the English muscle king – or rather 'Lord', in editing and taking over Brain's *Diseases of the Nervous System*, found muscle diseases following after neurological manifestations of distant neoplasms and peripheral nerves and before the autonomic nervous system, diseases of the skull bones and epilepsy. Bannister did somewhat better when editing Brain's *Clinical Neurology*, placing disorders of muscle at the end of a section of disorders of anatomical regions after disorders of nerve roots and peripheral nerves.

Inflammatory diseases followed in a new section. However, even after attempts to categorize muscle diseases into a tidy classification, those secondary to lower motor neurone and peripheral nerve lesions or to end-plate disorders are liable to be scattered elsewhere. Classification is not helped by the fact that facio-scapulo-humeral wasting – to give one example – can be either secondary to spino-muscular atrophy (a neurogenic condition) or due to a primary muscle dystrophy (myopathic); and both forms are linked to a gene defect on the long arm of chromosome 5.

In practice the approach can be much more logical. Is it secondary to a neural disorder (neurogenic atrophy, or myasthenic) . . . or a primary muscle condition? If myogenic, is it congenital or acquired? The clinical approach may seem relatively straightforward. The presence of a family history or the absence of a muscle or part of a muscle usually implies a congenital origin; tenderness, contractures, a high sedimentation rate and the presence of infiltrative cells on muscle biopsy suggest an acquired cause. Fatiguability with weakness on exercise suggests myasthenia: fatiguability with hardening of the muscles on exertion, a syndrome such as the McArdle's syndrome of lactate accumulation.

But there simplicity ends. Floppiness at birth can be due to drugs given to the mother or to maternal myasthenia. Myasthenia may be due to drugs such as the aminoglycosides, or secondary to carcinoma; and myasthenia can cause muscle wasting. The recognition of polymyalgia rheumatica, polymyositis or dermatomyositis can be relatively easy and these conditions can be treated with steroids, but the risks from prolonged steroid therapy must be weighed against the need to dampen down the condition over months or years. Advances in genetics, enzyme chemistry and mitochondrial metabolism can reopen assumed certainty and upset previous classifications. There is no better example than the rag-bag of conditions called opthalmoplegia plus. Weakness of the external muscles may be associated with muscle weakness elsewhere as in the Kiloh–Nevin syndrome, or with the mitochondrial myopathies which may involve the central nervous system; and it is always advisable to exclude ocular myasthenia before proceeding further.

For several decades, myasthenia* has been a topic of especial interest in the neighbouring centre of Manchester. Fergus Ferguson pronounced eloquently on the dangers of enemas and bowel procedures in causing what is often a dramatic worsening of myasthenia. Steroids can help but may also aggravate the condition and the Senior House Officer on the ward shared between the

---

*The southern U.S. Negro of old is said to have called myasthenia gravis 'mice in the gravy' and spinal meningitis 'smiling mightly Jesus'.

metabolic unit and neurology, doing routine potassium excretion studies on his patients, found that myasthenic patients on steroids also lost potassium. My wife (in Nuclear Medicine), Laurie Liversedge (the neurologist) and Harrison (the S.H.O.) showed that there was a loss in whole body potassium and that worsening of the condition could be prevented by giving potassium supplements along with the steroids.

Some years ago I had a patient, an artist from Manchester, who had worked on scaffolding doing murals and had illustrated many books, but her primary profession was as a medical illustrator. She very kindly provided me with beautiful pictures explaining her double vision with drawings of her brush held before her eyes. Her case-history is very typical of the ocular problems presenting to neurology.

At the age of nine she had poliomyelitis affecting her left leg and to a lesser degree her left arm. Aged eleven she started seeing double. By 35 she had to stop every few yards because of a frozen cold feeling and difficulty in voluntarily coordinating the movement of her legs. She had to give up painting when aged 40. She found herself becoming more and more cross-eyed and sleepy when attempting to conceive and execute book illustrations under pressure. She readily fatigued and would see double if she read for a while. She had to eat American style with her right hand, because her left hand let her down.

On examination, she was alert. Her speech was normal. There had never been any swallowing difficulty but she had fatiguing ptosis and double vision, a proximal weakness particularly of the neck and upper limbs, marked curvature of her back, with weakness and a little wasting of her left leg. Tests for myasthenia gravis were negative and the exact cause was never fully explained.

Patients handicapped by serious disabilities often arouse one's admiration. They are often very alert mentally and do their very best to live life to the full. One such patient, with advanced motor neurone disease in a wheelchair, organized a motley crowd of British holiday makers held up by a strike of French dockers at the Channel ports. They deserve all the support they get from Social Security and give back as much as they get. But they are all too often the victims of a crude system of administration claiming to eliminate fraud. They are in fact the last people guilty of such misdeamour, but in my experience they are victimized and rarely get accepted when they claim benefit on the first occasion. As a doctor I get bitter with the system and patients rightly must become very angry. I wish to illustrate this with the case of a patient I saw in 1971, but it could equally well have been in 1981 or 1991 or even, I suspect, in 2001.

He had muscular dystrophy from an early age with no affected relatives and had been fully investigated to confirm the diagnosis. He remained surprisingly well and was able to walk until aged 30. He dates a more serious deterioration from the few months he was in a Nursing Home in Fleetwood whilst his mother was in hospital for an operation. She was over 70 and since the operation was unable to push him in his chair. He had a wheelchair which he could lift and manipulate with his forearms up till the time of his recent deterioration. He could no longer lift himself from his shoulders and had to get from his chair to his bed by rocking along a board with a little help from his mother. There was no doubt that he could easily manipulate an electrically propelled chair. A disability grant was rebuffed by the Local Authorities and I advised him to apply again through the medical social worker and seek the aid of the district occupational physiotherapist, physiotherapist and local Muscular Dystrophy Group. Such is the lot of the average neurologist, but in 1989 the unusual occurred.

## Botulism

The outbreak of botulism in North West England and Wales in June 1989 was the largest in the U.K. affecting humans. Human botulism is a rare disease and most neurologists go through their career without ever seeing a case.

*The first two patients*
On Sunday the 4th June I was asked to see a 26 year-old patient by Nihal Gurusinghe, my neurosurgical colleague. The history given over the phone was that two weeks before admission he was involved in a fight with a neighbour, pushed against a wall and punched. He had bruising to his head, headache, and dizziness which lasted 24 hours. The previous day he had been admitted to a local hospital with blurred and double vision. He had could not swallow, had weakness of his right arm and a desire to close his right eye. He had difficulty in brushing his teeth. He could not move his tongue to the right. Food and drink spilt from the right side of his mouth. His speech was slurred as if he were drunk, and he staggered and felt drowsy. In hospital he was found to be alert and oriented with mild dysarthria. He had slight bilateral droopiness of the eyelids (ptosis), double vision on lateral gaze, and drooping of the right side of his mouth. Tongue and palatal movements were normal. There were no reflex changes.

He was transferred to our hospital for a CT scan. The scan was normal but Mr Gurusinghe was unhappy to transfer him back and requested my opinion. When I saw him, he had bilateral ptosis, bilateral VI and VII cranial nerve palsies, and a bulbar palsy affecting speech and swallowing. The weakness was more pronounced in his arms than in his legs, with diminished reflexes in the right arm and a right extensor plantar response. I noted that he was left-handed and it was just possible that the reflex asymmetry was congenital. I also agreed that he should be kept under observation and wondered whether he might have brainstem encephalitis or a cerebrovascular accident perhaps associated with a post-traumatic vascular dissection of an artery in the neck. Two hours later he had a respiratory arrest and was ventilated. A tracheostomy was performed and he was then transferred to the intensive care unit.

The next morning he was unable to move, having a flaccid paralysis of all four limbs. The right plantar remained extensor and there was a complete ophthalmoplegia (paralysis of eye movements) with dilated pupils. The electroencephalogram showed some slow wave activity. However the appearance of the EEG was not sufficiently abnormal to diagnose an encephalitis. In the next bed in ITU was another patient. He had also been admitted the previous day with a flaccid paralysis and in need of respiratory support.

The second patient was a 21 year-old student. He woke at three am, was violently sick and thought he had damaged his eye, causing double vision. His right eye blinked constantly, watered and was painful. He was not initially worried but had some hair-raising experiences when he went to the Eye Department, where they found mild conjunctival injection and double vision on upward and lateral gaze. An x-ray of his orbits was normal. He was just about to leave hospital, was given a drink and suddenly realised he couldn't swallow, choked and had to be dragged back by a nurse who sent him on to the Ear Nose and Throat Department. He could not breathe and hadn't a clue why this was happening. There he vomited three times with nasal regurgitation. His voice had deteriorated, his tongue was weak and he was unable to swallow. On further examination, his throat was red with pooling of saliva and he was unable to protrude his tongue. There was slow blinking of the eyelids and persistent diplopia to right and left. His ankle jerks were absent.

He was admitted to the ITU with a presumptive diagnosis of the Guillain-Barre syndrome (GBS). He looked tired with bilateral ptosis and bilateral facial nerve palsies. He was unable to shrug his shoulders, speak or swallow and had difficulty maintaining a respiratory peak flow of 200 litres/minute. The blood gases were normal as was the cerebro-spinal fluid. All four limbs were flaccid and areflexic. He felt scared as he couldn't move, couldn't see anything, couldn't do anything and did not know what was happening. He prayed it was recoverable and not going to last like this for the rest of his life. To exclude myasthenia gravis, 10 mg of Tensilon (edrophonium HCl) was given intravenously. His breathing noticeably improved. He could cough and clear his throat, lift his head from the bed, smile, frown and open his eyes but still had diplopia and was unable to speak. He deteriorated again within 30 minutes and a second dose of Tensilon was ineffective.

Two hours later he became weaker. Impaired breathing had altered his blood gases. He was intubated, ventilated and required a tracheostomy. Because of the absence of bowel movements (paralytic ileus), oral feeding was inadvisable and fluids were given intravenously.

Douglas Mitchell (Professor Mitchell) and I examined both patients. We considered the differential diagnosis. With a Guillain Barre syndrome there would be a peripheral neuropathy with slowing of conduction in the motor and possibly also in the sensory nerves. Repeat spinal fluid examinations might show a rise in the protein content without an obvious increase in the cell count. Because the cranial nerves were particularly involved, we felt that we could be dealing with the Miller Fisher variant of GBS with cranial nerve involvement, areflexia and ataxia. Cerebrovascular disease was also possible; but to have two young people with identical signs was most unusual. In the course of my clinical practice at that time I found myself treating a patient with the classical Miller Fisher syndrome and a diabetic patient with bilateral strokes, resulting in paralysis of all four limbs.

Very similar features, with the rapid development of numbness about the lips and tongue, accompanied by weakness affecting the extremities as well as the bulbar and respiratory muscles, can occur with various fish poisons. Poisoning with tetrodotoxin from puffer fish or with saxitoxin from shellfish such as clams and mussels, although an occasional cause of death, usually wears off with recovery over 5 days. These toxins cause blockage of sodium channels along the nerves, affecting nerve conduction at the nodes of Ranvier, where there is thinning of the myelin sheaths. Nerve conduction is slowed and prolonged but is unassociated with nerve degeneration. Ciguatoxin, found in semitropical fish and in salmon from fish farms, attacks the gastro-intestinal tract and the nervous system, but rarely embarrasses respiration or swallowing. However, neurological symptoms can last for 6 months or even two years. The sodium channels may either be slowed or excessively excited, depending on the form of ciguatoxin.

The initial positive response to edrophonium, although we had not seen it ourselves, raised the possibility of myasthenia gravis, a myasthenic syndrome or of a presynaptic block as in botulism or the Lambert Eaton syndrome of carcinomatous myasthenia. With myasthenia there would be normal nerve conduction but the electromyographic responses would display a decrease in the number and height of the motor neurone units with repetitive supramaximal stimulation. Such an impairment of the muscle response would indicate a block at the myoneural junction (neuro-muscular synapse) where the nerve ending lies on the muscle belly. Usually the response to Tensilon lasts about one minute. A prolonged response lasting 30 minutes is more probable with a presynaptic block at the nerve ending, where acetylcholine is released before crossing over the myo-neural junction. A presynaptic block can occur with the Lambert-Eaton syndrome, antibiotic toxicity, excess magnesium or manganese, decreased calcium levels, snake bite, spider venom or botulism. In such patients supramaximal stimulation may give a decremental response at low rates of stimulation but an increase in amplitude (a reversed myasthenic effect) during stimulation at higher rates. Dr Mitchell therefore proceeded to examine both patients neurophysiologically. The results in both patients were identical.

Repetitive neural stimulation did not show a defect at the neuromuscular junction, despite repeated testing. Instead, evidence of a reduction in amplitude of muscle action potentials at different stimulation sites along the peripheral nerves suggested a demyelinating block, as found in the Guillain-Barre syndrome. We were concerned with these findings and took advice whether our interpretation was correct in view of the very low motor action potentials. The tests were repeated on successive days but continued to show a demyelinating block and no increment or decrement following repetitive stimulation. Serological tests for botulism were negative. Furthermore a 5-day course of guanidine, said to aid recovery from a presynaptic block, did not help. My concern at the time was that they might have received food which had been criminally adulterated, producing a new syndrome. In July 1989 the deaths of 14 hamadryas baboons (Papio hamadryas) in Windsor safari park were also presumed to have been caused by an adulterant in food but the diagnosis proved to be that of botulism. However, we were confident that we could maintain life support until our patients recovered spontaneously from whatever was the primary diagnosis. We dismissed the use of antitoxin, which is only really effective if given before botulinum toxin enters nerves, as potentially dangerous, as horse serum which provides the immune globulin can cause a severe anaphylactic reaction.

We were initially unaware of other patients requiring admission with similar symptoms. Between the 2nd and 9th of June 10 patients were admitted to hospitals in Manchester, Liverpool, Oldham and Blackpool. Two children, from the same family, transferred from Blackpool to Manchester, caused Richard Newton, a Consultant Neuro-paediatrician, to suggest that botulism was the most likely diagnosis. Others, seeing patients with more classical features of botulism, were thinking on similar lines. On the 7th June, the mother of the first patient was admitted to Blackpool with similar, but less severe signs, She did not wish to be transferred to the same ITU as her son. However, from the information we received, the mother and son did not live in the same house and had not shared any meals.

The following Saturday (10th June) I was invited over to Blackpool for a meeting with the Public Health authorities. I came equipped with information on botulism but unable to explain the findings in our two patients. Before the meeting I was able to examine 5 other more mildly affected patients in the wards. Their stories and findings suggested botulism more clearly and the diagnosis was firmly agreed. The Public Health people then set to work. A Health Food shop in Fleetwood initially came under suspicion, and it was only after the second questionnaire to all affected – 27 patients spread across Lancashire and North Wales – that yoghurt appeared to be the causal agent.

Several clinical questions remained unanswered at this stage. We found a few rather unconvincing papers describing peripheral sensory and motor changes in human and animal botulism. Later we came across a paper from Cherington from Denver, Colorado – *Botulism: Ten-Year Experience*. Botulism is endemic in the Rocky Mountains because the boiling temperature at high altitudes is too low to destroy spores associated with home bottling of vegetable products. He wrote that electrical abnormality in botulism resembles that seen in the Eaton-Lambert syndrome, but may not be apparent early in the disease in the most severely affected patients. Moderately paralysed patients can show a greater potentiation, with rapid repetitive nerve stimulation, than those severely paralysed. Neurophysiological tests done by members of our department in Preston and Blackpool on 14 patients and elsewhere by other neurologists and neurophysiologists confirmed the veracity of Cherington's findings. Moderate to mildly affected patients had the more classical electrophysiological features of the disease. The other question was how our first patient and his mother both developed botulism.

I am now able to quote from the account which he gave his lawyer after he had recovered from the acute illness. He lived separately from his mother but visited her on the 1st June. He ate some yoghurt which his mother had purchased that evening, stating that he was very partial to yoghurt and had been known to eat as many as half a dozen pots consecutively. On this occasion he ate only half the pot and then told his mother that he thought it tasted revolting. She then had one spoonful of the yoghurt 'but she is not used to eating them and she was probably unable to tell whether it was good or bad'.

That night he worked as normal on the night shift as a machine operator. He got up early on the Friday to go shopping for a new suit to wear to a wedding the following day. He felt tired when he went to work from 4 to 8 pm (overtime) that day, but assumed that this was because he had worked the night shift and got up early to go shopping. The following day he got up at 6 am because he was intending to use his black BMW as the wedding car for his girlfriend's sister's wedding. He could hardly get out of bed because he felt so bad. His teeth and mouth were numb. After the wedding at 9 am he felt very tired. His eyes were uncomfortable and he was tired from driving the vehicle. He drove back to the house with some relatives but was unable to eat or drink because the muscles around his mouth and face were not working properly and his mouth seemed to be drooping. At around 11 am he went to his mother's house and said he was going to bed. She said she would wake him at 4 pm so that he could get ready to go to the evening wedding reception. However, he returned to his girlfriend's house and rang his doctor, who sent him to hospital. By that time he complained of double vision, inability to swallow and could not control any of his muscles.

The severity of symptoms in these two patients, compared to others who were affected at a later date, was reflected in the speed of onset. Whether it was dose-related we cannot tell. With poliomyelitis, activity during the incubation period can worsen muscular involvement. Our first patient was working on night shift and preparing to attend a wedding: the other patient had eaten hazelnut yoghurt at 1 pm, mowed a cricket pitch and scored 68 not out that afternoon.

They both required assisted ventilation for 25 and 53 days respectively. Fluids were given by means of a central venous line and later by naso-gastric tube. Afterwards we learnt that the first patient had had some hearing loss at the height of his illness. The probable cause of the hearing loss was paralysis of the tensor tympani and stapedius muscles affecting the state of tension of the ear drum. His girl friend bought him a Sony Walkman. He thought the Walkman was defective because he was unable to hear it clearly even at full volume. As he began to improve, he realised that his hearing had been impaired. Swallowing was slow to return and neostigmine was used to aid swallowing as soon as there was some improvement. After 43 days he left hospital with complete resolution of eye movements, speech, swallowing, and respiratory difficulties. His strength and reflexes were restored, the extensor plantar response cleared, and there was a mild residual right facial weakness. The second patient required prolonged feeding via a central venous line until bowel activity was restored. He needed antibiotics for a respiratory infection, became very depressed and required constant encouragement. Power returned partially to his lower limbs after eight days, (in his own account he says 10 days) but after 60 days breathing still presented difficulty and he could not swallow properly.

Intensive care, though life-saving, can be an horrendous experience. My justification for giving the patients' own accounts of their experiences and reactions is the need for greater awareness from doctors and nursing staff of how patients actually feel in these circumstances.

The first patient described the respiratory arrest vividly.

'I stopped breathing and had to be rushed to the intensive care department. I was effectively drowning because my lungs had filled with water. The doctors and nurses were unable to bring me round. All the time I thought I was dying, I felt as though I was going mental, and I was thrashing around in the bed. The doctors tried to hold me down to get oxygen on to my face and they put something down my throat so that I would not swallow my tongue. I really hate having anything over my mouth and face and this was really uncomfortable. All the time although I was unable to breathe I was fully conscious and aware of what was happening which made the whole incident even more frightening. I started to breathe on my own again and the large oxygen facial mask was removed for a smaller one as I was moved to the intensive care unit. Once there I was given a tracheotomy and placed on numerous drips.'

Being paralysed in the ITU was no less frightening:

'I was unable to move any muscle in my body, including my eyelids or my mouth, which meant I was unable to communicate at all. I cannot begin to describe the torture of being in a position where you know what people are saying about you but are unable to respond at all. My brain was functioning perfectly normally all the time but because of my paralysis, I was terrified. I hardly slept at all even though I was given liquid sleeping pills and had to be fed by a large drip, more like a hose pipe than an ordinary nasal tube, through the nose. Apart from the obvious physical discomforts of having a catheter, tracheotomy, nasal tube and numerous drips in one's body, which are actually physically painful, the emotional torture of being paralysed and not knowing why or how long it would last or what daily prognosis for the future would be was terrifying.

The tracheotomy had to be changed every week, which was very uncomfortable. In addition, the catheter had to be changed. This was acutely painful. It was terrible because I knew that these were due to be changed on the day when I had heard the doctors talking about what had to be done and I was nervous inside because I knew there would be pain. I never thought I was squeamish prior to having this botulism, but now I realise that I am. Throughout my incarceration in hospital and my illness, I lost two and a half stone in weight and have felt an incredible amount of sapping of my body strength.

Also during the first week that I was in hospital, whilst I was still completely paralysed, I was given electric shock treatments (electromyography to check the diagnosis). This again is acutely uncomfortable. However, I was paralysed so I was unable to move although the pain was acute. I am sure that this made the whole experience much worse. I could not even open my eyes. They were tight shut. After about ten days, I was able to nod which was the only way in which I could communicate. I thought that I was nodding my head vigorously when in fact it was barely perceptible to the visitors I had.

Once the paralysis gradually began to wear off, I could communicate by writing notes on a small pad of paper even though I was unable to speak because of the tracheotomy. Initially, when the tracheotomy was removed, I had to hold my hand over the dressing on my neck to enable me to speak at all and my voice sounded very different. It was a full five weeks before I was able to see clearly and even then I had been through a series of phases where I could open my eyes only partially, and then fully, and then suffered from double vision.'

How much he actually heard during the acute phase of the illness is not clear. He was aware of the doctors discussing the need to change his tracheotomy and his catheter and said that the doctors explained that he could be left with some paralysis. How accurate this was is unclear, but it does emphasize the need for caution in what is said near the bedside. In an addendum he explains about the faulty Walkman and realizes that his hearing was affected. The Walkman became more useful as he began to improve, shutting out the noise from the ventilators and other machinery in the ITU. As he could not manipulate the Walkman himself, or change the tapes, he had to find ways to draw attention to get the nurses to change the tape for him.

It became a game for me to invent different ways of doing this to get their attention. Using my mind in this way kept me sane. I would rattle the bars at the side of my bed or wave. Other ruses I invented to get the attention of the nurses were things like pulling out my life support tube, which caused a bell to ring. I also found that if I put my hand on my heart where the monitor was, it would make a noise which again caused attention. These small and insignificant things cheered me up no end and kept me from getting bored.

I do not have a verbatim record of the other patient's reactions, but from my questioning it was apparent he had similar problems. For a lot of the time he was pretty scared as he couldn't move, couldn't see anything, couldn't do anything and did not know what was happening. He prayed it was recoverable and not going to last like this for the rest of his life. By the second week he was able to listen to the news when they talked about botulism. He knew he had had yoghurt, he couldn't tell anybody and they heard somebody had died. This would be about the fourteenth day. He couldn't do anything and things were not getting better and he wondered whether this was going to be permanent or temporary. He complained of quite a lot of pain. First of all he got bad headaches. He had never previously had headaches and had pain when lying there, the mattress was uncomfortable, he slept in one position, he couldn't tell anybody. He had pains in the left then the right hip and a deadening down the leg as though it had fallen asleep. What he had to do was answer about fifty questions which he tried to do by wriggling his toe sometimes, but sometimes it was too weak. He had a very definite feeling of fear and was convinced at one stage that he was going to die until he was able to open his eyes. He also felt depressed up to the time that his friends would visit. He had nobody to talk to. Of course he could not talk for most of the time. His eyes were fully closed and he was on support. He looked forward to people coming in and couldn't sleep at nights. It felt really bad. He had a weird feeling with the tracheotomy. He had no idea what it was until he was able to see it and there were pipes which tended to leak over his shoulder and were constantly dripping. When the tracheotomy cuff was not fully inflated, air seemed to escape and resonate every few seconds and that really got him. For the first three weeks he was imagining himself in a different place or room. Every time he was moved slightly he felt he had been wheeled or hustled somewhere else in a different place each night until eventually he could see a little. There was a feeling of pressure building up and a painful irritation as regards his bladder. He had no control over defecation: if it happened, it happened. He had problems with constipation and the bowel was painful. He wasn't aware of chest problems except that physiotherapy to his chest was quite painful, and eventually he was sitting out in a chair. His head was spinning after lying for such a long time.

   What was most frustrating throughout the illness was not being able to get through to people, to communicate what he wanted, particularly when he had pain. It would take five or ten minutes to explain where the pain was. Particular problems were with the nasal drip. He vomited a lot of the time and stuff came out of his mouth. Changing the tracheotomy could be very uncomfortable and painful and sometimes lying on his arm or feet hurt a lot. The EMGs were extremely painful. When he had a talking tube in his tracheotomy, it was such a relief and his chest seemed to improve. Hearing was unaffected, he thought, but he heard better later on and there was one time when the shutting of bins in the ITU became unbearable. The problem was listening to people talking if he was lying on one ear and couldn't watch them. Various drips were painful as were the intramuscular injections.

## The Public Health Story

The Saturday meeting was followed by a second survey of the 8 known patients, seven of whom had had hazelnut yoghurt while the 8th was too ill to be interviewed. The outbreak was unusual in that the vehicle of intoxification was widely distributed before sale and patients presented singly to several different hospitals. The following afternoon they visited a factory farm producing hazelnut yoghurt, where they found 15 unopened cartons of hazelnut yoghurt, all of which were contaminated. They also obtained Clostridium botulinum from one sealed but badly blown can of hazelnut conserve. In total, 27 people were involved in the outbreak. The serum was negative in all of them. In addition Clostridium botulinum type B was detected in faeces from one patient and two opened cartons recovered from patients' homes were also positive. All other tests were negative. Furthermore, only 25 of the 27 patients affected were known to have obtained hazelnut yoghurt indirectly from producer 1 at the factory farm. Two other producers were investigated who might have supplied yoghurt containing hazelnut conserve from the same source but a link with the outbreak was not established.

The premises of producer 1, on the factory farm, were inspected and were of an adequate standard for the production of yoghurt. 150-200 gallons of skimmed pasteurised milk are transported by tank from the dairy to outbuildings 400 yards away. The milk is then pumped from the transporting tank to a batch pasteuriser before being heated to 110°F, when skimmed milk powder and starch is added. The temperature is then raised to 180°F (82°C) and the mixture held for 30 minutes whilst being agitated Sugar is added when the mixture reaches 180°F. The pasteurised mixture is pumped through a plate cooler into the inoculating tank and is held at approximately 110°F. The starter culture is added and mixed for 20 minutes, following which it was poured into ten gallon churns and placed in an incubator for 2-3 hours until 'set'. To make hazelnut yoghurt, one can of puree is emptied into each churn and the yoghurt gently mixed. The fruit yoghurt is then poured into the holding tank of a mechanical dispenser and cartoning machine. Approximately 360 cartons are filled from one 10-gallon churn.and each carton has a 'sell-by' date 25 days after production. Advice was given on the cartons that the yoghurt should be refrigerated and consumed within 2 days of purchase. The fact that each batch consisted of 360 cartons left many unaccounted for. Some might have been withdrawn from shops after the Department of Health's announcement and some thrown away after purchase following the radio warning. There was a fear both among clinicians and the public health authorities that other consumers could have been affected. However, there appeared not to have been any additional awareness of unexplained illnesses or deaths during that period.

The Public Health Enquiry was taken further. Hazelnuts were imported from several countries and roasted in a factory near Birmingham. Afterwards they were sent to a factory near Eastbourne where hazelnut puree (or conserve) was prepared from a mixture of pre-roasted hazelnuts, water, starch, and other ingredients, which was heated in a steam jacketed vat with a half ton capacity to a temperature of 90°C for 10 minutes. The mixture was pumped into metal cans which were closed at the top using a manually operated scamer and then placed in a retort of boiling water for a minimum of 20 minutes. Most of the hazelnut conserve manufactured contained sugar but a consignment of 36 cans sweetened with aspartame rather than with sugar had been received by producer 1 and stored at ambient temperature. Customers had reported to the conserve manufacturer that cans of the aspartame-sweetened hazelnut preparation had blown and, following this, just before delivery to producer 1, potassium sorbate was introduced into the mixture in an attempt to control yeasts. It is possible, but not established, that two other producers in the North West had received similar cans of conserve, but blown cans or contaminated cartons were not found on their premises.

Contamination of the conserve had occurred because of the use of low acid fruits (pH greater than 4.6); though only one other outbreak, associated with peanuts in Taiwan, had been caused by nuts, and, secondly, because there was insufficient heat used in the manufacturing process to destroy spores of Clostridium botulinum.

## The Other Affected Patients

I was able to act as clinical co-ordinator of the outbreak, seeing most of the patients at some time during or just after the outbreak. Various patterns in the development of symptoms emerged. The interval between consumption and the onset of symptoms was between 2 hours and 5 days, with a median of one day. The amount of yoghurt consumed varied from a couple of spoonfuls to three cartons and the Public Health officials were able to estimate from the cartons recovered the amount of toxin in the contaminated yoghurt. Yoghurt was popular among the children, among younger adults, most of whom were health fanatics, and as a convenience food for the elderly. Some, but not all, commented that the yoghurt had a different taste from usual and that the nuts tasted bitter. Those admitted within 48 hours of the first symptom had a combination of bulbar and ocular palsies. Seven required ventilatory support and two patients admitted to other hospitals had electrophysiological tests similar to the atypical findings already mentioned.

Where the presentation was oculo-bulbar in type, with double vision, droopy eyes, a nasal or slurred speech and difficulty in swallowing, the symptomatology was unequivocal. Thereafter, there was a progressive, and sometimes rapid, development of neurological deficits, usually spread over 3 days. The sequence of events varied. In most patients, difficulty in swallowing was the first symptom, with the development of a nasal voice after a few hours. In the more severe cases, visual symptoms developed simultaneously with the dysphagia. The severity of the ophthalmoparesis proved to be a good indicator of the risk of respiratory paralysis, overall disease severity and progression. Double vision occurred on lateral gaze before cranial nerve palsies became manifest, and three patients had nystagmus on lateral gaze at some stage of the illness. A partial ophthalmoplegia was usually associated with pronounced bilateral ptosis. When complete, there was a total external and internal ophthalmoplegia with widely dilated pupils. When there was ventilatory failure, it developed within 12 hours of the onset of ophthalmoplegia.

Other forms of presentation involved weakness of the legs. Three patients, including two children, had difficulty walking and going upstairs. One child was unable to hop two days before the onset of other symptoms. Two adults were noticed to have an alteration in speech before they themselves were aware of the problem. Those with the least severe onset complained of difficulty with saliva and a dry mouth. Approximately 40% of patients had more protean parasympathetic symptoms preceding the development of weakness with abdominal cramps, vomiting, diarrhoea or constipation, difficulty focusing, dizziness, paralytic ileus or urinary difficulty.

**Illustrative histories:-**
*A. Parasympathetic onset*
Two hours after having yoghurt, a policeman developed bloating of his stomach, coming on so abruptly and severely that he couldn't do up his trousers and he was unable to answer a call from his police sergeant to attend to his police duties. Afterwards he was reasonably well for two days until he went to work on the Saturday. He was working nights and had become over-

tired, especially as he had been doing a lot of sports. He developed double vision. He took a panda car to get some petrol and had to abandon it because he was misjudging distances. That day his speech became slurred as though drunk, he had difficulty swallowing and a dry throat and attended the Accident and Emergency department of a hospital. The diagnosis was made of tonsillitis although the doctor noticed that his pupils were dilated and asked him whether he had been on drugs. On Monday he couldn't get out of bed, the room was spinning, he had double vision, saliva could neither be swallowed nor spat out and was stringy. His speech was muffled and unintelligible. His wife had heard on the radio about botulism and sent him into hospital.

*B. Initial disturbance of speech*
A 74-year old lady purchased some yoghurt on the 7th and ate a carton the next day. Another yoghurt, kept in her house, proved to be positive for botulinum type B. On the day of eating the yoghurt, she went on a bus tour in the company of a number of friends, some of whom commented that she was not talking properly. She herself noticed nothing in particular until Friday evening, 9th June, when she came to eat her evening meal and was unable to swallow solids and was having difficulty even swallowing liquids. She felt listless and was worried though not particularly ill in other respects. By Saturday morning her legs felt peculiar. She went to church on Sunday but felt rotten and remained in bed for the rest of the day. On the Monday she went to see her general practitioner, who thought that there was nothing wrong with her and gave her some soothing medicine for her throat. That evening she heard about botulism and her right eye had become blurred. She rang the emergency doctor and was admitted to hospital via the Casualty Department.

*C. A lady aged 55 who took 10 days before admission to hospital*
She was a healthy lady regularly cycling to work. On the 1st June she had some hazelnut yoghurt after her normal evening meal and didn't have any immediate symptoms until the following evening, when after a roast dinner she felt she had an acid stomach upset. She had to go to bed, had acute stomach ache and indigestion-type pains which were not relieved by tablets. About 1 am she went to the toilet, was violently sick, and this eased the pain so that she was able to go back to sleep. She felt unwell the next day and her husband persuaded her to remain in bed. She did not eat that day and then had diarrhoea and was weak afterwards. At that stage she looked out of the window and noticed that the doors of the houses opposite were out of focus

and didn't fit in the doorways with the appropriate house. In fact, her vision was affected for seven days. At 4.30 the same day she had great difficulty swallowing a poached egg, couldn't stand the taste of a cigarette and went back to bed feeling unwell. On Sunday she went downstairs to make a cup of tea and was unable to stand up without wobbling. She noticed her balance was affected, couldn't talk, felt as though she had marbles in her mouth, and one of her neighbours thought she had had a stroke for these reasons. She was not able to eat dinner, her speech was still slurred, her eyes were running and she had to wipe them with tissues all the time. It was as though she had pieces of goo in her eyes like a dog. There was a feeling as though she had a film over her eyes that couldn't be peeled away.

She was seen by her general practitioner on the Monday morning. At that time her tongue had a nasty yellow fur. She no longer had any diarrhoea; in fact she had been constipated for nine days after the diarrhoea already described. She didn't feel her throat was sore and the doctor felt she had had gastroenteritis. Later on the 9th he diagnosed tonsillitis.

On the Tuesday she felt as though she had mouth ulcers. All food was blocked She gargled, put some ointment in her mouth and then when she tried to bring the stuff up she found she was bringing ream after ream of elastic-like tissue from her mouth in long strips and this was very worrying. She sat down on the settee and was too weak to get up. She had to drag herself bodily by the banisters to get upstairs. She was given antibiotics on the Wednesday and her husband had to open the capsules and pour them into hazelnut yoghurt to try to get the large tablets down. She found herself choking on this, her husband had to bang her back and she couldn't swallow the pieces of hazelnut yoghurt. There didn't appear to be any lump or anything in her throat – just that she couldn't swallow. She was most frightened about what could be the problem with her. She had to use a whole box of tissues on the eyes and by Friday she was unable to eat at all except for some Oxo and water. She couldn't even have tea or coffee and remained in bed most of the time. She couldn't watch television because of blurring of vision. On one occasion she spoke into the telephone and had to be bodily lifted because she was so ill and weary. It was at this time that the doctor gave her penicillin for tonsillitis.

She spent the entire weekend in bed. Her eyelids were very heavy and semi-closed and by Monday she heard a bulletin about botulism but others wouldn't believe that this was the problem, though her step-children were extremely concerned about her general weakness. She was unable to wash herself, he daughter had to wash her physically in the bathroom from top to toe. She was unable to take the lid off toothpaste and had to be helped with this. Eventually she was taken to Casualty on 13th June and when she got to the ward, she was found to be dehydrated. On the 15th neurophysiological tests confirmed a pre-synaptic block with post-tetanic facilitation. She was given a saline drip for three days. When she left hospital after ten days, she left in a wheelchair and it was another week before she could swallow things properly.

*D. Children*

There were six affected children, including two pairs of siblings. Their ages ran from 14 months to 14 years The most severely affected was 3 years of age. She awoke early on the morning of June 6th with a headache and vomited. She thought her nose was running, which was not so, but she had a marked halitosis. Later that day her speech became slurred. She became unsteady with increasing drowsiness and had difficulty in swallowing and drinking. She choked on drinks. On admission to hospital, she was floppy and weak. A diffuse encephalopathy, predominantly involving the brainstem, was provisionally diagnosed. Because of deterioration in her conscious level, she was transferred to Booth Hall Hospital the following day. On arrival she seemed to be confused with a diffuse encephalopathy, hypoventilation, and hypoxia. She had a total external opthalmoplegia, aphonia, aphagia, areflexia, a paralytic ileus, and required assisted respiration. Intracranial pressure was normal. Admission of her 24-month old brother 48 hours later, alert but with a similar clinical picture, led to the provisional diagnosis of botulism. Botulinum antitoxin was given and her condition improved. Symptoms resolved over three weeks.

All 27 patients complained of fatiguability, difficulty in swallowing and slurred speech, with weakness, often more pronounced in the legs than in the arms. Vision was blurred in 21 with droopiness of the eyes in 15 and double vision in 8. Ten had abdominal pain and vomiting; two with diarrhoea and 9 with constipation. Difficulty in breathing was experienced by 9 and sore throat by 7 and a dry mouth by 5. Less expected symptoms were drowsiness affecting 16, fever in 8 and headache in four. At the height of the illness eye movements were completely lost in 2, partially so in 14; pupil reactions lost in 12 and partially affected in 9. Breathing was severely affected in 13, partially in 6, requiring artificial ventilation from 8-53 for 8 patients. Arm and leg movements were lost in 8 and reflexes in 14. A disturbance of speech was present in 20 patients and of swallowing in 12. Six had a paralytic ileus and 9 secondary infection. One patient died and this has to be recorded as a preventable death.

*E. The patient who died*
A 74 year-old lady was admitted. The GPs. letter read as follows:-

This lady had hazelnut yoghurt 4 days ago, developed malaise, dry mouth, weakness, nausea two days ago. Seen yesterday. Diagnosed as a viral illness. Now complaining of inability to swallow, weakness and blurred vision. Past medical history: two hip replacements and well controlled hypertension. On examination, pulse 82/min., temperature 37°C, blood pressure 150/90. Drowsy, dehydrated and dysarthric. Chest contained a few crepitations but basal expansion good. pupils dilated but reacting. Uniform muscular weakness. All reflexes are O.K. except right ankle jerk absent and right plantar extensor. Abdomen normal. No neck rigidity. Takes moduretic daily. Diagnosis: Cl botulinum ingestion. P.S. Having rechecked reflexes 40 minutes after the above. Right and left diminished but present. Plantars extensor. Chest expansion still good. Respirations 15-18 per minute. (An excellent letter.)

On arrival in hospital she had bilateral ptosis, VI and VII cranial nerve palsies, limited upward gaze, and diplopia in all directions. She was aphonic without gag reflexes, and palate and tongue were immobile. Power and reflexes were reduced and both plantars flexor. Blood gases were normal and respiratory peak flow measured hourly. She was given antitoxin, intravenous fluids, and humidified oxygen. A nasogastric tube was passed. The next morning she seemed to improve but suddenly regurgitated and aspirated through the tube, stopped breathing, became cyanosed, and required intubation and positive ventilation. A paralytic ileus and an aspiration pneumonia with bilateral basal shadows on x-ray. Despite antibiotics and corrective measures, her blood pressure fell and the chest infection did not respond.

**Historical Aspects**
Paralytic illness following the consumption of sausages (Latin. botulus) was described in the early 19th century by Justinius Kerner, a German physician, and for many years was known as 'Kerner's disease'. In 1896 Van Ermengem isolated an anaerobic organism when investigating an illness affecting 23 musicians, three of whom died, all of whom had eaten raw salted ham after playing at a wake in the Belgium village of Ellezelles. A recurrent theme in the case-reports has been that others have died tragically after the initial diagnosis has been missed. For example, a 20 year-old Kenyan nomad had prepared soured milk in a gourd for a ceremony and sampled the contents through a straw. She became ill and died within 12 hours. After the funeral the attendants were given refreshments including the soured milk

preparation. Between one and four days later 10 fell sick and five died. Similarly in Colorado, a woman died after eating home-canned (bottled) mushrooms and two other members of her family became ill from tasting the mushrooms after they had attended the funeral.

Delayed recognition of an outbreak may also occur when patients are widely dispersed and present singly. In a Canadian outbreak, the diagnosis of botulism in two teenage sisters in Montreal led to the identification of 36 previously unrecognized victims of the same outbreak of type B botulism who had eaten garlic bread prepared from chopped garlic in soybean oil in a restaurant in Vancouver, British Columbia, during the preceding 6 weeks. The misdiagnoses included myasthenia gravis, psychiatric disorders and stroke.

The symptoms of food-borne botulism are caused by the ingestion of preformed neuro-toxins produced by strains of Clostridium botulinum, an anaerobic spore-forming gram positive rod-shaped bacillus widely distributed throughout the world in soil and marine sediments. The toxin-producing spores are heat resistant, requiring temperatures above 80°C for 30 minutes for their destruction, and are able to persist in a viable form as a contaminant of improperly processed foods. At high altitudes, as in the Rocky Mountains, the boiling point is too low to destroy spores. In an acid milieu, spores remain dormant but will germinate at room or body temperature under anaerobic conditions at a pH of 6 or above. The types of toxin most often associated with human disease are types A,B and E (rarely F and G). Type A is probably the most toxic and is found in North America west of the Mississippi and in Africa. Type B is found principally east of the Mississippi and in Europe. Contaminated seafood is the usual vehicle for type E intoxication. Types C1,C2, and D, associated with animal botulism, are probably not absorbed by the human gastrointestinal tract.

Botulism is one of the most powerful toxins known. It is indistinguishable from tetanus but 1,000 times more potent. It is most active as a dichain composed of a heavy chain which binds with specific sites on the nerve terminal and light chain which contains the region responsible for paralysis. Proteolytic enzymes such as trypsin may nick the single chain proteins to form dichains and even trichains with a resultant increase in toxicity. Thus, when isolated from cultures, type A is a fully toxic dichain protein, type E is a mildly toxic mixture with a majority of single chains and type B a mixture of single and dichains and nearly fully toxic. The toxin binds to the nerve terminals, enters by a process known as endocytosis and causes permanent damage affecting the presynaptic release of acetylcholine. Muscle fatiguability and paralysis result, with secondary destruction of the nerve terminal.

Recovery is possible several weeks later as a result of the sprouting of new nerve terminals with the formation of new neuro-muscular connections.

Food-borne botulism in man is rare in the United Kingdom. Five incidents relate to the ingestion of home-prepared dishes – rabbit and pigeon broth, jugged hare, vegetarian nut brown, minced meat pie and macaroni cheese – and was unknown before the Loch Maree incident in August 1922. The *Campbelltown Courier* described it as a 'Highland Tragedy': six visitors and a ghillie died. Obscure type of disease. Eventually 8 people died They had gone fishing on the loch taking with them freshly prepared duck paste sandwiches from the hotel.

From *The Times* report of August 19th 1922.

> In the evening the guests dined at the hotel. It was only about breakfast time the next day that the first and not very pronounced symptoms were experienced. Young Mr Talbot excused himself from breakfast, saying that he had double vision and was not quite fit. Later Mr Williams, another guest, made practically an identical complaint. For a time 'seeing double' was regarded as a joke, but before long symptoms pointing to some disturbing agency were more clearly discovered in dizziness among the guests, cases of actual sickness, and later a distressing form of paralysis which affected the muscles of the throat ultimately making speech impossible. Consciousness persisted to the end in each case, and the sufferers, unable to speak, communicated their wishes and explained their symptoms in writing... The distress deepened, although there was very little pain, and general collapse followed.

The *Campbelltown Courier* concentrated on the ghillie's death.

### The Ghillie's Farewell

A pathetic feature of the death of Kenneth Maclennan is that on Wednesday, knowing he was on his deathbed, he expressed his wish to end his days at home. On Thursday he was taken to the croft at Opilin where he lived with his widowed mother, but only lived half an hour. Just before passing away, he managed to write the simple word, 'Goodbye'.

MacLennan had been out on the loch on Monday with Major and Mrs Anderson, of London. At lunch time, the Major said he did not care for paste, and handed over his share of the sandwiches to MacLennan. He thus narrowly escaped the fate of his wife and the ghillie.

The Birmingham outbreak in 1978 was almost as dramatic. Two couples in their mid-60s and 70s took afternoon tea together, consisting of tinned salmon salad, fruit and cream at 5 pm on the day before admission. Nine to eleven hours after the meal all four developed nausea, vomiting, a dry mouth, dizziness and blurring of vision. The younger couple were admitted semiconscious to the Casualty Department, where the Casualty Officer, who had been reading for an exam, made an immediate diagnosis of botulism. The Casualty sister asked if they had shared the meal with anyone and getting a positive reply, tried to contact the other couple. The police broke into their house finding them both comatose.

At 7 am all had evidence of extrinsic ocular muscle paralysis and rapidly developed paralysis of the facial, pharyngeal, truncal and peripheral muscles, resulting in difficulty with vision, speech, swallowing and respiration. Despite the ashen appearance, their blood pressure was normal. Paralysis rapidly progressed and within 4 hours all had to be transferred to the intensive care unit. Progressive hypoventilatory respiratory failure followed and all four patients were intubated and ventilated within 6 hours of admission. The clinical diagnosis of botulism (later shown to be type E) was provisionally confirmed on the day of admission by the demonstration of circulating neurotoxin, lethal to mice, in the serum of all four patients. Treatment with trivalent equine antitoxin was commenced within 4 hours of admission.

Supportive intensive care and antitoxin therapy were complemented by the use of aminopyridine, with no detectable effect on the respiratory muscles. Two patients developed fits. Two survived but the other two (one from each couple) died.

In 1989 a 49 year-old man was ventilated for 173 days after developing botulism following a shelf-stable Kosher meal of rice and vegetables with an offensive smell and taste on a French Airline. He ate only two mouthfuls, 9 to 10 hours later he had blurred and double vision followed by nausea and vomiting, difficulty in swallowing and speech, dryness of the mouth and arm weakness. He was on total parenteral nutrition for 158 days, catheterised for 111 days, discharged from hospital walking with the aid of sticks after 237 days and the tracheostomy was closed on day 265.

**Toxico-infective Forms of Botulism**

Botulism, like tetanus, may result from the germination of spores of Clostridium botulinum within the tissues of the body. Wound botulism may occur in young males with compound fractures, in abscesses of drug abusers and with contaminated traumatic wounds, allowing anaerobic multiplication and germination of clostridia. The diagnosis may be made electrophysiologically, serologically or by recovery of spores from infected wounds. Thorough debidement of wounds and the use of antibiotics (other than aminoglycosides which can potentiate the neuro-muscular blockade) is required.

Food-borne botulism can occur in young people, as in the 4-year old boy from Flat Lick near Red Bird Kentucky, described by McQuillen and Josifek in 1972. But even with family outbreaks of food-borne botulism, infants are usually spared because they are commonly fed on special diets that reduce their risk of exposure to foods containing botulinum toxin. Not until 1976 was infantile botulism described. Most of the documented cases (95%) have occurred in the United States, two-thirds of them being in California.

Infant botulism occurs in the first year of life, usually between 2 and 5 months of age. Study of the intestinal micro-flora has suggested that there may be a delay in the establishment of normal flora, colonization by organisms that promote Clostridia, the absence of organisms that inhibit Clostridia and a change in diet that results in constipation and stasis, allowing the germination and out-growth of spores. Symptoms may start insidiously with constipation preceding other manifestations by as much as three weeks. Thereafter the child becomes lethargic, weak and floppy with a weak cry and inability to suck. Infants may present as failure to thrive, or with feeding difficulties, or may die without premonitory signs of illness. There is some evidence that botulism may be a rare cause of the sudden infant death syndrome, with the presence of Clostridia in post-mortem faecal specimens from infants who have died suddenly. Progressive weakness and hypotonic serum can arise from excessive secretion of antidiuretic hormone in affected infants. The diagnosis is often more readily made from the faeces than from the sera. Treatment not only involves giving the antitoxin, preferably as human botulism immune globulin (BIG, but should always include sterilizing the gastro-intestinal tract with antibiotics. Some patients may require assisted ventilation and parenteral feeding.

At least a third of the California cases are linked to feeding honey* which may contain spores and provides a non-acid environment in which they can germinate. Approximately 10% of U.S. honey contains spores. 6% of samples of raw sugar or molasses for apiculture are contaminated by soil containing spores and multiplication of Clostridia can occur in pupae and dead adult bees (but not in bee larvae). Advice is given suggesting that it is prudent not to feed honey to infants under 12 months of age.

---

*Honey has been implicated in disease in another way. Cyrus defeated Pompey's troops at Trebizond in 401B.C. by persuading the peasants to feed Pompey's forces with 'mad honey' from mountain laurel (Rhododendron ponticum). 'All the soldiers that ate from the combs lost their senses, vomited and were affected so that none of them was able to stand upright; such as had a little were like men greatly intoxicated.' Those not slain in the subsequent battle recovered rapidly. Honey gathered from bees feeding on certain strains of Rhododendron contains Grayanotoxin. Within a few minutes to three hours, patients develop dizziness, weakness, sweating, nausea and vomiting. They may faint with hypotension, shock and a slow pulse. In addition to the original report by Xenophon, there have been more recent outbreaks in the United States and in Turkey.

Adult toxico-infection is unusual but has occasionally been reported in association with a compromized gastric acid barrier due to achlorhydria, with gastro-intestinal operations and with stagnant loops of bowel. Relapses can occur and the bacillus and toxin may be recovered from the faeces long after serological tests become negative.

## Long-term Symptoms Following Botulism

After the acute phase of botulism, survival is greeted with considerable relief. Most outbreaks involve few individuals and reports of subsequent morbidity are largely anecdotal. But three papers reviewing some of the larger outbreaks report continued symptoms: some for as long as five years.

I was able to follow up 21 of the 26 surviving patients: 16 were seen for legal reports between January and March 1990. After the legal proceedings were completed, I sent a questionnaire to all 26 patients (or their parents) in January 1992 and all but 4 replied. I also sent a more selected questionnaire in 1996, 7 years after the outbreak. I was concerned to find out whether the late symptoms had a physical condition with features which could be measured, and whether the recognition of late symptoms adds to our understanding of post-viral fatigue syndromes.

Because the whole question of M.E. (myalgic encephalomyelitis; chronic fatigue syndrome) is surrounded with so much emotion, I will give an internationally accepted definition of chronic fatigue syndrome before proceeding further. It is a chronic illness of uncertain aetiology, characterized by at least six months of debilitating fatigue and associated symptoms. The symptoms of the syndrome are all non-specific and some (but not all) are also seen in psychiatric illness. The symptomatology suggesting an organic component to the illness includes its abrupt onset with an 'infectious-like' illness, intermittent unexplained fevers, arthralgias and 'gelling' (stiffness), sore throats, cough, photophobia, night sweats, and post-exertional malaise with systemic symptoms. The illness can last for years and is associated with marked impairment of functional health status.

Sixteen of the 22 patients replying to my first questionnaire of January 1992 complained of late symptoms. Grading the severity of the acute phase into those with mild symptoms, those requiring hospitalization for more than 15 days, and those requiring ventilation, I found no direct association between the initial severity and the persistence of symptoms. Thus prolonged symptoms were reported at 38 months by 3 of the 7 patients who had been ventilated, 5 or the 6 moderately affected and 8 of the 13 mildly affected. I commented at the time that the younger patients tended to show the best improvement. Among the elderly, it is possible that secondary factors may have combined to delay recovery but there was little to suggest that the expected life-span had been shortened by the illness. The middle group represented those who were most active and included 4 sports fanatics. They may represent the most introspective or intelligent group but it is also probable that a mild reduction in exercise tolerance would more readily be recognized.

If we seek to analyse the complaints, we can take into account that after paresis, respiratory difficulty, pains from tracheotomies, drips and catheters, return to physical fitness would be a prolonged affair and far from smooth. Some symptoms would be expected on the basis of natural anxiety:-

a) A 15 year-old girl seen in March 1990 remained tired all the time, with backache and is unable to do PE and badminton. If she plays badminton for five minutes she has to sit and rest for three quarters of an hour. The previous May she had played tennis for two hours at a stretch. She also finds that her social life has been affected as she is very tired the next day if she stays out at all. By July 1990 she felt some improvement but, doing Saturday work in a supermarket, her eyes get tired working the till and she has not been going out at night, so has had very little social life.

b) A 74-year old complained that she gets odd difficulties focusing and has lost sweetness of taste. She used to enjoy cooking but has to cook by the recipe book because what tastes well for her, for example a curry, no one else can eat. She has to chew things well as they can catch when eating and she has to put her head forwards and retch slightly and take sips of water with her food. She has problems going up and down stairs, getting shortness of breath, palpitation and is unable to clean the house now. She feels as though there is a lump at the bottom of her back which hurts if she does too much. On a good day she is able to walk on the flat round, for example, a supermarket, but on a bad day she will stay in bed until midday and then try and get up and do something.

c) Another elderly person aged 74 complained of unsteadiness on her feet, urgency of micturition and loss of hair. The new glasses have not really improved matters when driving. She has difficulty getting off to sleep, and finds that she is much more reluctant and weak when doing housework, whereas previously she used to enjoy it.

d) A 40-year old woman explained that she was very weak after returning home but matters improved, levelling out about December 1990. She tires or fatigues after physical activity, cannot walk far and after walking up two flights of stairs, is jiggered. She can walk upstairs in her own house unless she has done something energetic such as washing the floor. If she is going up longer stairs, as in a shop, her legs ache and her whole body, particularly her chest, aches. It is not a pain but a feeling of exhaustion. When kneeling for Communion she has to pull herself up afterwards. When walking the dog, she finds herself slowing down and, if she is tired, the right eye goes bloodshot. After the evening meal she feels fit for nothing. When she goes driving, she does not like driving for more than 30 minutes as she feels stiff and has to stop. There are times when she gets cramp in her feet. She used to do swimming to keep herself fit but she has had to give up because the pressure of water on her chest disturbed her.

There are many reasons why a person should have a sub-acute fatigue syndrome on recovery from either botulism or an infection:

a. myalgic pains, tiredness and depression are well recognized as following a viral or rickettsial disease for many months, as with glandular fever and dengue (break-back fever);

b. feelings 'why should this happen to me?' lead to feelings of paranoia and depression;

c. athletes, e.g. ballet dancers, are prepared to put up with various aches and pains whilst achieving, but similar aches and pains when no longer achieving are poorly tolerated.

All such symptoms are from time to time seen in the chronic fatigue syndrome, unnaturally prolonged, and can be difficult to separate from other forms of the chronic fatigue syndrome. When challenged, patients may react adversely, making an empathic relationship with their medical adviser extremely difficult.

Thirty-eight months after the acute phase, I recruited 8 adult patients on the basis of accessibility, and excluding children and elderly patients, and asked them to volunteer for further investigation.

The tests involved were: psychological tests based on a U.K. proforma for the post-viral fatigue syndrome; laboratory screening; pulmonary function tests and repeat electromyography. Previous testing at this stage, reported in earlier papers, had failed to show any association with the chronic fatigue syndrome or any objective impairment. I had intended, particularly by repeating the pulmonary function tests in a swimming pool with the weight of the water on the diaphragm and after exercise, to see whether more exacting tests could reveal further information. I also wished to look at mitochondrial enzymes. These are enzymes present in cells throughout the body which involve cell activity and respiration. Unfortunately none of the more exacting tests were performed due to a breakdown in communication, leading to inadequate preparation for testing and I was left with the same negative results as reported by previous workers. By 1996 all patients had shrugged off their residual symptoms. This last questionnaire was combined with the opportunity to send blood away for sophisticated antibody measurement, the results of which are still awaited.

The main complaints were carefully analysed.

Changes in life style affected four patients who were forced to change their careers because of lack of stamina. One patient gave up business studies and a girl complained of losing time from school and inability to make up her grades. One lady who had a full-time job now has to employ a cleaner. A taxi driver says he can only work three hours in the morning, must sleep in the afternoon and can then resume for a few hours in the evening. Although he was at one time a builder, he no longer possesses the energy to decorate and renovate his house. Another changed from an outdoor job to a desk job and a policeman complained that it has taken nearly 2 years to rekindle enthusiasm for his job, which involves a great deal of stamina.

Sleep difficulties which affected 7 patients tended to resolve within 6 months. One explanation was a fear of falling asleep. For several months a patient who had been tetraplegic and required ventilation complained of not being able to lie on his stomach. Three of the four elderly patients continued to experience impaired sleep patterns. Four patients experienced dreams and flashbacks but these tended to lessen and clear within 1 to 2 years.

Breathing problems did not reflect the degree of respiratory involvement in the acute phase, and overall there were fewer complaints than expected. Most breathing troubles were related to lack of stamina; thus some patients were unable to walk and talk at the same time.

The cricketer complained of poor eye-hand coordination affecting a range of sporting activities. One child was regarded as more clumsy and the two eldest patients became increasingly unsteady. Most patients had lost considerable weight in the acute phase. This weight loss was slowly regained by most patients. Those rendered relatively inactive often had to be content with an unacceptable gain in weight, which accentuated any residual clumsiness.

Various complaints were made that the voice had changed. It was more nasal, would tire, lacked strength, was affected by poorly coordinated breathing, or sounded different. One patient complained of a stammer. Most of these problems tended to improve: the nasal speech within 2 months, speech volume and fatiguability within a year, but at times of stress speech problems could return.

Symptoms concerning choking, chewing and swallowing often continued. There was probably both a psychological and an organic component to these symptoms, with the complaint that the mouth still felt paralysed and stiff, the jaw would fatigue with chewing, there would be gagging on certain foods, and a fear that food may go down 'the wrong way'. Some patients reported a late improvement after twelve months, whilst others continued to be wary of certain foods, which they would help down with sips of water. Complaints of ulceration within the mouth or nasal passages tended to persist.

Visual symptoms were frequently complained of and could take several forms, varying from photophobia and difficulty in focusing to squints and double vision. One elderly patient complained of a rapid deterioration of vision. Improvement in the co-ordination of binocular vision could be slow, imperfect and liable to worsen with fatigue.

Mental symptoms tended to be more prominent in the medico-legal reports and in supplementary reports from psychiatrists than in the follow-up surveys. Two patients complained of increased irritability, three of lack of concentration and two of memory difficulties, but the overall impression was of an excellent degree of adjustment to morbidity of their illness.

**Ecological factors and animal botulism**
The rarity of human botulism, particularly in Great Britain, meant that the 1989 outbreak took everyone by surprise. Many questions can be asked. Can we take comfort in the fact that no lives were lost when full life-support procedures were inaugurated? The answer must be an emphatic NO. Even so I stand by the decision not to use antitoxin several days after the two most severe patients were admitted to the intensive care unit for two reasons: that the toxin was already fixed within nerves and because of the risk of an anaphylactic reaction to horse serum. For these reasons it is questionable whether the same lives would be saved without antitoxin in circumstances similar to the Birmingham outbreak or with type A botulism. Our hope is that the publicity we have given to the outbreak will mean that botulism is more quickly recognized, were it to break out, that, as in California, human antiglobulin becomes available, and that in future people are not misled by negative serological tests and atypical neuro-physiological findings. Perhaps the most important lesson of all is that any patient with swallowing difficulties, impaired ventilation, the sudden onset of ophthalmoparesis or paralytic ileus must be under constant observation. The airway needs to be protected and with any form of intestinal stasis a naso-gastric tube is not an adequate treatment.

There is an economic impact to any botulism outbreak which increases sharply with the scattering of affected individuals. Jonathan Mann, who was later to work for the World Health Organization, estimated that an outbreak of food-borne botulism involving 34 victims in 1978 resulted in costs to the community in excess of $5.8 million. As botulism is one of the rarest of the food-borne illnesses affecting humans, the public health impact of food safety must affect all national budgets. In the past botulism has been associated with sausages, hams, and fish. Fish still remains a hazard, as in Alaska with the preparation of dried, salted or fermented fish. Fish are not only eaten in the country of origin but may be sent great distances by air commercially or to meet individual demands. Muslims buy fish in Manchester flown in from India. Uncooked fish from Japan is eaten worldwide. And freshwater whitefish (ribbitz, kapchunka fish) soaked in brine and then air-dried has been the cause of outbreaks of botulism in New York City and in Israel. Poor packaging and lack of refrigeration have contributed, but it is also possible that sodium chloride does not necessarily penetrate the intestinal contents of the fish. Vast changes in dietary habits have occurred throughout the civilized world and recent outbreaks of botulism have involved modern foods such as sautéed onions, chopped garlic, canned peppers, soft cheeses and cheese sauce.

Food exposed to view in delicatessens, if allowed to heat or remain unused for several days, has a high risk potential. My colleague in Preston, David Hutchinson, wrote a leading article outlining the public health hazards which can give rise to botulism. The increasing use of modified atmospheric packaging and the dependence on refrigeration to extend the shelf life of raw meat, fresh fish, coleslaw, and several processed products without preservatives has added to the potential danger. Vacuum packaging may result in an environment conducive to the growth of anaerobes, which, combined with the ability of non-proteolytic strains to grow at refrigeration temperature, has led to concern that toxin may be produced and released before spoilage is obvious to the consumer. Adequate processing and storage must be the primary objective of preserving foods. The spores of all strains of Clostridium botulinum are destroyed by heat at 121°C for two and a half minutes, but not all food is suitable for such heat treatment. Canned (or bottled) products such as cured meats rely on salt and nitrite to inhibit the growth of spores and a reduced heat treatment to kill vegetative cells. Acidic fruits and acidified vegetables are subjected only to pasteurisation and depend on the low pH to inhibit production of toxin. The survival of aerobic spore-bearers and yeasts in tins of tomatoes or soft fruits may alter the pH and allow growth of Clostridium botulinum. The recognition of blown containers should prevent their use. Foods in modified atmospheric packaging have been available with a good safety record but the possibility that ambient temperatures may be too high to inhibit toxin production has led to calls for additional safety controls, including low dose irradiation, co-inoculation with lactic acid bacilli and heat treatment after packaging. Food and Drug Administrations have advised that mushroom packaging should be pierced with air holes to prevent botulinum toxin forming. It would also seem sensible to take similar measures with the packaging of all fresh vegetables if they are not for immediate use.

Almost in direct contradiction to hygienic requirements, consumer demand is for convenience foods with minimal or no preservative and extended durability. Storage at or below 3.3°C is perhaps the single most important safety factor, but this is not always achieved under retail or housekeeping conditions. Nor can one rely on the recommended heating times for such products to inactivate botulinum toxin completely. Vigilance is always necessary because food-borne botulism is a preventable disease.

Human botulism is a rare disease which could readily burgeon into a serious menace. In the first 50 years of the 20th century only 5,635 persons were reported with botulism and just 1,714 died. But thousands, if not millions, of animals and birds die each year from botulism and there are many lessons and implications to be learnt from animal botulism. There is a cross-over in that during the 1989 outbreak two children shared a carton of hazelnut yoghurt with their cat. They became ill but not the cat. I had been in close contact with the neighbouring veterinary research station, sharing the platform on several occasions in discussions on Creutzfeld-Jacob disease and Bovine Spongioform Encephalopathy and therefore approached them for as much information as possible on the presentation of botulism in animals. The importance of environmental and ecological factors swiftly became apparent.

James Lovelock, in Gaia – *A New Look at Life on Earth* – states that when life first began, it was anaerobic. When the atmosphere became poisoned with oxygen, anaerobic organisms sought refuge in the soil, in marine deposits and in the guts of the new aerobic creatures. However, from time to time they take their vengeance on the second generation of living organisms.

The Clostridia are but one of the anaerobic organisms disseminated by being carried, for the most part harmlessly, as vegetative forms within the guts of herbivores, but they can cause such diseases as necrotizing enteritis, gas gangrene, and tetanus as well as botulism. As stated, toxins from Clostridium botulinum are responsible for the deaths of hundreds, if not thousands, of wild, domesticated and exotic species of bird and animal each year. On one lake in Canada 50,000 birds died in 1971, 100,000 sheep died in Australia in 1933, and for many years 100,000 cattle died annually in South Africa. Outbreaks have occurred in pheasant, mink and trout farms, among horses, foxhounds, turkeys and broiler chickens and in zoos, affecting birds, big cats (in zoos and circuses), New World monkeys, and sea lions.

Most intoxications are food-borne but toxico-infective and wound botulism also occur. Some outbreaks, particularly involving ducks on the Norfolk Broads, have been described as water-borne, with winter and spring outbreaks. It has since been realized that these outbreaks are not due to persistence of toxins in the frozen water, but to changes in the water level affecting invertebrates harbouring Clostridia.

Among animals and birds the first intimation of an epidemic may be of deaths for no apparent reason. But where one can study the clinical features, they differ little between medical and veterinary practice. Birds, such as ducks, chickens, turkeys, and wildfowl, initially appear dull and reluctant to move. As the illness progresses, their eyes shut, their wings and neck are stretched out and the legs tucked underneath. Similar observations apply to a wide variety of mammals: cattle, lions, foxhounds, baboons, sheep, and pigs. A good example is the horse. It will appear depressed and dull, the eyes closed. If the lids are opened, the pupils will be seen to be dilated. It will be reluctant to move, to rise from the ground or take food. When trying to eat it will dribble and drop food from the mouth. There is a progression of symptomatic features: abdominal distension, colic, vomiting, inability to swallow, diaphragmatic breathing, weakness, muscle tremors, and stumbling – with the development of a flaccid paralysis starting in the hind quarters, giving an abnormal lying posture and splaying of the legs when trying to stand. Later the weakness affects the fore-quarters and head posture. Characteristically the tongue can be grasped and pulled out from the mouth.

The biggest risk factor, causing epidemics of botulism especially in birds, is the imbibing of contaminated water. Water is most likely to be contaminated in drought and hot weather, lying in shallow stagnant pools, or where water has seeped from alkaline soils. Overgrowth of pond weed may lead to oxygen depletion with rotting vegetable and organic matter and decomposing carcasses in the water. Aquatic invertebrates, blowfly larvae maggots, and all types of carcasses may contain Clostridia.

Destruction of livestock is usually associated with unnatural necrophagia, e.g. from the presence of rodent carcasses in fodder. Lamsiekte among cattle in South Africa develops in times of drought when the parched grass is deficient in phosphorus. They develop a craving, seeking to replenish the phosphorus from the shells of dead tortoises. A similar condition, called Dry Bible, occurs among sheep and cattle in Western Australia. Malnourished and undernourished animals develop pica and are susceptible to botulism from carrion. Livestock on farms – horses, cattle, pigs, poultry – particularly in winter – depend on man to supply foodstuff. Grass harvested for silage is inevitably contaminated with soil. Properly dried big bale silage is safe, but, if damp, heavily moulded samples are hermetically wrapped in plastic and sealed, fermentation can occur and the pH can be as high as 8.5. In an alkaline pH with increasing temperature spores may germinate with the production of toxin. Infected meat scraps may be added to animal feed not only on traditional farms but in the wider context of farming, for example in mink farms. And botulism among trout in fish farms has occurred after feeding with spoiled marine fish scraps. Man may thus be an inadvertent and indirect cause of serious outbreaks of animal botulism.

Man's pollution of the environment can also be an important factor. Seepage of alkaline waste from factories and thermal effluence as from power stations can enhance bacterial proliferation where there is oxygen depletion. Diversion of water from streams for domestic purposes may alter the flora with an overgrowth of pond weed, rotting matter, stagnation and oxygen depletion. Cannibalism can occur among factory-farmed poultry, associated with overcrowding, inadequate trough space and an unbalanced diet. Failure to remove dead birds, pecked when alive and after death, may lead to an outbreak of botulism.

Although immunization has been used to protect cattle, horses, mink and exotic animals, few animals in their natural surroundings ever develop antibodies to botulism, and there is considerable species variation. Cattle and sheep are less susceptible than horses, and what may kill a horse may not kill a mouse. Predators who eat carrion are least affected and probably have a genetic reduced susceptibility to the symptoms of botulism. In a zoo outbreak, infected carcasses did not affect coatis or jaguars and caused only mild ataxia but no respiratory paralysis in lions. Repeated infections may occur in susceptible animals and it is presumed that unrecognized mild botulism may occur quite frequently in non-domestic carnivores, particularly if food hygiene is bad. Because of the extreme potency of Clostridia botulinum toxin, it is likely that sub-lethal doses are too small to stimulate an immune response. However, with repeated mild infections, it is possible that immunity does develop, as is suggested by the presence of antitoxin in carrion-eating birds, such as the turkey vulture, fish-eating gulls and crows.

Differences in the toxicity of the various botulinum toxins were clearly shown by some experimental work performed by Japanese scientists in chickens. Injected into a vein, toxin A is 1,000 times more toxic than toxin C, but given by a tube into the duodenal part of the intestine, the toxins were equipotent with the absorption of toxin C 100 times greater. Ten spores of types A, C, and D were given by mouth to different batches of chickens, all of whom died. However, when the spores were given after the caecum (the lower bowel) was tied off, they did not die. Thus, in chickens the site of spore germination and the production and absorption of toxin from germinating spores is the caecum.

Other forms of botulism may also occur in animals. A comparable example of wound botulism from veterinary practice occurred as a sequel to open castration performed in a barn at a local racetrack. Two weeks after surgery, the horse seemed stiff after galloping and was seen dropping food from its mouth. It became tremulous, the tone in the eyelids, tail, and tongue was markedly diminished, and the eyelids and tail could be lifted with minimal resistance. The tongue could be pulled out of the side of the mouth and the horse was unable to swallow. Under anaesthetic the scrotal incisions were reopened, exposing a necrotic foul-smelling remnant of the spermatic cord. Debridement was performed and Clostridium botulinum B isolated. Antitoxin and penicillin were given. The horse was fed gruel via a nasogastric tube. Hydration was monitored and oral toilet performed The horse gradually improved over 10 days' hospitalization. Drainage from the surgical site ceased on day 4, muscle tone in the tongue and tail improved on day 5, and swallowing returned on day 8.

A very definite insight into toxico-infective botulism comes from work on shaker foal disease. I mentioned that whilst in Kentucky two colleagues of mine at the University of Kentucky Medical Center in Lexington, Mike McQuillen and Harvey Cantor, had confirmed the pre-synaptic nature of the neuro-muscular block in shaker foal disease. Swerczek in 1980 was able to establish that shaker foal disease was due to botulism. Furthermore he was able to show how and why the disease occurs. It most frequently develops in fast growing foals between 2 and 4 weeks old. Their mares are usually fed on an excessively nutritious diet and produce an above-average yield of milk with a high fat content. The foals are particularly at risk after periods of stress to the lactating mares. As a result of stress, the fat content of the milk contains an excessive amount of corticosteroids. Excessive outpouring of corticosteroids which are fat soluble give rise to steroid 'stress' ulcers, classically sited in the stomach. When the foals begin to explore other sources of food, clostridial spores are ingested from contaminated soil and faecal material. Whereas in normal circumstances the spores are harmless, passing unaltered through the gut, they are held by, and able to proliferate in, the necrotic gastric ulcers. Swerczek was able to reproduce and confirm this sequence of events experimentally.

### Putting Botulinum to Good Use

For more than seven years I, along with many other neurologists, have been running dystonia clinics using botulinum toxin type A therapeutically to treat twenty or more patients per clinic. Scott in California found botulinum toxin more suitable than bunglotoxin (derived from snake venom) and other chemical agents for the correction of squints by altering the balance between the external ocular muscles responsible for the abnormal position of the eye. Neurologists and ophthalmologists may use botulinum toxin in the treatment of blepharospasm (inability to keep the eyes open fully) and as an alternative to tarsorraphy (stitching the eyelids to keep the eye closed) to protect the eye, as, for example, following a Bell's Palsy. Botulinum toxin, marketed as Dysport or Botox, is also used in the treatment of other focal dystonias, and for spasticity and writer's cramp. The indications for its use are expanding rapidly, and its application is currently being explored in yet more medical and surgical procedures. Small doses of botulinum, which, if given orally could induce severe disease, are injected directly into specific muscles, inducing temporary muscle weakness and easing previously untreatable, often painful, and functionally devastating muscle spasms.

The two commercial forms of botulinum differ in the ease with which antibodies develop and in their potency, so that an adjustment has to be made in the units used before interchanging them. They also share a common drawback – expense. To treat blepharospasm costs about £100, for spasmodic torticollis £300, and for spasticity £500-600. Furthermore the treatment will probably need repeating 3 or 4 times a year. For this reason, as well as for the need to develop expertise, its use is concentrated in various regional centres. Concentration in regional centres has other advantages. The results can be monitored and compared. The aetiology can be studied, and investigations arranged to exclude alternative diagnoses. Treatment failures can be reassessed and other therapeutic measures taken, including the use of type C botulinum where antibodies have developed.

The term 'dystonia' refers to sustained or repetitive muscle contractions, which may be generalized throughout the body or focal at one particular site. Until the 1970s, most patients with dystonia were referred to psychiatrists in the belief that dystonia was an hysterical manifestation. As Robert Whyte said in the 18th century, 'Physicians have bestowed the character of *nervous* on all those disorders whose nature and causes they were ignorant of'. Some neurologists have always believed that the dystonias have an organic basis and earlier I mentioned my surprise when at Maida Vale Hospital in the 1960s R.T.C. Pratt, an otherwise very organic, practical and pragmatic psychiatrist, had patients walk round and round a table whilst receiving electric shocks to their neck to treat spasmodic torticollis. John Walton in 1977, in Brain's *Diseases of the Nervous System*, still felt that most cases were hysterical in origin; and even in the 1990s we can say little more than that they are a poorly understood group of conditions believed to be due to neurochemical abnormalities in the basal ganglia. With upwards of 20,000 people affected in Britain alone, they form a sizeable group requiring treatment, even if the treatment is essentially symptomatic. An aetiological association for these movement disorders can be found by investigation in approximately 20% and there may be a genetic basis for some of the others, but most cases are sporadic and their cause unknown.

Generalized or multifocal dystonia mainly occurs in children before the age of 13; only about 3% develop after the age of 20. This type of dystonia is the one most likely to have a defined genetic background. The legs are commonly affected first before spreading elsewhere. One form of generalized dystonia, Segawa's disease, can respond to quite small, regular doses of L-dopa; and I have seen some dramatic responses with L-dopa. Thus, though only a small proportion respond to dopamine, it is always worthwhile trying L-dopa before embarking on other treatments. The alternative treatment has been high doses of atropinic drugs such as benzhexol. Benzhexol (Artane) has also been used for spasmodic torticollis. Atropine poisoning, as with belladona from deadly nightshade, makes one 'as hot as a hare, as blind as a bat, as dry as a bone, as red as a beet, and as mad as a hen'. Even building up the dosage of benzhexol to 80 mg daily in slow stages causes many side effects, such as dryness of the mouth, blurred vision, restlessness, high temperatures, and hallucinations. I have rarely had the courage to use this drug in the advised dosage. For generalized dystonia relatively little can be done and botulinum is usually an impractical treatment for this condition. In the early 1970s I tried amantadine for 6 patients with spasmodic torticollis with slight improvement and have continued to use other drugs such as acetazolamide (diamox) for repetitive tremulousness of spasm and clonazepam to produce relaxation and some improvement in posture, which unfortunately tends not to be sustained.

By contrast, essential blepharospasm can respond to botulinum dramatically in up to 90% of patients. Blepharospasm usually comes on after the 4th decade of life and is characterized by involuntary closure of the eyelids, leading to impaired vision. The closure may be semi-permanent or occur periodically throughout the day, especially with fatigue. Thus reading and driving may be especially affected, and the frequency increased in bright sunlight. The differential diagnosis includes ocular myasthenia and apraxia of eyelid opening which may be a serious problem later in life. Treatment is very simple. 60 to 140 units of dysport are injected, divided between 4 sites around the eye. Improvement occurs after 5 to 10 days and any side-effects – temporary weakness of the upper lid with ptosis, grittiness of the eyes, double vision or mild facial weakness – will occur along with the improvement, but rarely persist for more than 1-2 days. Initially the injections were sited below the eyebrow, at the lower, outer corner of the orbit and near the nose, avoiding the lachrymal duct. However the upper injections commonly caused temporary ptosis and it was found that injections above the eyebrow were equally effective. More recently the use of a minute dose given pre-tarsally into the lower, fleshy part of the upper lid, can prolong the effect of the injections. Improvement may persist for months.

Facial tic (hemifacial spasm) has features similar to blepharospasm and may be socially highly embarrassing with the constant risk of accusations of winking in a suggestive manner. Muscle spasms usually begin around the orbit in the orbicularis oculi muscles and then spread to affect the brow, lower face and platysma muscle below the chin. Unlike blepharospasm, which may affect both eyes simultaneously, the movements are invariably unilateral and may continue in sleep. Chewing and talking characteristically aggravate hemifacial spasm. There is some controversy as to the best treatment for hemifacial spasm. It is claimed by some neurosurgeons that microvascular surgery, separating a blood vessel in close proximity to the facial nerve (and presumably irritating it) as it emerges from the brainstem, can cure 90% of patients. But this involves a major operation and one can never be sure that a blood vessel pressing upon a nerve will be found. In practice a Magnetic Resonance (MR) scan of the back of the brain is performed and unless there is clear evidence of an aberrant blood vessel, most clinicians prefer to treat the condition symptomatically with botulinum. A similar dosage is used to that for blepharospasm but given at three sites, two above the eyebrow and one laterally and below the eye. A small dose can be given into the platysma muscle but injections lower in the cheek or near the mouth are to be avoided because of the risk of drooping of the side of the mouth and dribbling.

There are several rarer types of dystonia around the mouth, affecting the jaw (oro-mandibular), the tongue (lingual) and swallowing (pharyngeal dystonia). The combination of these spasms with blepharospasm is named Meige's syndrome or, more aptly, Brueghel's syndrome after a famous depiction of a peasant woman by Pieter Brueghel the Elder. I have had little experience of treating these. The patients I have had with spasmodic or laryngeal dysphonia, with a strangled or whispered speech, have been treated successfully with the help of an ENT surgeon.

Spasmodic torticollis presents in several ways: as a wry neck with the head turned to one side, with spasmodic twisting or jerking to the side, or thrusting of the head and neck forwards (antecollis) or backwards (retrocollis). The abnormal postures or spasms can be painful, disabling, affecting function such as driving, walking across roads, or be socially embarrassing. Patients will use various tricks or 'gestes' to overcome the problem. One schoolmaster used to wear a hat in class; more commonly a hand or a finger is held lightly touching the chin, not necessarily antagonistically to the involuntary movement. After examination, it is important to exclude potentially treatable underlying problems which may set off the dystonia by irritation. These include brachial cysts, anomalies of the upper vertebrae in the neck, wasting conditions affecting the musculature, and Wilson's disease involving disorders of copper metabolism. I have referred to the unsatisfactory drug treatment of this condition. Many surgical treatments have also been in vogue but proved unsatisfactory – stereotactic surgery, root resection, cutting the sternocleidomastoid muscle, and nerve stimulation. Botulinum toxin, perhaps supplemented by drugs, can help over 80% of patients, limiting the movement and/or restoring posture.

Patients usually develop spasmodic torticollis in middle age and come for treatment 2-3 years later. They may have assumed that the onset of the condition followed a traumatic incident such as a road traffic accident or developed when working in poor lighting conditions, thereby relating it to 'crabs', which coal-miners used to get from working long hours in damp, ill-lit mines. But there is really no convincing mode of onset. Even today, when dystonia clinics have been going for some years, patients present having had traction applied to the neck by orthopaedic surgeons, received anti-depressants from psychiatrists or G.P.s, and given reassurance from those who do not have the faintest idea what the condition is. They may have tried a series of remedial exercises or devised a treatment frame themselves. Particularly in the early days of dystonia clinics, when patients did not know what to expect, some patients could appear very jittery and psychologically unbalanced; but a remarkable change would occur in their general demeanour once they experienced the beneficial advantage of an effective therapy. After a few years of continual spasms, spontaneous remission may occur in a small proportion of the patients, irrespective of treatment. Unfortunately, about 5% treated with botulinum will become refractory to the injections and the overall success rate for symptomatic treatment with botulinum is around 80%.

The most commonly involved muscles are the sterno-mastoids, arising from the mastoid process and attached to the sternum and clavicle (sterno-cleido-mastoid). The right sternomastoid will produce torsion of the head to the left, and if both sternomastoid muscles are in spasm the head will be pulled forwards or tilted backwards. The trapezii and paraspinal muscles will tilt the head backwards and the splenii and scalenes will cause a lateral tilt.

The decision has to be made which muscles to inject. This can be approached scientifically, using electrodes over the muscles (surface polymyography), providing a 'write out' on reams of paper of the activity of each muscle group. The results are rarely more exact than using clinical judgment. However some departments prefer to use a form of deep myography with hollow needles, via the needle injecting electrodes in order to try to deliver the botulism as near as possible to the muscle motor end plates. About 500 units of Dysport, divided between two, or perhaps, three muscles, may be needed to correct the dystonia. The more muscles are injected at any one time, the greater the risk of side effects. Difficulties in swallowing occur at about the time of a positive response, usually at around 10 days. It may be necessary to advise the patient to take liquids only for a day or two but the dysphagia may be more persistent. The other common side effect is to weaken the muscles of the neck so much that posture is adversely affected. It is felt that injecting pairs of muscles at the same time, e.g. the sternomastoids, will increase the risk of dysphagia, but which muscles are particularly sensitive is disputed. Greatest relief comes from injecting into a painful muscle. As pain may be caused by pulling on a muscle antagonistic to the over-active muscle causing the torsion, it may be necessary to inject both agonist and antagonist. Success may be measured by relief of an abnormal posture. But the greatest benefit comes from a reduction or cessation of torsion and jerking. Sometimes injection into a relatively quiescent muscle may prove as successful in bringing relief as an injection into an apparently overactive muscle. The injections can be carried out in other groups of muscles within a week of the first injection, minimizing side effects and adding to the correction of the disability, but the success of injections for cervical dystonia has to be measured in weeks rather than in months.

Injection into spastic muscles is to correct deformities and prevent contractures. It permits the fuller use of muscle relaxants and physiotherapy to improve function. In the same way botulinum is now used in stroke victims to correct the deformities of hemiplegia and if possible to obtain an earlier return of function to the fingers and hand of an affected limb. I find that the successful application of botulinum to writer's cramp and in repetitive strain injuries can never be guaranteed. In my experience writer's cramp is not a uniform condition and on examination, there may be a variety of underlying pathologies and physical findings.

The question remains, particularly when injecting into the neck muscles for various forms of cervical dystonia, as to the extent of localization or dissemination of the toxin. Where exactly does the toxin get to? Is it all attached to the nerves entering a particular muscle or does it track down the muscle sheaths, seep into capillaries, accumulate in fat and supporting tissues and find its way into neighbouring or even distant muscles? The neck 'righting' reflexes are complex and changes occur in apparently untreated muscles. The swallowing difficulties suggest some tracking down of toxin, possibly along nerves. I tried to devise a method, which I was unable to put into practice, whereby the toxin could be labelled with a radionuclide and its dissemination traced. There has been a classical paper, which, perhaps because of the eminence of its authors, has not been confirmed by repetition (nor by conventional electromyography), using the technique of single fibre electromyography, which showed that the performance of muscles remote from the site of injection has been altered due to diffusion of toxin. There have also been a few isolated reports in which the repeated use of therapeutic doses of botulinum toxin for spastic paraparesis and for spasmodic torticollis have resulted in patients developing a syndrome which resembles clinical botulism. No fatalities have occurred and it is presumed that some of the toxin was inadvertently injected directly into blood vessels. However, in one of the reported cases, systemic botulism did not develop until 21 days after a repeat injection into the neck; a situation which does not support the explanation of a leakage into the blood stream.

### Future Experimental Applications of Botulinum Toxins

Besides the immediate therapeutic use of botulinum, which has yet to be fully explored, botulinum, as one of the clostridial neurotoxins, has excited the interest of experimental physiologists. Why, with food-borne botulism, is there a march of symptom development? The orofacial involvement occurs early, before that of the respiratory muscles. Is it purely a matter that a larger dose is required to impair respiration? Why in animals are the hind limbs weakened initially and do the other symptoms follow later, not in the same order as in humans? Why in certain predators do symptoms such as ataxia and weakness occur but very rarely do the symptoms progress to include respiratory weakness? There are two explanations to these questions. The first involves the manner and routes whereby the toxin is disseminated; the second suggests an active process of adjustment by the nervous system.

The explanation that there may be an adjustment by the nervous system itself receives support from examination of the effects of intramuscular injections of toxin. When using injections for the correction of squints, there is commonly an overcorrection, followed later by a finer adjustment so that the eye assumes a central position which does not depend on whether or not sight was retained in that eye. Treatment for blepharospasm or hemifacial spasm weakening the ocular muscles also leads to a helpful reduction of the blink rate. And when treating spasmodic torticollis, even though one rarely injects more than three muscles, changes in activity may be apparent, possibly via the mechanism of the 'righting reflexes' involving the untreated muscles. Therefore we may reasonably ask whether the toxin response is followed by a separate central nervous system response, and are we, by the use of botulinum, learning something of the compensatory functions of the non-cortical parts of the central nervous system?

These questions occurred to me when attending an international conference on the clostridial neurotoxins in Oxford. The ostensible purpose of the conference was to examine our present knowledge of the properties of the neurotoxins and to assess how they might be used in genetic engineering and for transporting useful substances into selected sites within the central nervous system. The toxins are already produced commercially in highly purified crystalline form as a high molecular weight protein of 900,000 and distributed as a stable freeze-dried product composed of two molecules of neurotoxin bond to a haemagglutinin or non-toxic complex.

Two disulfide chains link the heavy chain of 100 kDa to the light chain of 50 kDa The heavy chain is involved in neuro-specific binding and penetration of the neurones; the light chain damages the neurone and blocks the pre-synaptic release of neuro-transmitter. The initial stage of penetration of the neurone (endocytosis) with passage of the toxin from the neurone's surface into its cytoplasm (cytosol) takes about 5 hours. Part of the heavy chain, the C-terminal, binds to the cell membranes and the other part, the N-terminal, forms pores which enable the toxin to cross the endosomal membrane. This act of translocation is dependent on the pH. Once within the neurone, the heavy chain may have a further function, namely aiding transport to the pre-synaptic terminal and also in a centripetal, retrograde direction along the axon to the cell body and even (particularly with tetanus – and to a lesser extent with botulinum) from the lower motor neurone across synapses to upper motor neurones and to Renshaw cells. Renshaw cells are smaller, lower motor neurones cells which fire back on the larger motor neurones (anterior horn cells), inhibiting them from further activity. Thus once an anterior horn cell has fired in response to a stimulus from an upper motor neurone it will stop firing until a further impulse is sent. If not turned off by Renshaw cell activity, it will continue to discharge independently of other stimuli. In tetanus, failure of Renshaw cell activity leads to the grimacing and muscle spasms which characterize that disease.

Muscle contraction depends upon the release of acetylcholine from the nerve on to the muscle across the myo-neural junction at the motor end plate. Acetylcholine is secreted (formed) in the lower part of the nerve and held as vesicles until required. An insoluble core of three presynaptic proteins, collectively termed SNARE proteins, are responsible for vesicle docking and neuro-transmitter release. SNARE proteins developed at an early stage of evolution and form alpha-helices which function as a uniform complex. Similar substrate proteins are found elsewhere in the body where they mediate a number of vesicle-dependent functions. The light chains of the clostridial toxins contain zinc-endopeptidases that specifically target the SNARE proteins to block vesicle docking and neuro-transmitter release. Whether they also impair the secretory activities of these cells is unclear. The different strains of clostridial toxins act at various sites on the SNARE proteins splitting open (cleaving) their peptide bonds.

Tetanus toxoid, more so than botulinum, is the vehicle of choice for bioengineering. by reason of its ease of retrograde transport up nerve axons. The heavy chain can fulfil its present functions providing access into the nerve. It then releases an altered light chain engineered to contain other substances. Bioengineering could thus provide access to peripheral nerves, navigation across synapses and retrograde transport within the central nervous system. Through retrograde transport to anterior horn cells, without the need to cross synapses, the formation of free radicals within the cells could be inhibited, and enzymes such as superoxidase dismutase, important in motor neurone diseases, could be targeted to useful sites. An Anglo-American group working at Imperial College, London and the University of Maryland were able to present the results of experiments at the Oxford conference involving the transmission of superoxidase dismutase bound to tetanus toxoid into anterior horn cells after injecting the hind limbs of rabbits. Thus the clostridial toxins, previously known only as poisons, have shown their potential as a probe or vehicle for the treatment of disease.

PART IV

# THE FINALE OF THE NEUROLOGIST'S TALE

**Looking Back**

PROGRESS IN MEDICINE takes advantage of advancing technology, not necessarily by anticipated steps. The development of antibiotics did not eliminate the need for surgery; it opened up a new era of cardiac surgery, not possible without antibiotic cover. In fact advances in technology have had more impact on Medicine than on any other sphere of human activity. Technical advance in aeronautical and military research was given pride of place by various governments, paid for by selling arms to foreign belligerents, and their peaceful value withheld due to official secrecy. But doctors have had to adjust to the frequent changes of developing technology, more so than those in any other occupation: ... more so than the military, more so than even those in communications. We enter an era of molecular biology, of advances in transplantation, immunology, biophysics, seeking to introduce and make changes within the cell. Neurology in particular has had to adjust to newer and newer imagining techniques – gamma cameras, computerised tomography, magnetic resonance scanning, proton emission tomography, and SPECT. Diseases are being tackled by new methods using cytokines, interferons, etc. The learning process in medicine is continuing and each doctor must be a perpetual student. There is no end!

We may relax only to be alerted by a new achievement which excites us, which we cannot ignore. Medicine, and especially neurology, which allows exploration of the workings of the human brain, cannot rest. Man may explore the heavens:-

> ... thro' vast immensity can pierce,
> See worlds on worlds compose one universe,
> Observe how system into system runs,
> What other planets circle other suns,
> What vary'd being peoples ev'ry star.

Man can explore the depths of the oceans where there is still much that is unknown.

> Go, wond'rous creature! mount where Science guides,
> Go, measure earth, weigh air, and state the tides.'

But it is the great chain of being, as Alexander Pope declared, that provides continual excitement.

> Know then thyself.
> A mortal man unfold . . .
> . . . such wisdom in an earthly shape,
> And shew'd a NEWTON as we shew an Ape.

What is the great potential which man has yet to realize? Why is it that man is all confused, the glory, jest and riddle of the world?

How the brain works. Every little advance that provides a tantalizing glance, but not the full picture, excites our enthusiasm. How an encased blob of jelly, a sponge seeping with liquids in the form of neuro-endocrine, transmitter and inhibitor substances, which only has true anatomical shape when fixed in mordants, can direct and control the more substantial parts of our bodies, our joints and muscles, is a surprising and enthralling mystery. That it is capable of thought, language, emotion, sensitivity, kindness and humour as well as harm deepens creation's puzzle. In neurology we come up against the central physiology controlling the whole body. We try to overcome pathological changes which affect its function. We try, along with organic psychologists, to link the substantive brain with its abstracted essence, the mind.

I have been obsessed with two extensions of this thought process: the development of language and the boundaries of what we see as reality. Language has evolved by a series of unanticipated steps from grunts which have established meaning, into a method of active or empathic communication, through vocabulary, grammar, syntax, into music, prose and poetry, recorded as writing, typing, and on disc, broadcast with all the inflexions of the human voice, providing computer languages, computer graphics, the computation of mathematical symbols, and the methodology of virtual reality. Through the evolution of language we can pool the 'brain-power' of the human race; both those alive today and those who have gone before.

The neurological boundaries of reality are tenuous, transgressing into the realms of philosophy and psychiatry. To quote Kant, 'We see things not as they are: but as we are'. Our sensations are limited:- by the makeup of our body, the sensitivity of our peripheral sensors, for example able to detect certain colours but not ultra-violet or infra-red; by the modulation imposed on them at various levels of the nervous system; and by our interpretation, muddied and transmuted by previous experiences or emotional reactions. Our body image can be tricked, as all forms of awareness can be tricked, by weightlessness or disturbances of balance and tilt. Our body image may be extended when we hold a pen in our hand, drive a car, ski, or plug ourselves into a computer. The body image, damaged by deformity or trauma, may impose itself upon us, affecting our actions and our self-esteem. Our capacity to fantasize – to act out a situation, the role of play in childhood in preparation for an adult existence, our ability to create, as in art, that which can never be truly real, our drives, sexuality, inter-relationships – all underline the insubstantiality of our existence; but without which 'we would be as nothing'.

Can we therefore emparcel and tie up clearly defined boundaries of reality, thereby ending the neurologist's tale with a wry twist and press a firm seal on its contents? The answer is an emphatic 'No'. Our world of reality is one of shifting contours, demanding of us frequent adjustment. The future burgeonings of virtual reality and the internet are unrevealed. New drugs, new methods of diagnosis, treatment and management, new understandings of the human mind and frame, will continue to excite us until we ourselves are no longer capable of awareness. There is no end.

**Life After Neurology**

Retirement from the National Health Service occurs at 65. In fact many of my colleagues chose early retirement. It is possible to continue in private practice. Thus my uncle was still seeing patients with dyslexia in his 70s and wrote books on Hughling-Jackson and Oscar Wilde in his nineties. Others continue with medico-legal activities for years, having greater time to spend on each case but becoming medically more out of touch with time. Apart from examining and attending conferences, I decided to give up completely at 65 and to look for other forms of activity which I had been unable to follow before that time. The USA have apparently abandoned a cut-off period in one's career and rightly so, as the population becomes older and at the same time retains good health for a longer period. But it is also pleasing to be able to change one's direction, forego administrative responsibilities and concentrate in a more relaxed way on continuing for a few sessions rather than carry out the previous heavy schedule.

I chose to try out four different careers. The option of sessions in neurophysiology was not open to me. I would have liked to continue with my dystonia clinic, treating patients with botulinum. But neither were feasible. One realizes also that after a break of six months or a year, difficulties can arise in returning to clinical work in so far as treatments have changed.

One cannot rely on the information given by drug firms and it is difficult to marry well tried practice with what has since come to be required, using old and new drugs in a discriminating manner.

Each of these different careers unsurprisingly harked back to my experience over many years of neurology. Firstly, I returned to a life-long interest of mine which had been under wraps during my years in neurology, standing as a Liberal Democrat candidate at the General Election for Bolton North East. As I wrote a few months later when it seemed appropriate to broaden my C.V. '... This gave me further understanding of the inter-relationship between General Practice and Hospitals, into the role of Social Services involved with the elderly, with younger people and those statemented with learning difficulties. I also learnt more about the problems of drug addiction, Public Health and Green and Economic aspects of positive health.'

Later that year I became a Civil Servant working at the Medicines Control Agency licencing new drugs. This was a fascinating aspect of medicine, working closely with pharmacists and statisticians and learning much from them. My trainer, initiating me into the requirements of assessing drugs, was an interesting and pleasant personality, but one of the most demanding and schoolmasterly of all the departmental heads. I felt that if I could satisfy him, which I am glad to say I gradually succeeded in doing, I could satisfy all the others. One learnt that the demands made on the firms in their controlled trials were far more rigorous than the presentation of randomized controlled trials or meta-analyses accepted by medical journals.

Working at the MCA also meant attending meetings of the Committee for the Safety of Medicines and provided an opportunity to improve one's IT and statistical skills. They were going through a period of change and expectation that NICE, the agency for determining priorities in the use of expensive procedures and medications, was being planned and harmonization of drug licencing throughout Europe was developing. Alas, they took me on for only four months, expecting a vast increase in applications before European harmonization of licencing came into effect. The anticipated increase in work-load did not occur and the handover from Market Towers, overlooking the MI5 building, to Canary Wharf, occurred quietly. Therefore, as against those retiring in their 50s, I was not given a 3-year contract.

As I was leaving, the post of Professor at the University of Central Lancashire responsible for Postgraduate training, and overseeing the transfer of general practitioners to the new primary health trusts was advertised, I prepared thoroughly for this, even writing a booklet on the future of medicine, including such topics as the incoming government's plans, Health and the Pharmaceutical Industry, Evidence based medicine, and priorities within the NHS. I was considered to be the front runner for the post until it was realized that I was over the age limit for employment by the University of Central Lancashire.

I now sit as a Liberal Democrat councillor for Blackburn with Darwen unitary authority, acting as spokesperson for Social Services and Leisure and Culture. Working virtually as a social worker, dealing with problems within the ward I represent, maintains the human aspect which meant so much in Neurology. It is curious what people will do but the privilege of having worked in Neurology, able to study the brain and its workings in health and disease at first hand, lives on.

# Index

Aberdeen 80
Abetalipoproteinaemia and related syndromes 76-8
Abraham, E.P., Sir 2
Acanthocytes, Acanthocytosis 74, 75, 75, 77, 79
Accident and Emergency 33
Achondroplasia 70
Addison's disease 40
Agraphia 65
Akureyi, Iceland 54
Albuquerque 5, 210
Alexia 64
Almuree, Lord 55
Alvarez on 'small strokes' 147
Amantadine 46f., 221, 256
Aminoff, Michael 75
Amish, Amish Old Order 81f.
Anaesthetics, anaesthetists 33, 116
Angina 116
Anglesey, Marquis of 114
Anthrax (woolsorter's disease) 21
Anticonvulsants 111, 112
Aphasia, aphasiology 21, 65, 121-6, 144, 214
Aphonia 192f.
Appalachia 10, 69, 83, 92
Apparition of Roman soldiers to apprentice 132
Appenzeller, Otto 5
Apraxia 151
Arbil 23
Argyll-Robertson pupils 55
Aristotle 114
Art, aspects of 195-199
Arteriosclerosis 129, 144, 150
Astigmatism in Modigliani and El Greco 196
AT (ataxia telangiectasia) 56
Aylesbury 17-18
Ayurvedic medicine 211

Baboons, death of from botulism 228
Baghdad 19-24
Bailey, Percival 104
Bakthavathsalam, Dr 211
Bannister and Brain, *Clinical Neurology* 4
Bannister, Dr Roger 3, 4
   ed. *Diseases of the Nervous System* 222-3
Barnard, Robin 42
Bassen-Kornzweig syndrome 73, 76
Bath 12-13
Bedford 66-7
Behcet's disease 146

Belladona 47
Bender, Morris 220
Benzhexol (Artane) 256
Berrios, G.E. 127
Beta-blocker 49
Bethesda, Maryland 50
Betts, Professor 75, 101
Bible Belt 69-42
Bickerstaff, Edwin 158
Biffin, Lord 183
Biffin, Sarah 181ff.
Binswanger syndrome 147
Bioelectrical phenomena 160-3
Blackburn with Darwen, Liberal Councillor for 267
Bladder, dysfunction of in multiple sclerosis 220
Blepharospasm 255-7, 261
Bletchley 18
Bletchley Park 17
Blyton, Dr Gifford 93
Bolton, N.E., candidate 226
Bombay 33
Botulinum 42, 254f., 257, 259
   two commercial forms of 255
   antitoxin 239, 253
   used as treatment for stroke 259
   to correct deformities of hemiplegia 259
   used in treatment of dystonia 254f.
   in correcting squints 255
   in treating essential blepharospasm 256
   in treating Wilson's disease 258
   localization and dissemination of toxin 260
   Future experimental applications of 260-262
   antitoxin 239, 253
Botulism 79, 229-254
   Case histories of 225-7
   Outbreaks in Manchester, Liverpool, Oldham and Blackpool 229
   Birmingham outbreak of 242f.
   Endemic in Rocky Mountains 229
   Symptoms of 230f.
   Onset and progress of 230f.
   Horrendous experience of described by patients 230f.
   Public Health measures 234-5
   Illustrative histories of 236-240
   Historical aspects of 240-242
   toxico-infective forms of 243-245
   Long-term symptoms following 245-249
   In infants 244

Botulism *(cont.)*
  In animals 249-254
  Ecological factors 249-254
Bradley, Helen 196
Bradley, Tom 195
Brain's *Diseases of the Nervous System* 54, 222, 255
Brain death 100
Brain, Lord 41f., 43
Brain, questions raised concerning working of 264
Brainstem 192f.
Brauner, Victor 197
British Epilepsy Association 101, 106-7
British Medical Journal 64
British Military Hospital, Singapore 33f.
Broca's area 124
Brown, Christy 180
Brown, D.I., (Stowe School) 16
Brueghel's syndrome 257
BSE (Bovine spongiform encephalitis) 100, 251
'BTA' (Been to America) 57, 66
Buchanan, Dr 67
Buckinghamshire 7f., 13-19
Burden, George 107
Bures St Mary 8
Burn, J., Professor 2
Burnfield, Alexander 218
Burnley 5
Bury St Edmunds 5-7, 11f.

Caisson's disease in divers and tunnellers 216
Calne, Donald 50, 57
Campbell, M. 54
Cantor, Harvey 68, 79, 84, 254
Cardiff 11
Carleton, Alice 2
Carroll, Lewis 157
Castle, Barbara (née Betts) 18
Cataplexy 201
Causalgia 116
Caution, need for when discussing patients 232
Cawthorne, Sir Terence 29
Cerebral cortex, 6
Cerebro-vascular disease 144-9
Cervical spondylosis 206-7
Charcot 84, 85, 86, 87, 156
Charcot's Hysteria renaissant 83-90
Charington, Denver, Colorado on botulism 229
Children of deaf patients, role as interpreters 62
Children's Hospital, Great Ormond Street 54
Chomsky, Noam 125
Choreo-athetosis 165
Chronic fatigue syndrome 42, 54, 246ff.
Chuke, Dr Paul 70
Clark, David 62, 67, 69, 71, 79, 84
Clioquinol 168
Clostridia 244, 251
  Botulinum toxin 241, 253
  Clostridial neurotoxins,

Oxford International Conference on 250-3, 260, 261, 262
  Future applications of 260f.
CME (Continuing Medical Education) 190
Cocks, Seymour, Dr 111
Cohen, Henry, (Lord Cohen) 31
Coimbatore 211f.
Colchicine 168
Colour blindness in artists 195f.
Coma 214
  Causes of 215
Comatose patient, management of 215
Cooper, Irving 44
Corpora quadrigemina 5
Cotzias, C.G. 47
CPAP (Continuous positive airway pressure) 202
Creed, J., Dr 3
Creutzfeld-Jakob Disease, (CJD) 43, 100, 192, 251
Crichton-Brown, James 6
Christ-Siemens syndrome 91
Critchley, Professor A. Michael (father) 11, 15, 16-18
  Appointment in Baghdad 19-24
  Published works of 20
Critchley, Dr Doris (mother) 12, 17, 18, 21
Critchley, Giles, FRCS (son) 67
Critchley, Helen, Ll.B. (Mrs Barfield, daughter) 96
Critchley Dr Hugo (son) 5
Critchley, Dr Jane (sister) 12, 15
Critchley, Julian, Sir, M.P. (cousin) 183
Critchley, Macdonald (uncle) 5, 7f., 16, 26, 32, 44, 48, 106, 149, 265
Critchley, Dr Mair (wife) 55, 90, 224
Critchley, Tom, Australian High Commisioner in Malaya 39
Croft, Peter 42
Crown of thorns 10f. See also Neuroacanthocytosis
Cummings, Professor 75
Cutforth, Robert 25
Croce, Benedetto 197
Cunningham, D. 3
Cytowic, R.E., 118

Daggett, Bill 29
Danish Neurological Association 111
Darcus, D., Dr 2
Darwin, Charles 103, 119
David Lewis Centre 108
Davies-Jones, Alwyn 128
Daws, Alex 97
Dawson van Bogaert disease 70, 100
Dayime sleepiness index, cases of 199
D-dopa 47
Deafness and education 61
Deafness and hearing children of deaf parents 27, 52, 57-62

# INDEX

Deaf parents, children's protective attitude towards 61
Deaf segregation of 60
Deafness and social responsibility 60
Deaf unit for the 136
Delinquency as influenced by dyslexia 62-66
Denmark, Dr John 136, 137
Denny-Brown, D. 5
Dent, C.E., Professor 81
Deepdale Hospital 97
Diagnostic puzzles 221-2
Dialects, oldest, where found 94
Difficulties in diagnosis, case history 222
Difficulties in finding suitable patient subjects for examinations 191
Dimsdale, Helen 42f., 54, 55
*Diseases of the Spinal Cord*, see Eisen, A.A.
Domiciliary visits 217
Donovan, J. 120
Dopamine 47, 48, 50, 122, 256
Doppelganger sensations 157
Dostoyevski, F. 105
Down's syndrome 153
Drug-induced neurological disease 163-9
Drug reactions 16
Drug tolerance 164
Dry Bible disease among sheep 252
Duff, Brian 40
Dulwich Hospital 26
Dumas, Alexandre 148
Duncan, Rod 134
Dupuytren 113
Dupuytren's disease 110-11
Dyslexia as giving rise to delinquency 62-66
Drummond, General Sir Alexander 33
Dyck, Peter 54
Dysentery 35
Dyslexia 62-6
Dyspnoea 53
Dysport 259
Dystonia 254, 255f., 258

Early American English 92-95
East Anglia and Huntingdon's disease 7f., 11f.
East Terence 25
Easton, Dr 66
Eaton-Lambert syndrome 229
Eccles, Sir John 2
ECG 66, 87
Ecological factors and animal botulism 249f.
Edinburgh 5
EEG 53, 54, 57, 68, 70, 78, 86, 87, 96, 97, 98, 99, 100, 102, 104, 105, 110, 209
Ehlers-Danlos syndrome 146
Eisen, Andy, Professor 170
Eisen, A.A., jnt author of *Diseases of the Spinal Cord* 221
Elithorn, Alick 42
Elizabethan English 94, 95
Elliott, Frank 105

Ellis-Van Creveld type of dwarfism 82, 83
Emergencies, poorly managed 215
Emery, Alan 81
EMG 79
ENT (Ear, nose and throat) 7f., 40, 74, 226
Epilepsy 85, 86, 96, 99, 101-113, 111, 112
    definition of 101
    hot water epilepsy 106
    laughter epilepsy 104
    and multiple sclerosis 217
    musicogenic epilepsy 106
    reading epilepsy 106
    reflex epilepsy 105, 106
    treatment of 107
Epileptic Colony, Epileptic Centre 96, 101
Erastus 104
Espionage by governess 15
Esquirol, J.E.D. 127
Estes, Dr Worth 75
Esssential Tremor 48, 149
Excessive sleepiness, causes of 199

Facial tic 257
Failure rates in examinations for the Royal College of Physicians 189
Federal Narcotics Institute 70
Feral children 57
Ferguson, Fergus 223f.
Ferguson, Maynard 47
Ferguson-Smith 81
Ferrier, Sir David 5, 6
Finger spelling 58, 59, 62, 137, 139, 140
Fish poisons 227
Flashbacks 12
Florey, Sir Howard 2
Foerster, F.M. 104
Ford, Frank 67, 69
Foster, Stephen 90
Fox, Harold 40
Friedreich's ataxia 73, 76
Frontal lobectomy 3
Fugue, hysterical 89

Galton, F. 127
Gamstrop, Professor Ingrid 81
Ganser syndrome 89
Gastaut, Henri 112
Gate control theory 114
Gelineau's syndrome 200
Gerstmann's syndrome 150
Gilles de la Tourette syndromes 72, 80, 122
Gilliatt, R., Professor 48, 54, 75
Glasgow 112
Glasgow coma scale 214
Glees, Paul 2
Godlee, Sir Rickman 6
Gordon, Dr Neil 97, 101
Gorman, Pierre 58
Gower, Sir William 51, 153
Goya, F. 29-30

Grand mal 72
Grant, Hilary 42
*Gray's Anatomy* 2
Grays, Essex 33
Guillain-Barre syndrome 68, 117, 226, 228
  Miller-Fisher variant of 227
Gurkha 35, 40
Gurusinghe, Nihal 171, 225
Gynaecology 26

Hallpike, C.E. 48, 57
Hallucinations 127-133, 137, 139, 196f.
  and art 211
  Musical 133f.
  Prelingually deaf schizophrenic patients 135
  Unusual auditory 133f.
  Specific to schizophrenic 140
Hammersmith Hospital 50, 111
Handicapped patients badly treated by Social Security 224-5
Hansford-Johnson, Pamela 155
Harding, Anita 55, 75
Harper, P.S., Professor 11
Harris College 75, 102, 155
Harrison, Senior House Officer 224
Hayward, Harry, Chief Nurse 108
Head, Henry 47
Headington 52
Head injury in American football 205
Head injuries, inadequate treatment of 204
Head injury of National Hunt jockey 205
  in road accident: case history 205
  from being trampled by cows: case history 207
Hearing 27f.
Heatley, Dr A. 2
Heilman, K.M. 150
Henson, Ronnie 42
Herne Hill 30
Heroin addiction 145
Herpes simplex encephalitis 78
Herxheimer reaction 38
Hesling, Gordon 76
Hewitson, John 70
Hexamethonium 57
Hierons, Raymond 150
Highlands Hospital, North London 45
Hill, Sir Denis 26, 107
HIV testing 193
Holmes-Adie pupils 55
Holmes, Ted 76
Holstein, Judge Huno von 63
Honey and disease 244
Hope Hospital, Manchester 4
Hornykiewicz, O. 47, 49
Horowitz, M.J. 130
Horsley, Victor 56
Hospital for Epilepsy and Paralysis, Regent's Park 6
House Physician 31-32, 41

House Surgeon 27-31
Hoyle, Clifford 25
Hughlings Jackson, J. 122
Humoral influences on human speech 121
Huntington, Drs, father and son 7, 10
Huntington's chorea, Huntington's disease 7f., 8, 71, 151-2
  Macdonald Critchley's sign in 9f.
Hurwitz, Louis 45
Hutchinson, David 250
Hyoscine 47
Hyperbaric oxygen 216-7
Hypertensive encephalopathy 56
Hypoglycaemia in insulin dependent diabetic 215
Hysteria 83, 86, 87, 88, 221-2
Hystero-epilepsy 72

Idioglossa of schoolchildren 93
Ill health associated with poverty 192
Image, William Edmund 5
India, Wilson's disease in 51
Indiana 82
Infirmary, Preston 97
Inner language of deaf children 58
Inner speech 125
Intercranial pressure raising of 215
Interferon 221
Intra-thecal chlorocresol 113
Intra-thecal phenol 113
Irish MRCP, examining for 194
Ironside, Redvers 104

James I 57
James, Philip 216
Jamieson, Doug 68
Japan 39
Jefferson, Sir Jeffrey 96
Jellinek, Ernest 43
Jesperson, O. 120
Jewesberry, Eric 150
Johns Hopkins Hospital 44, 67, 68, 79, 83
Johnston, Alan 61f.
Johore-Baru 40

Kamunting, British Military hospital 33, 36, 37
Kant, Immanuel 264
Kartagener's syndrome 55, 56
Kayser-Fleischer ring 51
Kelly, Reg 42, 43, 218
Kentucky 10, 17, 71-76, 78-9, 83, 84, 90-92, 93, 105
Kerner, Justinius 240
Khartoum, External Examiner for MD in Sudan 194
Kiloh-Nevin syndrome 223
Kinefelter syndrome 80
King's College Hospital 4, 5, 6, 24-26, 43, 51
Kingsley, Charles 2
Kinnear Wilson, S.A. 51, 103, 104

## INDEX

Klawans, Harold 1-2
Klee, P. 131
Klein, M. 130
Kluang, British Military Hospital 40-41
Knapp, Elizabeth 8f.
Kocen, Roman, S. 35, 37
Kurdish porters 20, 21

Laevodopa, L-dopa 46, 47, 48, 50, 51, 53, 80, 101, 122, 161, 202, 256
La Grande Hysterie, phases of 84f., 86
Lambert-Eaton syndrome 227f.
Lamsiekte, South African cattle disease 252
Lancashire, see also Preston and district 53
Lancashire Moor 96
Lancaster University 125
Langho Epileptic Colony 96, 108, 112
Language 119, 151
    Development of 264
Laycock, Thomas 5
Lecture tours 209-213
    in Canada and the USA 209-10
    in India 210-11
    in South Africa 212
Lederhose disease 110
Leeds 107
Lees, Andrew 45, 57
Legal system, defects in 203
Le Gros Clark, Sir Wilfred 2
Lenneberg, E.H. 58
Leonidakis, Mary 68
Leptospirosis 36-38
Le Quesne, Pamela 167
Lesch-Nyham syndrome 79
Levine-Critchley syndrome 74-76
Lewis, David 666
Lewis, G.E.D. 38f.
Lewis, 'Tiny' 38
Lexington 67, 70, 78
L'Hermite's peduncular hallucinosis 131
    'barber's chair' sign 220
Liberal Democrat 266
Liddell, Professor 2, 3
Life after Neurology 265-267
Linnaeus, own migraine attacks 157
Littlehampton, Mandy 2
Liversedge, Laurie 165, 224
Lloyd, June 77
Logue, Valentine 41-2
London Chest Hospital 50
London Hospital 41
Louis-Bar, D. 56
Lovelock, James 251
Lowestoft, Suffolk 33
Lucknow 105
Lumbar puncture can lead to coning 216
Luttrell, Colonel Walter 183, 186

McArdle's syndrome 223
McCarthy, John 120

McCusick, Victor 81, 83
MacDougall-Hawthorn diet 29
McEwen, Sir William 6
MacDougall, Roger 219
Mackay-Dick, J. Col. 38
MacLennan, Kenneth 242-3
McQuillen, Mike 78-9, 254
Maghull 108
Magnetic Resonance Imaging 212
Magoffin County, Kentucky 93
Maher, Dr Robert 113, 115f.
Maida Vale 41, 43, 44, 45, 51, 52, 54, 104, 170, 255
Malacca 212
    National Service in 32-6
Malaria in Khartoum 195
Malaya 32ff., 36, 37, 213
Malaysia 212
Manchester 97, 213f.
Mann, Jonathan 124, 249
Manson-Barr, Sir P. 25
Marfan's disease, Marfan's syndrome 80, 81, 145
Marshall, John 42
Martin, Archie 112
Martin, John 130
Martin, Purdon 45, 104
Matisse, H. 128
Matthews, Bertie 31
Matthews, Professor Bryan 166, 169
*Mayflower*, voyagers on 7f.
Medical aspects of art 195-199
Medical emergency, poor management of 192
Medicine, Committee for the Safety of 266
Medicine, progress in 263-265
Medicines Control Agency 266
Medico-legal work 203-209
Meige's syndrome 257
Melzack, R. 114, 116
Memory 123
Meniere's disease 28f.
Meningitis 52
    tuberculous 51
    viral, grave error in treatment of 14
Methods of examination for the Royal College of Physicians 188f.
Midwifery 26
Migraine 4, 67, 87, 101, 128, 148, 153-60, 209
Miller Fisher, C. 148
Mills, A., Professor 20
Milward, Sheila 218
Misuse of medical opinions by lawyers 203
Mitchell, Professor Douglas 133, 169, 227
Monteiro, Dr Brendan 136
Montuschi, Elio 31
Motorneurone disease 11, 169-72, 223, 228
    Association 169
    groups 217
    Madras form of 211
    patient in wheelchair, leadership of 224

Mouth- and foot-painting artists 172-186
  aims of 172
  achievements of 173, 181f.
  Association of with criticisms 172-3
  case histories of 273ff., 174ff.
  motivation of 173, 181f.
  self-esteem, financial and other independence 173-77
  spectrum of 179-182
MR scanning 143, 170
Muller, Max 120
Multiple Sclerosis 70, 101, 113, 115, 116, 171, 192, 204, 217-221
  Diagnosis of through Charcot's triad 219
  Onset, course and general trend 218,
  Patients' own account of and questions concerning 218
  Causation of still unclear 219
  Possible treatments of 219-220
  and decompression 216f.
  Multiple Sclerosis Society 218
  Suggested trigger factor in 219
Multiple subluxations 207
Murray, Jock 218
Muscle Neurology 222-225
Muscular dystrophy 224-5
Muscular Dystrophy Group 225
Myalgic encephalomyelitis 42
Myasthenia 223, 227
Myography, deep 259

Narcolepsy 201
National Health Service 17f. 18, 24-5, 267
National Hospital for Nervous Diseases 3, 16, 51
National Service, Army 4, 32-36, 41
Negus, David 3
Negus, Sir Victor 3, 30
Neuro-acanthocytosis 71-4, 101
Neurological boundaries of reality 264
Neurological emergencies 213-17
  brain damage in leading to loss of physical control 213
  causes of death in, 213
  history taking, importance of in 214
  impairment of faculties in 213
Neurological disease induced by drugs 163-9
Neuological trauma resulting from electric shock 208
Neurologists and neurosurgeons, collaboration between 170, 204
Neurologist, role of the 141-144
Neurologist's view of homo sapiens 187
Neurology 1-3, 11, 16f., 27, 28, 41, 44, 96f., 98, 112, 123, 125, 133
  formerly combined with psychiatry 141
Neurology and Neurosurgery, Midland Centre for, Birmingham 170, 204
Neuropaediatrics 57, 63, 67, 68, 228
Neurology, Retirement from 265-267
Neurophysiology 53-4, 98, 100

Neuropraxia 205
Neurosurgery 78, 91, 96, 97, 146f.
Nevin, Sam 6, 29, 32, 43, 54
Newton, Richard, Dr 228
Nicholson, J.T., Professor 75
Northern Ireland, Deafness in 59

Obstructive apnoea 202
Obstructive sleep apnoea, mechanical aids beneficial to 202
Ohio 82
Oldfield, Dr Josiah (father of Josie) 16
Oldfield, Dr Josie (the author's godmother) 16
Olszewski-Steele-Richardson progressive supranuclear palsy 49
Ondine's curse 202
Oneirism 132
Ophthalmoplegia plus 223
OPCA (olivopontine cerebellar atrophy) 56
Oram, Sam 25
Oswald, Lee Harvey 63
Owen, Vivian 109
Oxford University 4

Paediatrics 16-17, 76, 125
Pain 113-118
Pampiglione, G., (Pep) 54
Pappworth, M. 31f.
Parietal lobes, rehabilitation and disability 149-153
  Macdonald Critchley on 149
Parkinson's disease, Parkinsonism 10, 11, 27, 44-51, 53, 57, 80, 101, 111, 122, 142, 153, 202, 203
Parsonage, Maurice 106
Parsons, M. 34
Patients examined for medico-legal purposes 203
Patients' societies 217
Patient subjects in examinations 190
Pearson, Bruce 25
Pearson, Hubert 31
Pelham, Herbert 8
Pendle 5
Pennsylvania 82
Pennybacker, Joe 3
Perforated appendix 209
Peri-Sylvan language zone 64, 123
Perkin, D. 34
Perspective in childhood 12
PET (Positon Emission Tomography) 99
Peters, R., Professor 3
Petit mal 99, 102, 105, 106
Peyser, Dr Nathan 63
Phantom limbs 117, 130
Phantom phenomena 117f., 130
Phillips, Charles 3
Pink disease 167
Plymouth 7
Poacher 11
Poliomyelitis 176, 217, 224, 230

# INDEX

Pollution of environment as possible cause of botulism 253
Popper, Karl 2
Pond, Sir Desmond 57
Polunin, Ivan 41
POSSUM device 172, 178
Post-war restrictions 18-19
Pranesh, Dr 211
Prankeard, Professor 57
Pratt, R.T.C. 42, 255
Prelingually deaf, communication skills among 140
Prelingually deaf schizophrenic patients 135-140
Preston and surrounding area 40, 50, 51, 75, 78, 91, 96, 101, 169, 171
Prioritizing of expensive treatments 143f.
Prosody 124f.
Professor at University of Central Lancashire 266
Pseudo-hallucinations 129, 135
Pseudo-parkinsonism 44
Psychiatry 1, 4, 33, 57, 74, 87, 88, 107, 125, 126, 127
Psycholinguistics 126
Psychology 123
Psychotherapy 4
Punch-drunkenness 206
Puritans voyaging on *Mayflower* 7
Putnam, T.J. 216
Pylonephrosis as cause of death in multiple sclerosis 220

Qadim, testicular tumour with secondary in frontal lobe of brain 19
Qassim, Colonel 22
Queen Square 54, 57, 67, 75, 106, 114
QWERTY typewriter keyboard 65

Rabies 20
Radcliffe Infirmary, Oxford 3
Radiology 78, 83, 170
Ramsay, Melvin 54
Ramsbottom 113
Ransome, Arthur 156
Reed, Graham 127
Reid Report 108
Refsum's syndrome 43
Renshaw cells 261
Renwick, M. 81
Retirement 265f.
Richardson, A.R. 54
Rickettsiae 35f.
Rift Valley Fever 195
Riluzole 11
Ritchie Russell 3, 128
Robinson, Roger 70
Rochdale 113
Rosetti, Dante Gabriel 134
Ross Russell, Ralph 36, 37
Royal College of Physicians 113, 141, 152
    Examiner for membership of the 187-195

Royal Free disease 54
Royal Free Hospital 11, 42, 53-6
Royal National Institute for the Deaf 58
Royal National Orthopaedic Hospital 54
Royal Victoria Hospital, Belfast 194
Russia, visit to 210

Sacks, Oliver 1, 2, 3, 4, 46
St Mary's Hospital 4
St Pancras Hospital 55
Salem, witches of 8f.
Salvador Dali 162
Samson's Tower, Abbey ruins 12
San Francisco 56
Schizophrenia 125, 126, 135-139
    in the deaf: case histories 138f.
Schneider, K. 136
Schott, G.D. 116
Sedgwick House School for Epilepsy 112
Segawa's disease 256
Selegiline 49, 50
    Data top Study, North America Multicentre Study U.K. 50
Sewell, Joseph 63
Shaker foal disease 254
Shaw, Professor Ian 169
Sheffield 96
Sherlock, Professor Sheila 53
Sherrington, Sir Charles 2
Sherrington, Andrew 3
Shy-Drager syndrome 50
Sicuteri on central biochemical dysnociception 159
Sign in Huntington's chorea discovered by Macdonald Critchley 9
Sign language 58, 59, 137, 138, 139, 140, 171
Sinclair, David C. 2
Singapore 33f.
Sleep apnoea 201
Sleep disorders 199-203
Sleep singing 160-163
Smith, The hon. Honor V. 52
SMON (subacute myelo-optico-neuropathy) 167f.
Snake handling 92f.
South Africa 212-13
Spasmodic torticollis 256, 257, 258
Spasticity 113, 115
SPECT (Single photon emission tomography) 99
Speech 119-127
See also Early American English
*Speech: Origins and Development of* by Edmund Critchley 57
*Speedwell*, companion ship to *Mayflower* 7f.
Spinal cord 1, 6, 115, 169-72, 171, 172, 217
    cervical, radiculopathies of 171
Spy 15
SQUID (Superconductivity quantum interference device) 162-3

Status epilepticus 102
Steele-Richardson-Olszweski syndrome 160
Stegmann, Arnulf Erich, founder of Worldwide Association of Mouth- and Foot-painting Artists 174, 186n.
Stern, Gerald 50, 57
Storr, Anthony 2, 129
Stroke 27, 101, 144
    at altitude: case histories 145f.
    lacunar 147
    treatment of 146
Stuart, Jesse 69
Stuttering 122
Swash, Michael 169
Symonds, Sir Charles 111
Synaesthesia 118

Tabes dorsalis 6, 55
Taiping 38-9
Takayushu's disease 146
Tanner, Selwyn 31
Tarsh, Michael 4
TENS machine 115
'Terry': case history 71f.
Tertiary-neo syphilis 55
Tetanus 261
Tetanus toxoid 262
Thalassaemia 41
Thalidomide 167, 174
Thomas, P.K., Professor 10, 54, 114
Thompson, Dr George 108, 219
Tinnitus 52
Tizard, Professor Jack 71
Todd, Richard Bentley 102
Tolstoy, L. 197
Toole, James 148
Townsend, Horace 54
Toxocara 109f.
Toxoplasma 109f.
'Tralee': case history 73
Trevor-Roper, Patrick 195
Tropical Medicine Department, St Pancras Hospital 55
Tuberculosis, neurological aspects of 51-3
Tuberculous meningitis 52
Turnbull, Wing Commander Gordon 130
Turner-Warwick, Dame Margaret 187f.
Tutton, Ken 96, 97

Uhthoff's phenomena in multiple sclerosis 220
Uncontrollable inner speech 124
Underwood Speed Training Group 65
United States 81-2
    concentration of Huntington's Chorea in 7f.
University of Central Lancashire 169

University College Hospital 54, 55-7
University of Kentucky 83
Upper Chine School, Isle of Wight 16

Vakil, Dr Sarosh 50, 109, 111
Vancouver, British Columbia 50
Vascular Hypothesis 156
Vasoconstrictions 5
Vessie, P.R. 9
Vogt-Koyanagi syndrome 29
Vollum, Dr 36, 38

Wain, Louis 130
Wakefield Asylum, Yorkshire 6
Wakeley, Sir Cecil 25
Wakeley, Richard 28f.
Walker Brian 81
Walker, Joan 31
Wall, P.D. 114
Wallace, Alfred R. 119, 120
Walton, John, (Lord Walton of Detchant) 5, 222, 255
Warren, Frank 137
Watches and bioelectrical phenomena 160-3
Watson, Lyall 161
Weatherall, Sir David 41, 75, 81
Weddell, G. 2
Weir Mitchell 116, 117
Wernicke's aphasia 123
West London Hospital 6
Whaddon Chase hunt 14f.
Whiplash injuries 206-7
Whittingham Psychiatric Hospital 108, 136
Whittingham Hospital 31
Whitty, C. 128
Whyte, Robert 255
Wikler, Professor Abe 71, 92
Wilkie 8f.
Will, Bob 43
Williams, Dr Cratis 93, 94
Williams, Roger, Rev. 10
Wilson, Kathleen 137
Wilson's Disease 51, 53, 258
Woodcock, Susan 97
World Health Organization 88
Written examinations for MRCP 193

Yahr, Melvin 44
Yes and no 21
Yoghurt as cause of botulism 229f.
Young, Alistair, Col. 34

Ziel-Nielsen Stains 52
Zilkha, K. 219

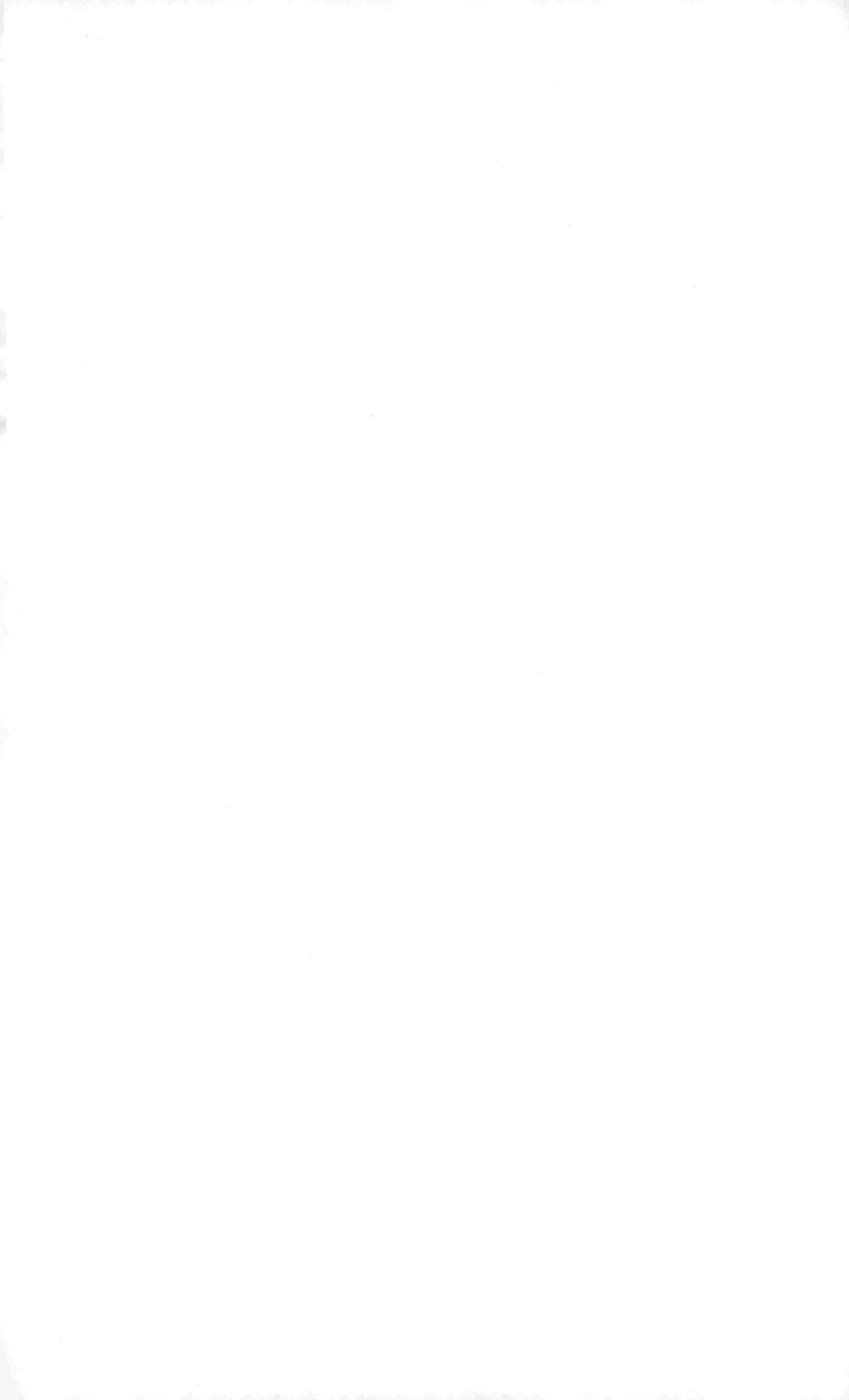